practical laboratory
DIAGNOSIS of DISEASE

CLINICAL
CHEMISTRY

A Core Course for Health Sciences Students & Pathology Residents

David N Bailey, MD
Distinguished Research Professor of Pathology and Pharmacy
University of California, San Diego

Robert L Fitzgerald, PhD, DABCC
Professor of Pathology
University of California, San Diego

Publishing Team

Aimee Algas Alker (editorial/proofreading)
Jennifer Brinson (design)
Erik N Tanck (production)
Joshua Weikersheimer (publishing direction)

Notice

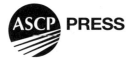

ISBN 978-089189-6548

Printed in the United States of America

21 20 19 18 17

CLINICAL CHEMISTRY

David N Bailey, MD and
Robert L Fitzgerald, PhD, DABCC

Acknowledgments

The authors gratefully acknowledge the contributions of many colleagues who, over the years, have contributed material that was included in the numerous editions of the course manuals that were forerunners to this book. These individuals include, first and foremost, Alfred Zettner (the founding head of the division of laboratory medicine at the University of California, San Diego), who had the vision to write a course manual for students and prepared earlier versions of it. Individuals who contributed to specific sections of the manuals include Nicholas M Alexander (thyroid disease), Wolfgang Dillmann (adrenocortical disease), Anna Dreilinger (statistics), Wendy Frankel (cardiac disease), and Richard McPherson (protein abnormalities). Others contributed by reviewing and editing the manuals during their teaching of the course over the years: David A Herold, Michael J Kelner, and Norbert W Tietz. Michael Kelner also provided helpful discussions on current state of the art technology.

This work has indeed been a labor of love by these individuals, whose overarching mission was simply to improve the teaching of introductory clinical chemistry.

David N Bailey and Robert L Fitzgerald

contents

Foreword vi

1 Clinical laboratory statistics 1
2 The effects of hemolysis, icterus, lipemia, refrigeration, diurnal variation, and drugs on laboratory tests; pediatric clinical chemistry 11
3 The laboratory diagnosis of myocardial infarction and congestive heart failure 16
4 The laboratory diagnosis of gastrointestinal disease. 25
5 The laboratory diagnosis of renal disease 37
6 Urinalysis 47
7 The laboratory examination of body fluids 55
8 The laboratory diagnosis of electrolyte and acid-base disturbances . . 65
9 The laboratory diagnosis of calcium, phosphorus, and magnesium disorders. 85
10 The laboratory diagnosis of iron disorders. 95
11 The laboratory diagnosis of pancreatic disease 101
12 The laboratory diagnosis of liver disease. 109
13 Tumor markers 119
14 The laboratory diagnosis of protein abnormalities 127
15 Reproductive clinical chemistry 149
16 Clinical toxicology 156
17 Therapeutic drug monitoring 177
18 The laboratory diagnosis of thyroid disease. 189
19 The laboratory diagnosis of diabetes mellitus 201
20 The laboratory diagnosis of adrenocortical disease. 213
21 The laboratory diagnosis of lipid disorders 225

Appendices

A Preparation of laboratory sessions. 235
B Outline of the differential diagnosis for selected abnormal clinical chemistry tests. 239
C The differential diagnosis of some of the most common clinical chemistry abnormalities encountered by pathology residents taking night call 247
Index. 260

©2017 ASCP   ISBN 978-089189-6548   v

Foreword

This book is the product of an introductory course in clinical chemistry for medical students at the University of California, San Diego (UC San Diego), which was taught first as a required course for 30 years (1982-2011) and, following a revision of the curriculum, as a popular elective course (2012 onward). A required companion course in clinical chemistry for UC San Diego pharmacy students has been taught since the school's inception more than 10 years ago. For both courses, a manual has been prepared and updated annually, and a set of PowerPoint lecture slides has been made available for each session. Most sessions include illustrative clinical cases. In addition, 2 laboratories (blood drawing with subsequent discussion of the panel results; urinalysis) have been integrated into the course, and preparation of these sessions is described in this book. Since 2010, the authors have also included this core material in teaching UC San Diego pathology residents and medical technology students during required rotations in clinical chemistry.

The course focuses on the laboratory diagnosis of the most common diseases by organ system and relates diagnostic testing to the pathophysiology of the diseases in development of the differential diagnosis. Analytical methodology is not discussed unless essential to interpreting the test result.

Based on more than 30 years of teaching this course, we believe that we have identified the clinical chemistry "core" material that should be taught to health sciences students and pathology residents. Accordingly, we emphasize that this book is not a reference textbook but rather a course handbook complete with PowerPoint lecture slides and cases.

Learning objectives and key terms are defined at the beginning of each chapter. In addition, key terms are **bolded** when they are first used in the text so that the reader can refer to them easily. Key points are <u>underlined</u> in each section. It should be noted that the terms "serum" and "plasma" are used interchangeably, since many clinical laboratories use both for analyses. Where there are differences between the 2 specimens, we make this clear.

Students indicate that this course has prepared them well for their respective licensing examinations and clinical rotations. Residents indicate that the material has helped them prepare for board examinations.

We hope that you will find the book, the associated PowerPoint slides, and the laboratory sessions helpful in conducting an introductory course in clinical chemistry for health sciences students and pathology residents.

David N Bailey and Robert L Fitzgerald

chapter 1

Clinical laboratory statistics

1.1 Objectives

At the end of this session, the learner should be able to

- ➤ describe the sources of variation influencing laboratory tests (ie, analytical, intraindividual, and interindividual)
- ➤ discuss the approach to establishing reference ranges for laboratory tests
- ➤ describe the use of the parametric and nonparametric methods for calculation of reference ranges, and the requirements for applying each method
- ➤ calculate percent of false positives from the number of tests performed on a patient
- ➤ calculate the number of patterns of test results from the number of types of results and the number of tests performed on a patient
- ➤ calculate clinical sensitivity of a test
- ➤ calculate clinical specificity of a test
- ➤ calculate positive and negative predictive values of a test
- ➤ discuss the effect of disease prevalence on predictive values
- ➤ calculate efficiency of a test
- ➤ describe the difference between intraindividual and interindividual variation
- ➤ describe preanalytical factors and analytical factors affecting analytical variation
- ➤ define accuracy and precision
- ➤ differentiate random error from systematic error
- ➤ define a receiver operating characteristic and how it is used in the evaluation of a test

1.2 Key terms

accuracy: closeness of agreement of a measured value and the true value

analytical variation: observed differences in the value of a laboratory result arising during the analysis

coefficient of variation: a relative measure of precision, determined by dividing the standard deviation by the mean, usually expressed as a percentage

efficiency: the fraction of subjects correctly classified by a test, usually expressed as a percentage

Gaussian distribution: the classic "bell shaped" curve, with 95% of the values occurring within ±2 standard deviations of the mean (2.5% occurring above, and 2.5% occurring below the mean); the skewness and kurtosis are 0, and the mean, median, and mode equal one another

interindividual variation: differences in the true value of an analyte among individuals

intraindividual variation: differences in the true value of an analyte within the same individual

kurtosis: the measure of peakedness (vs flatness) of a distribution curve

mean: the arithmetic average

median: the value of the middle observation when a dataset is arranged in rank order

mode: the most frequently observed value in a dataset

negative predictive value: the fraction of negative values that are correct; determined by dividing the true negatives by the sum of the true negatives and false negatives, usually expressed as a percentage

nonparametric reference range calculation: calculation of the reference range as the middle 95% of values (at least 120 values required to define population) that do not display a Gaussian distribution

parametric reference range calculation: calculation of the reference range as mean ±2 standard deviations (for a Gaussian distribution)

positive predictive value: the fraction of positive values that are correct; determined by dividing the true positives by the sum of the true positives and false positives, usually expressed as a percentage

preanalytical variation: the combination of factors that affect a laboratory result prior to the analysis itself (eg, sample collection, sample contamination, hemoconcentration, hemolysis, lipemia, icterus)

precision: the closeness of agreement between independent measurements; generally expressed as coefficient of variation or standard deviation

random error: an error occurring by chance such that 95% of the results fall within 2 standard deviations of the mean

receiver operating characteristic: a plot of the sensitivity (true positive rate, Y axis) vs 1 – specificity (false positive rate, X axis) at different thresholds (cutoffs) for a diagnostic test; the area under the curve indicates how well a test distinguishes between 2 groups (eg, diseased vs nondiseased); the greater the area, the higher the ability to properly classify disease state

reference range: generally the inner 95% of values for a laboratory test as measured in a defined population; the subject population is typically disease free ("normal") with respect to the test of interest

sensitivity: the ability of a test to detect a true positive; determined by dividing the true positives by the sum of the true positives and false negatives, usually expressed as a percentage

skewness: the measure of asymmetry of a distribution curve

specificity: the ability of a test to detect a true negative; determined by dividing the true negatives by the sum of the true negatives and false positives, usually expressed as a percentage

standard deviation: a measure of precision (square root of the variance)

systematic error: an error occurring due to a change in the system, creating a bias in the measurement

variance: the average of the squared differences from the mean

1.3 Background/significance

Utilization of clinical laboratory results is based upon knowledge of their accuracy, precision, and reliability. Interpretation of the data is usually performed by comparison with established reference ranges for the population. Thus, a basic understanding of clinical laboratory statistics and how reference ranges are established is important.

1.4 Sources of variation

Laboratory test results can be affected by a variety of variables. **Preanalytical variation** refers to the combination of factors that affect a laboratory result prior to the analysis itself, which include effects of improper blood drawing (eg, hemolysis, hemoconcentration from prolonged tourniquet application) as well as how the sample is processed and stored prior to analysis. Additional variables include **interindividual variation** (eg, variation among individuals based on age, gender, diet) and **intraindividual variation** (eg, diurnal variation of analytes such as cortisol within an individual). In contrast, **analytical variation** refers to differences in laboratory results based on the imprecision or imperfections in the analytical process itself. Total variation is the sum of preanalytical, interindividual, intraindividual, and analytical variation.

1.5 Establishing reference ranges

Reference ranges are established in order to permit comparison of individual test results to those from a relatively large number of individuals in the same population (eg, same age range, same gender).

The following steps are generally followed when establishing a reference range:

1. select the analyte for which the reference range is to be established

2. select the analytical methodology and instrumentation to be used for measurement of the analyte

3. define the reference population; demographically it should match the population whose test results will be compared with the reference range (eg, age range, gender)

4. choose the selection method for the reference population such that it will yield a random sampling (eg, the first 100 individuals presenting for a wellness checkup)

5. collect, process, and test the samples

6. organize the results into a frequency histogram **f1.1**, displaying the numerical value of the test result, the number of observations with that result, and the rank (cumulative number of observations)

Value		Number of observations	Rank
1	4	xxxx	4
2	15	xxxxxxxxxxxxxxx	19
3	23	xxxxxxxxxxxxxxxxxxxxxxx	42
4	25	xxxxxxxxxxxxxxxxxxxxxxxxx	67
5	22	xxxxxxxxxxxxxxxxxxxxxx	89
6	19	xxxxxxxxxxxxxxxxxxx	108
7	12	xxxxxxxxxxxx	120
8	2	xx	122
9	0		
10	0		
11	0		
12	0		
13	1	x	123

f1.1 Frequency histogram

7. eliminate any values (outliers) that are so far away from the rest of the data that their inclusion might alter the results; in general, if the distance between the most extreme datapoint and its nearest neighbor is >1/3 of the total range covered by the dataset then the datapoint should be discarded [ISBN9781594251023]

Reject the largest value (n) when:

$$\frac{X(n) - X(n-1)}{X(n) - X(1)} > \frac{1}{3}$$

Reject the smallest value X(1) when:

$$\frac{X(2) - X(1)}{X(n) - X(1)} > \frac{1}{3}$$

Once an outlier has been eliminated, the dataset should be reevaluated for additional outliers, which may become apparent only after elimination of the first outlier.

1. Determine whether the resulting dataset has a **Gaussian distribution**, which is characterized by having the classical "bell shaped" curve **f1.2**. A perfect Gaussian distribution has the same value for the **mean** (the arithmetic average), the **median** (the value of the middle observation), and the **mode** (the most frequently observed value). It also has **skewness** (a measure of asymmetry) and **kurtosis** (a measure of peakedness) equal to 0. In practice, skewness and kurtosis ranging from –1 to +1 are acceptable in evaluating whether a Gaussian distribution exists [ISBN9780323036580c].

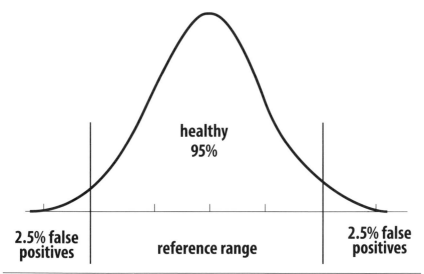

f1.2 Gaussian distribution

2. Select a method for calculating the reference range:

If the distribution is Gaussian the **parametric reference range calculation** can be used:

Reference range = mean (X) ± 2 standard deviations (SD)

If the distribution is not Gaussian the **nonparametric reference range calculation** must be used, and there must be a minimum of 120 datapoints [ISBN9780323036580b].

Reference range = the inner 95% of values
(excluding the upper 2.5% & the lower 2.5% of values)

This exclusion is due to the fact that, by definition, a reference range represents 95% of the values of a reference population excluding 5% of the healthy population (2.5% with values above the 95% and 2.5% with values below the 95%) [ISBN9780323036580b; ISBN9781416061649]. The values for the 5% of the healthy population whose test results lie outside the calculated reference range are considered to be false positives (FPs), regardless of whether they fall above or below the reference range, since they indicate positivity or negativity for disease (eg, hemoglobin above and below the reference range can be suggestive of disease). It should be noted that the nonparametric method may also be used to calculate reference ranges for a Gaussian distribution as long as at least 120 datapoints are present.

1.6 **False positives**

Since a reference range represents the inner 95% of values of a healthy population, excluding 5% of the healthy population, it follows that the more tests performed on a healthy population, the more FPs will result:

$$\% \text{ FPs} = (1 - 0.95^n) \times 100\%, \text{ where n = number of tests performed}$$

Thus, for 1 test, there will be 5% FPs; for 2 tests, 10%; for 3 tests, 14%; for 4 tests, 19%; for 5 tests, 23%, etc, as 0.95 is raised to the second, third, fourth, and fifth power, respectively. This should be appreciated whenever ordering a panel of tests on apparently healthy individuals. Results falling outside the reference range cause concern for the patient and provider alike, and frequently necessitate follow-up testing.

1.7 **Patterns of test results**

Individuals who evaluate laboratory results must be familiar with the numerous patterns of test results in order to make diagnoses. Mathematically, the number of patterns that can result from performing a battery of tests is given by the following:

$$\text{number of patterns of test results} = X^n, \text{ where n = number of tests performed } \&$$
$$X = \text{number of categories of results appreciated by the observer}$$

Thus, for 3 categories of results ("low," "normal," and "high") and 2 tests, there would be 9 patterns. For 5 categories of results ("very low," "low," "normal," "high," and "very high") and 3 tests, there would be 25 patterns.

1.8 **Clinical sensitivity & specificity**

Sensitivity and specificity are performance characteristics of a test. Determining each requires figuring out whether or not a disease or condition is present in a population through use of an independent (reference) test. The test is then applied to 2 populations: one that does not have disease (as defined by the reference test) and another in which the reference test has established disease.

Sensitivity is defined as the proportion of diseased subjects correctly classified by the test (ie, the ability to detect a true positive [TP] in a person with the disease). If a subject is known to have disease, as established by a reference test, and has a positive test result, it is classified as a TP. If the test result is negative for a subject with the disease, this result is classified as a false negative (FN):

$$\text{sensitivity} = 100\% \times (TP)/(TP + FN)$$

Specificity is defined as the proportion of healthy subjects correctly classified by the test (ie, the ability to detect a true negative [TN] in a person without the disease). If a subject is known to not have disease, as established by a reference test, and has a negative test result, this result is classified as a TN, while, if the test result is positive, it is classified as a FP:

$$\text{specificity} = 100\% \times (TN)/(TN + FP)$$

It should be noted that enhancement of sensitivity occurs at the expense of specificity and vice versa. Often in screening tests, the desire is to optimize the detection of disease, which is done by lowering the cutoff level for the test, thereby increasing the number of FP results and decreasing the specificity of the test. This maximizes the predictive value of a negative result (see next section), which in screening, usually does not present a problem since a second (more specific) test is performed to determine which presumptive positive results are in fact TPs. An example would be a screening test for human immunodeficiency virus infection, which is set to optimize detection of disease at the expense of specificity. A second, more specific confirmatory test is then performed to "rule in" a disease diagnosis.

In other situations it may be more important to enhance the specificity of a test. This is done by increasing the cutoff level for the test, thereby decreasing the number of FPs and decreasing the sensitivity of the test, both of which maximize the predictive value of a positive result (see next section).

1.9 Predictive values

Predictive values reflect the odds that the results of a test will correctly classify an individual with the disease or condition. Thus the predictive value of a positive test result (PV+; **positive predictive value**) indicates the percent of positive results that correctly classify an individual as having the disease:

$$PV+ = 100\% \times (TP)/(TP + FP)$$

The predictive value of a negative test result (PV−; **negative predictive value**) indicates the percent of negative results that correctly classify an individual as not having the disease:

$$PV- = 100\% \times (TN)/(TN + FN)$$

It is important to appreciate the effect of disease prevalence on predictive values. In general, as the prevalence of disease increases, the PV+ increases. As the prevalence decreases, the PV− improves.

1.10 Efficiency

The **efficiency** of a test reflects the fraction of subjects that are correctly classified by a test, whether or not the result is positive or negative:

$$efficiency = 100\% \times (TP + TN)/(TP + TN + FP + FN)$$

1.11 Examples

t1.1 depicts these calculations in a population of subjects with disease (as determined by a reference test) and in a population of subjects without disease (as determined by the reference test).

1.12 Analytical variation

As previously noted, variation among laboratory results is the sum of preanalytical variation, interindividual variation, intraindividual variation, and analytical variation. The laboratory has little control over the first 3, but utilizes procedures to minimize analytical variation (variation that occurs during the analysis itself).

t1.1 Examples of calculations

	Number of subjects with positive test	Number of subjects with negative test	TOTALS
Number of subjects with disease*	TP	FN	TP + FN
Number of subjects without disease*	FP	TN	FP + TN
Totals	TP + FP	FN + TN	TP + FP + FN + TN
	Number of subjects with positive test	**Number of subjects with negative test**	**TOTALS**
Number of subjects with disease*	68	32	100; sensitivity = 68%
Number of subjects without disease*	2	98	100; specificity = 98%
	PV(+) = 97%; PV(−) = 75%; efficiency = 83%		
Totals	70	130	200

*The presence or absence of disease is established by an independent test (eg, reference method, imaging study, biopsy, etc)

In practice, clinical laboratories analyze commercial control samples of varying concentrations along with the patient samples. The mean and standard deviation for the control samples are determined. **Random error** will cause the results to fall within 2 standard deviations of the mean 95% of the time, indicating that the control is acceptable. However, results that exceed established quality control rules suggest possible **systematic error**, which must be identified and corrected (eg, a faulty sampler in the instrument, a defective reagent) **f1.3**.

The way to determine if a patient's laboratory values have actually changed is to determine if the difference between the first and the subsequent measurement is >3× the standard deviation of the assay. Differences >3× the standard deviation of the assay are likely to represent a real change in the patient [ISBN9780323036580a].

low accuracy	high accuracy	high accuracy	low accuracy
high precision	low precision	high precision	low precision
small random error	large random error	small random error	large random error
large systematic error	small systematic error	small systematic error	small systematic error

f1.3 Accuracy & precision; random & systematic error

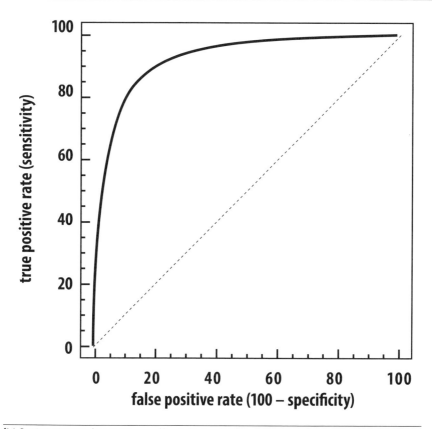

f1.4 Receiver-operating characteristic: curved line (indicator with high predictive power); dashed line (indicator with no predictive power)

1.13 **Accuracy & precision**

The **accuracy** of a test determines how close the measured value of an analyte is to the true value. This is generally determined by analysis of certified reference material with values traceable to the National Institute of Standards and Technology, as well as by use of external quality control check samples.

The **precision** of a test determines the reproducibility of the result. It follows that results can be accurate and precise, accurate but not precise, and precise but not accurate. Of course, results can also be inaccurate and imprecise **f1.3**.

A commonly used measure of precision is the **coefficient of variation**, which is calculated by dividing the **standard deviation** (the square root of the **variance**) by the mean and expressing it as a percentage. Laboratory tests aim to keep both within run and between run analytical precision as low as possible.

1.14 **Receiver operating characteristic**

The **receiver operating characteristic f1.4** is a plot of the TP rate (sensitivity) on the Y axis vs the FP rate (100% − specificity) on the X axis at different cutoff (threshold for determining a positive result) values. The area under the resulting curve is a measure of how well a test can distinguish between 2 groups (eg, diseased vs nondiseased).

1.15 **References**

ISBN9780323036580a Blick KE, Passey RB [2010] Quality control for the clinical chemistry laboratory. In: Kaplan LA, Pesce AJ, ed. *Clinical Chemistry: Theory, Analysis, Correlation*, 5e. Mosby; 462

ISBN9780323036580b Horn PS [2010] Reference intervals and clinical decision limits. In: Kaplan LA, Pesce AJ, ed. *Clinical Chemistry: Theory, Analysis, Correlation*, 5e. Mosby; 444-445.

ISBN9780323036580c Jandreski MA, Kahn S [2010] Laboratory statistics. In: Kaplan LA, Pesce AJ, ed. *Clinical Chemistry: Theory, Analysis, Correlation*, 5e. Mosby; 418

ISBN9781416061649 Horowitz GL [2012] Establishment and use of reference values. In: Burtis CA, Ashwood ER, Bruns DE, ed. *Tietz Textbook of Clinical Chemistry and Molecular Diagnostics*, 5e Elsevier Saunders; 95-118

ISBN9781594251023 Bertholf RL [2011] Statistical methods in laboratory medicine. In: Clark W, ed. *Contemporary Practice in Clinical Chemistry*, 2e. AACC Press; 23

The effects of hemolysis, icterus, lipemia, refrigeration, diurnal variation, and drugs on laboratory tests; pediatric clinical chemistry

2.1 Objectives

At the end of the session, the learner should be able to

- ➤ describe causes of in vitro hemolysis in laboratory samples
- ➤ discuss the effect of hemolysis on serum potassium, sodium, calcium, folate, and aspartate aminotransferase
- ➤ describe the effect of icterus on analysis of samples
- ➤ describe the effect of lipemia on analysis of samples
- ➤ describe the effect of refrigeration of uncentrifuged blood samples on plasma and serum potassium
- ➤ describe the diurnal rhythm of serum cortisol, growth hormone, serum iron, and thyroxine
- ➤ describe methods by which drugs can interfere with laboratory tests
- ➤ discuss differences between analytes in neonates/children and adults and the mechanisms underlying them

2.2 Key terms

analyte: a substance measured by an analytical technique

artifact: altered condition of a material resulting from artificial, rather than natural, processes

diurnal variation: changes in analyte concentrations within an individual in the same day

hemolysis: rupture of red blood cells, releasing hemoglobin and other contents into the surrounding plasma or serum, often causing interference with analysis of a sample

icterus: the presence of increased concentration of total bilirubin in a specimen, often causing interference with analysis of a sample

lipemia: the presence of increased concentrations of lipid in a specimen, often resulting in light scattering and interference with analysis of a sample

2.3 Background/significance

Laboratory testing is affected by the quality of the specimen submitted for analysis. Inadequate specimen quality contributes to preanalytical variation. Major contributors to specimen inadequacy include hemolysis, icterus, and lipemia. Modern laboratory instrumentation measures these potentially interfering factors prior to analysis and flags affected results as invalid. Medications also frequently alter laboratory results as a direct effect or a side effect, while laboratory values in neonates and children frequently differ from those in adults.

2.4 Hemolysis

Hemolysis of blood samples results from disruption of red cell membranes, permitting leakage of red cell contents into the surrounding plasma or serum. This may occur via mechanical means (eg, vigorously shaking an uncentrifuged sample or drawing it through a very small gauge needle while applying a large amount of suction as with a syringe), chemical means (eg, introducing a hyperosmolar or hypoosmolar solution such as water or isopropanol into the uncentrifuged sample), heating or freezing the sample, or allowing the uncentrifuged sample to sit for several days before analysis.

Hemolysis can affect the results of laboratory analyses by increasing the concentration of those constituents of plasma or serum that are higher in the red cell matrix than in the plasma or serum. Such **analytes** include potassium, aspartate aminotransferase, and folate. Conversely, hemolysis can decrease the concentration of those constituents of plasma or serum that are lower in the red cell matrix than in the plasma or serum by diluting them. These analytes include calcium and sodium. Finally, measurement of analytes that depend on detecting spectrophotometric absorption in the visible region near the absorption bands for oxyhemoglobin (410 nm, 540 nm, and 575 nm) may be perturbed. The degree of interference depends upon the analytical methodology utilized.

Modern laboratory instrumentation detects hemolysis by measuring absorbance of the serum or plasma at 570 nm and 600 nm (near the major absorption bands for oxyhemoglobin; the hemolysis index) and will flag the sample as hemolyzed if the absorption exceeds the permitted threshold for a given analyte.

Obviously the contamination of other body fluids by whole blood can also affect laboratory results. For example, a traumatic lumbar puncture that introduces blood into cerebrospinal fluid (CSF) will greatly increase the total protein concentration in the CSF since the plasma protein concentration is several hundredfold greater than that in CSF. The contamination of amniotic fluid by maternal blood will decrease the measured lecithin:sphingomyelin (L:S) ratio in the fluid since the L:S ratio in blood is lower than that in amniotic fluid obtained during the third trimester of pregnancy.

2.5 Icterus

Elevated bilirubin (eg, in a patient with hepatitis or cirrhosis) can also affect certain laboratory results by causing absorbance at 450 nm. Analytes whose measurements depend on detecting absorption near this wavelength can be affected. Modern laboratory instrumentation detects **icterus** by measuring the absorbance of the sample at 480 nm and 505 nm (near the major absorption band for bilirubin; the icterus index) and will flag the sample as icteric if the absorption exceeds the permitted threshold for a given analyte.

2.6 Lipemia

Excessive lipid concentrations in a serum or plasma sample can cause light scattering, thereby interfering with analysis. Modern laboratory instruments detect **lipemia** by measuring the absorbance of the sample at 660 nm and 700 nm, wavelengths that are sufficiently removed from those used to detect hemoglobin and bilirubin interference (the lipemia index). If absorption exceeds the permitted threshold for a given analyte, the sample is flagged as lipemic.

The measurement of hemolysis, icterus, and lipemia in serum and plasma samples is commonly known as serum indices. Most modern instrumentation measures serum indices prior to reporting results. Results from samples that exceed established serum index thresholds for individual laboratory tests are suppressed in order to prevent erroneous results from being issued.

2.7 Refrigeration of uncentrifuged samples

Refrigeration (4°C) of an uncentrifuged blood sample inhibits the sodium-potassium ATPase pump, which pumps 2 potassium ions into the red cell and 3 sodium ions out of the red cell. Refrigeration disrupts potassium transport into the erythrocytes, leading to increased plasma or serum potassium without hemolysis, also known as an **artifact** as it results from the refrigeration process itself. Since no hemolysis results, the laboratory instrumentation will permit analysis of the sample, and an erroneously elevated potassium measurement will occur. To preclude this event, samples for electrolyte analysis should not be refrigerated and ideally should be centrifuged prior to delivery to the laboratory if coming from an external location.

2.8 Diurnal variation

Diurnal variation of analytes contributes to the intraindividual variation in laboratory results. In normal individuals, certain serum and plasma analytes (eg, cortisol and iron) are higher in the morning than in the evening, while others (eg, thyroid stimulating hormone and thyroxine) are higher in the evening than in the morning. Growth hormone is elevated during sleep.

2.9 Effects of drugs

Medications can affect laboratory results by exerting their intended pharmacological effects (eg, aldosterone receptor blockers will cause elevation of serum or plasma potassium and loss of sodium), while others can have side effects that alter laboratory results (eg, increase in serum cortisol and transferrin after use of oral contraceptives due to an increase in binding proteins, decrease of total thyroxine by aspirin due to displacement from binding proteins). Still other drugs can directly interfere with analytical measurements (eg, Digibind interference with the serum digoxin assay). If drug interference with a laboratory result is suspected, the user should consult the clinical laboratory issuing the result.

2.10 Pediatric clinical chemistry

Reference ranges for many analytes in neonates and children are very different than those for adults. While practitioners will refer to reference ranges when interpreting results for these populations, general knowledge of some of the major differences is important.

Concentrations of some analytes that are <u>higher</u> in the serum and plasma of neonates and children than in adults include the following:

➤ alkaline phosphatase [PMID17012488] and phosphorus [PMID3402068] (due to rapid bone growth and increased osteoclastic activity)

➤ α fetoprotein (produced by the fetal liver) [PMID15469851] and hemoglobin F (fetal hemoglobin production)

➤ ammonia [PMID7600690] and bilirubin [PMID12691874] (due to neonatal hepatic immaturity, resulting in decreased conversion of ammonia to urea and decreased conjugation of bilirubin)

➤ aspartate aminotransferase (may be due to release of placental aspartate aminotransferase into the fetal circulation) [PMID10213291]

➤ creatine kinase (may be due to neonatal muscle exertion during delivery) [PMID10074896]

➤ γ glutamyl transferase (may be maternal in origin) [PMID22958834]

➤ potassium (due to lower glomerular filtration rate and decreased urinary clearance of potassium in the neonate) [PMID12691874]

➤ proteins in cerebrospinal fluid (due to immature blood-brain barrier in neonates) [PMID12691874]

➤ thyroid stimulating hormone (due to postdelivery surge) [PMID12691874] and total thyroxine (in response to surge of thyroid stimulating hormone) [PMID12691874]

Concentrations of some analytes that are <u>lower</u> in neonates and children than in adults include the following:

➤ albumin (presumably due to reduced synthetic capability of the neonatal liver) [PMID3402068]

➤ amylase (neonates produce little pancreatic amylase) [PMID12691874]

➤ bicarbonate (may be due to decreased renal reabsorption of bicarbonate in the neonate) [ISBN9780721646619]

➤ cholesterol (due to low cholesterol in diet) [PMID12691874]

➤ copper (may be due to low serum ceruloplasmin in newborns) [PMID3402069]

➤ haptoglobin (essentially absent in newborns) [PMID7536645]

➤ immunoglobulins IgG [PMID3261214], IgA [PMID3261214], IgM [PMID3261214], and IgE [PMID8595709] (small amounts of IgG are maternal; IgA, IgM, and IgE do not cross the placenta so that the infant is born without these immunoglobulins; immunoglobulin synthesis begins after birth)

2.11 **References**

2.11.1 **Journals**

PMID10074896 Soldin SJ, Murthy JN, Agarwalla PK et al [1999] Pediatric reference ranges for creatine kinase, CKMS, troponin I, iron and cortisol. *Clin Biochem* 32: 77-80

PMID10213291 Knapen MFCM, Van der Wildt B, Sijtsma EG et al [1999] Glutathione S-transferase α 1-1 and aminotransferases in umbilical cord blood. *Early Hum Dev* 54:129-135

PMID12691874 Ghoshal AK, Soldin SJ [2003] Evaluation of the Dade Behring Dimension RxL: integrated chemistry system-pediatric reference ranges. *Clin Chim Acta* 331:135-46

PMID15469851 Bader D, Riskin A, Vafsi O et al [2004] α-fetoprotein in the early neonatal period – a large study and review of the literature. *Clin Chim Acta* 349:15-23

PMID17012488 Corathers SD [2006] The alkaline phosphatase level: nuances of a familiar test. *Pediatr Rev* 27:382-84

PMID22958834 Melkie M, Yigeremu M, Nigussie P et al [2012] Robust reference intervals for liver function test (LFT) analytes in newborns and infants. *BMC Res Notes* 5:493

PMID3261214 Lockitch G, Halstead, Quigley G et al [1988] Age and sex specific pediatric reference intervals: study de sign and methods illustrated by measurement of serum proteins with the Behring LN nephelometer. *Clin Chem* 34:1618-21

PMID3402068 Lockitch G, Halstead AC, Albersheim S et al [1988] Age and sex specific pediatric reference intervals for biochemistry analytes as measured with the Ektachem-700 analyzer. *Clin Chem* 34:1622-25

PMID3402069 Lockitch G, Halstead A, Wadsworth L et al [1988] Age and sex specific pediatric reference intervals for zinc, copper, selenium, iron, vitamins A&E, and related proteins. *Clin Chem* 34:1625-28

PMID7536645 Kanakoudi F, Drossou V, Tzimouli V et al [1995] Serum concentrations of 10 acute-phase proteins in healthy term and preterm infants from birth to age 6 months. *Clin Chem* 41:605-8

PMID7600690 Diaz J, Tornel PL, Martinez P [1995] Reference intervals for blood ammonia in healthy subjects, determined by microdiffusion. *Clin Chem* 41:1048

PMID8595709 Soldin SK, Morales A, Albalos R et al [1995] Pediatric reference ranges on the Abbott IMX for FSH, LH, prolactin, TSH, T_4, T_3, free T_4, free T_3, T-uptake, IgE, and ferritin. *Clin Biochem* 28:603-6

2.11.2 **Book**

ISBN9780721646619 Weisberg HF [1984] pH and blood gases. In: Hicks JM, Boeckx RL, ed. *Pediatric Clinical Chemistry*. WB Saunders, 88

The laboratory diagnosis of myocardial infarction & congestive heart failure

3.1 Objectives

At the end of the session, the learner should be able to

➢ discuss the use of serum cardiac troponins I&T in the diagnostic workup of suspected myocardial infarction

➢ discuss the use of serum creatine kinase MB in the diagnostic workup of suspected myocardial infarction

➢ discuss the use of serum myoglobin in the diagnostic workup of suspected myocardial infarction

➢ discuss the time course for elevation, peak, and return to baseline for the cardiac troponins, creatine kinase MB, and serum myoglobin

➢ describe conditions other than myocardial infarction in which serum creatine kinase MB may be elevated

➢ discuss the calculation of creatine kinase index, its use, and how to interpret the results

➢ discuss the use of serum B type natriuretic peptide (BNP) and N terminal-pro B type natriuretic peptide (NT terminal-pro BNP) in the diagnostic workup of congestive heart failure

➢ discuss copeptin and its potential use in ruling out myocardial infarction

3.2 Key terms

acute coronary syndrome: a wide range of acute heart conditions including ST segment elevation myocardial infarction (STEMI), non-ST segment myocardial infarction, and unstable angina.

acute myocardial infarction: blockage of circulation to heart tissue, causing necrosis (myocyte death) and frequently associated with pallor, diaphoresis, substernal chest pain radiating down the arms and up to the jaw, nausea, dyspnea, dizziness, and electrocardiographic changes

B natriuretic peptide (BNP): an active hormone cleaved from a promolecule that is released from the left heart ventricle with cardiac overload and myocardial stretch

cardiac biomarkers: proteins released from myocardium that can be used to monitor cardiac injury

cardiac troponins I (cTnI) and T (cTnT): components of the muscle contractile apparatus that have amino acid sequences that are distinct from skeletal muscle, making them cardiac specific

congestive heart failure: cardiac dysfunction caused by insufficient cardiac output to satisfy the perfusion needs of the patient and characterized by dyspnea, sodium and water retention, and edema

copeptin: a 39 amino acid peptide derived from a hypothalamic preprohormone that increases within minutes of a myocardial infarction

creatine kinase (CK): an enzyme released from a variety of tissues, indicating nonspecific muscle tissue damage and catalyzing the phosphorylation of creatine

creatine kinase index: the ratio of CKMB (ng/mL) to total CK activity (U/L), multiplied by 100; helpful in differentiating CK elevations of skeletal muscle origin from those of myocardial origin

creatine kinase MB (CKMB): an isoenzyme of creatine kinase present in myocardium (~10%-20% of total CK) and in large skeletal muscle (~2%-5% of total CK)

dyspnea: labored breathing

isoenzyme: a group of proteins that have the same catalytic function but have different sequences

myoglobin: an early nonspecific biomarker of injury to skeletal and myocardial muscle

NT pro-BNP: a biologically inactive protein cleaved from a promolecule that is released from the left heart ventricle with cardiac overload and myocardial stretch

3.3 Background/significance

Acute coronary syndrome and **congestive heart failure** afflict millions of people each year, and the use of biomarkers, coupled with clinical examination and other studies, is required to diagnose these conditions.

Following ischemic injury to cells, cell membrane integrity is compromised, allowing intracellular constituents to leak into the blood. Important parameters that determine the usefulness of a cellular constituent as a biomarker include cellular location (cytosolic components reach the blood faster than structural components), molecular size (smaller components reach the blood faster than larger components), and tissue specificity (markers more specific for cardiac tissue provide more assay specificity than those that are less specific for cardiac tissue). Unfortunately, no biomarker is completely specific for diagnosis of myocardial infarction; thus a combination of biomarkers is usually used, although some clinical laboratories are now offering a "troponin only" approach due to the advent of "highly sensitive" troponin assays (see below).

3.4 Troponin

Of the biomarkers currently used, **cardiac troponin I (cTnI) and T (cTnT)** offer the highest degree of cardiac specificity. Troponin is a regulatory protein complex located on the thin filament of the contractile apparatus and consists of 3 protein subunits: troponin T (which binds to tropomyosin), I (which inhibits myosin ATPase), and C (which binds to calcium). Although troponin is present in skeletal muscle as well as cardiac tissue, the cTnI and cTnT cardiac isoenzymes have a different amino acid composition compared to skeletal muscle, and thus are cardiac specific. In addition to their use in detecting **acute myocardial infarction**, elevations of the cardiac troponins are also thought to be of prognostic significance, with mild elevations being associated with future adverse cardiac events [PMID18209672, PMID25545229]. A key indicator for the diagnosis of an acute event is a rise and fall of the biomarker over a period of hours to days (depending on the degree of myocardial cell necrosis).

A newer generation of highly sensitive troponin assays (not yet approved by the US Food and Drug Administration [FDA]) under development are sufficiently sensitive to measure concentrations in 50% of healthy adults [PMID22105197]. These assays, which measure concentrations <0.01 ng/mL, are reliable. In fact, most normal individuals will have serum concentrations <0.01 ng/mL. The percent change from baseline results appears to provide the best diagnostic for myocardial infarction, with changes >20% considered to be significant [PMID22205772].

Reference ranges for cTnI vary depending on the assay being used and the precision at the lower end of the reportable range. Reference ranges for cTnT are more standardized because only 1 manufacturer creates this assay, but they vary depending on the preferences of individual laboratories. With the currently available fourth generation cTnT assay, the reference range is <0.01 ng/mL. The timeframe for first elevation depends on the assay sensitivity. Classically, troponins start to rise ~4-6 hours following acute myocardial infarction, peak at 24-36 hours, and return to baseline after 72 hours. With the newer generation highly sensitive assays, troponin concentrations can be elevated within 1-2 hours of an infarction.

In microinfarctions, in which the amount of tissue necrosis is small, the degree and duration of troponin elevation may be considerably less **f3.1** [PMID12087146]. The key findings in these cases is a clear rise and fall of cTnT in the setting of symptoms consistent with a myocardial infarction. In those situations, CKMB may not be elevated [PMID12087146].

3.5 Creatine kinase

Creatine kinase (CK) is an enzyme that catalyzes the phosphorylation of creatine in muscle to phosphocreatine. CK is a dimer, consisting of 2 units (M, muscle; B, brain). Thus there are 3 isoenzymes: MM, MB, and BB. In skeletal muscle, the predominant form of CK is CKMM, while the highest percentage of **creatine kinase MB (CKMB)** activity (10%-20% of total CK activity) is in myocardium [ISBN9781416061649]. A small amount of CKMB (~2%-5% of total CK activity) resides in skeletal muscle [ISBN9781416061649]. Isoenzyme CKBB is not used as a cardiac marker. The reference range for CK activity depends on the laboratory performing the test but is generally <200 U/L. Since it is present in muscle, its activity is directly proportional to the amount of muscle mass, so

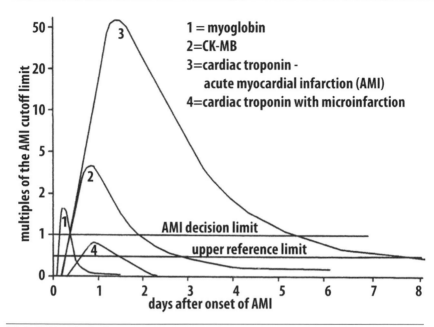

f3.1 Cardiac biomarker timeline

that individuals with larger muscle mass generally have higher CK activity than those with lower muscle mass [PMID17569697].

Concentrations of CKMB (ng/mL), in contrast to activity measurements (U/L, used for total CK), are helpful in the diagnosis of acute myocardial infarction, in which condition they are usually >10 ng/mL. The CKMB starts to rise ~4-6 hours following myocardial infarction, peaks at 18-36 hours, and returns to normal by 72 hours. Since CKMB is also present in skeletal muscle the use of the **creatine kinase index** can be helpful in differentiating CKMB elevations of skeletal muscle origin from those of myocardial origin. At least 3 samples should be obtained within the first 24 hours.

$$\text{CK index} = \frac{\text{CKMB mass (ng/mL)}}{\text{total CK activity (U/L)}} \times 100$$

(dimensionless—not a percentage)

Normal CK index is <2.5; CK indices >2.5 suggest cardiac damage
➤ CKMB <10 ng/mL; CK index <2.5 is considered normal
➤ CKMB >10 ng/mL; CK index >2.5 suggests cardiac damage
➤ CKMB >10 ng/mL; CK index <2.5 suggests skeletal muscle damage

The CK index is elevated with acute myocardial infarction as the elevation of the CK activity (denominator) is primarily due to the contribution from CKMB, so that the numerator (CKMB mass) is proportionately a substantial part of the total. In contrast, the CK index is not elevated with skeletal muscle damage as the elevation of the CK activity (denominator) is primarily due to the contribution from CKMM, so that the numerator (CKMB mass) is proportionately a small part of the total.

Elevations of CKMB can also be seen with myocarditis, polymyositis, dermatomyositis, muscle trauma, muscular dystrophies, malignant hyperthermia, shock, severe angina, rhabdomyolysis, and coronary insufficiency. Accordingly, CKMB is not recommended by the 2014 American Heart Association/American College of Cardiology guidelines for the management of patients with acute coronary syndromes [PMID25249586].

3.6 Myoglobin

Myoglobin is a low molecular weight oxygen carrying protein (16 Kd) present in all skeletal and cardiac muscle. Due to its small size, it appears in serum rapidly after release from injured tissue and is cleared into the urine. Because it is found in most tissues, it has the least specificity of the **cardiac biomarkers**, and for this reason it is not recommended by the 2014 American Heart Association/ American College of Cardiology guidelines for the management of patients with acute coronary syndromes [PMID25249586]. Myoglobin begins to rise 2-3 hours following myocardial infarction, peaks at 6-9 hours, and returns to baseline at 24 hours. An increase of ≥25% over 90 minutes is seen following acute myocardial infarction.

The timeline for rise and fall of cardiac troponin, CKMB, and myoglobin is shown in **f3.1**.

3.7 Copeptin

Arginine vasopressin (AVP; antidiuretic hormone [ADH]), produced in the hypothalamus and stored in the anterior pituitary, is involved in multiple cardiovascular functions. Its small size and short half-life make its measurement very challenging, and thus it is not widely used for diagnosis of acute myocardial infarction. **Copeptin** is a 39 amino acid peptide that is derived from a hypothalamic preprohormone consisting of vasopressin, neurophysin II, and copeptin. Thus, copeptin can serve as a vasopressin "surrogate," since it is produced stoichiometrically with vasopressin. It can be measured by immunoassay (which use is not yet FDA approved). It is increased within minutes of acute myocardial infarction and declines within a few hours. Recent studies [PMID19555842, PMID20447532, PMID21807867] suggest that the combination of troponin and copeptin biomarkers provides a remarkable negative predictive value that is independent of the time of onset of chest pain.

Clinical validation studies are still underway.

3.8 Congestive heart failure

With volume overload and myocardial stretch the left heart ventricle releases the promolecule pro-B natriuretic peptide (pro-BNP). During the release process, pro-BNP is cleaved into the active hormone **B natriuretic peptide (BNP)** and an inactive N terminal fragment (**NT pro-BNP**). Both of these are useful biomarkers for evaluating **congestive heart failure**.

In individuals without congestive heart failure, serum BNP is <100 pg/mL. In contrast, given its longer half-life, the NT pro-BNP is much higher. Both BNP and NT pro-BNP increase with age; however, most laboratories only report age related reference ranges for NT pro-BNP:

➤ NT pro-BNP (<50 years old): <450 pg/mL

➤ NT pro-BNP (50-75 years old): <900 pg/mL

➤ NT pro-BNP (>75 years old): <1,800 pg/mL

BNP has also been used in the diagnosis of myocardial infarction since it rises rapidly over the first 24 hours after myocardial infarction and then stabilizes [PMID12460861]. However, it lacks the sensitivity of the cardiac troponins for diagnosis.

3.9 Changing horizons

The field of biomarkers for myocardial infarction and congestive heart failure is rapidly evolving due to the improvement of the sensitivity of existing assays (eg, troponin) as well as development of assays for newer markers (eg, copeptin, galectin-3, ST2) that may be diagnostically and prognostically useful. This chapter focuses on those markers that are still most commonly used in the diagnosis of myocardial infarction and congestive heart failure.

3.10 References
3.10.1 Jounrnals

PMID12087146 Antman EM [2002] Decision making with cardiac troponin test. *N Engl J Med* 26:2079-82

PMID12460861 De Lemos JA, Morrow DA [2002] Brain natriuretic peptide measurement in acute coronary syndromes – ready for clinical application? *Circulation* 106:2868-70

PMID17569697 Brancaccio P, Maffulli N, Limongelli FM [2007] Creatine kinase monitoring in sport medicine. *Br Med Bull* 81-82:209-230

PMID18209672 Babuin L, Vasile VC, Rio Perez JA et al [2008] Elevated cardiac troponin is an independent risk factor for short and long term mortality in medical intensive care unit patients. *Crit Care Med* 36:759-65

PMID19555842 Reichlin T, Hochholzer W, Stelzig C et al [2009] Incremental value of copeptin for rapid rule out of acute myocardial infarction. *J Am Coll Cardiol* 54:60-68

PMID20447532 Keller T, Tzikas S, Zeller T et al [2010] Copeptin improves early diagnosis of acute myocardial infarction. *J Am Coll Cardiol* 55:2096-2106

PMID21807867 Giannitsis E, Kehayova T, Vafaie M et al [2011] Combined testing of high-sensitivity troponin T and copeptin on presentation at prespecified cutoffs improves rapid rule-out of non-ST segment elevation myocardial infarction. *Clin Chem* 57:1452-55

PMID22105197 Mahajan VS, Jarolim P [2011] How to interpret elevated cardiac troponin levels. *Circulation* 124:2350-2354

PMID22205772 Katus HA, Giannitsis E, Jaffe AS [2012] Interpreting changes in troponin – clinical judgement is essential. *Clin Chem* 58: 39-43

PMID25249586 Amsterdam EA, Wenger NK, Brindis RG et al [2014] 2014 AHA/ guideline for the management of patients with non-ST-elevation acute coronary syndrome – executive summary. *Circulation* 130:2354-2394

 ISBN 978-089189-6548

PMID25545229 Torre M, Jarolim P [2015] Cardiac troponin assays in the management of heart failure. *Clin Chim Acta* 441:92-98

3.10.2 Book

ISBN9781416061649 Apple FS, Goetze JP, Jaffe AS [2012] Cardiac function. In: Burtis CA, Ashwood ER, Bruns DE, ed. *Tietz Textbook of Clinical Chemistry and Molecular Diagnostics*, 5e. Elsevier Saunders, 1457-1522

3.11 Clinical cases

3.11.1 Case 1

A 53-year-old female presented to the emergency department with squeezing substernal chest pain radiating down both arms and accompanied by palpitations, diaphoresis, dizziness, and shortness of breath for 4 hours. She was a nonsmoker and nonrecreational drug user. She had no history of hypertension, diabetes, cardiac disease, or hypercholesterolemia. The electrocardiogram showed 0.5-1.0 mm ST segment depression.

Vital signs: blood pressure 163/102 mm Hg, heart rate 58 beats/min, respiratory rate 18 breaths/min, and oral temperature 37.0°C.

Cardiac examination showed a regular rate and rhythm. The remainder of the physical examination was normal.

t3.1 Laboratory results

	6 hr	12 hr	18 hr	24 hr	30 hr
CK (ref <200 U/L)	176	195	175	98	84
CKMB (ref <10 ng/mL)	8	14	10	6	4
cTnT (ref <0.01 ng/mL)	0.10	0.80	0.73	0.50	0.35

3.11.1.1 Questions

1. Calculate the CK index for each time point.

2. Did the patient "rule in" or "rule out" for myocardial infarction based on these laboratory findings?

3. Why is the total CK normal (<200 U/L)?

3.11.2 Case 2

A 57-year-old male presents to the emergency department with a 1 hour history of shortness of breath, coughing, and "chest tightness." He states that his symptoms appeared suddenly while he was watching television on his couch. He describes a constant "squeezing" sensation in his chest limited to the parasternal region and associated with a paroxysmal nonproductive cough. He describes his shortness of breath as "difficulty getting air," denying any pain on inspiration or expiration. He denies any similar episode in the past. His past medical history is significant for type I diabetes mellitus, hypertension, and severe peripheral vascular disease. 6 years ago his right leg was amputated just above the knee, and his left leg was amputated below the knee. He denies any syncopal episode or thigh or abdominal swelling. He sleeps on 1 pillow at night and usually does not wake up to urinate. He used to drink alcohol heavily but has not had a drink for more than 10 years. He denies any tobacco or illicit drug use.

Vital signs: oral temperature 97°F, heart rate 128 beats/min, respiratory rate 28 breaths/min, BP 179/102 mm Hg

Results of the physical exam are as follows:

➤ neck: no jugular venous distension (JVD)
➤ heart
  o sinus tachycardia, regular rhythm
  o grade I/VI nonradiating systolic ejection murmur at the left sternal border
➤ lungs
  o fine rales in the lower half of each lung field
  o no rhonchi or friction rubs
➤ chest wall: no tenderness to palpation
➤ abdomen
  o no ascites or hepatosplenomegaly
  o no tenderness

Chest X ray: bilateral fluffy infiltrates consistent with pulmonary edema

EKG: sinus tachycardia; no acute changes from previous EKG; no ST segment depression or elevation (on admission)

t3.2 Laboratory tests

	Admission	30 min	60 min	90 min	3 hr	8 hr	12 hr
CKMB (ng/mL; normal <10)	2.7	4.3	5.3	6.5	9.8	11.4	8.8
Troponin I (ng/mL; normal <0.07)	0.1	0.3	0.5	0.8	3.6	8.2	5.9
Myoglobin (ng/mL; normal <100)	49	98	165	184	129	86	56

3.11.2.1 Questions

1. How do you interpret these data? Are they diagnostic?

2. Given the above results, graph their relative crescendos, peaks, and durations of elevation.

3. What do the lab tests tell you about the chronology of events?

4. Why might the patient not have presented with typical chest pain?

3.11.3 **Case answers**

3.11.3.1 **Case 1 answers**

1.   6 hours: 4.5; 12 hours: 7.2; 18 hours: 5.7; 24 hours: 6.1; and 30 hours: 4.8

2.   Since cTnT showed an increase by 6 hours and continued to rise (>20% from baseline), the patient "ruled in" for myocardial infarction. In addition, the CK ratios exceeded 2.5, and the CKMB exceeded 10 ng/mL. It should be noted that, in this case, both the CKMB and cTnT peaked a little earlier than the classic 18-36 hours and 24-36 hour timeline, respectively, demonstrating the interindividual variability in myocardial infarctions related to size and degree of the infarction.

3.   The patient could conceivably have low body mass, resulting in a low baseline CK. Also, CKMB (which contributes to total CK) is less sensitive for myocardial infarction than cTnT.

3.11.3.2 **Case 2 answers**

1.   The CKMB peaks >10 ng/mL, the troponin I peaks >0.07 ng/mL, and the myoglobin peaks >100 ng/mL. In addition the myoglobin exceeds an increase of 25% over 90 minutes, and the troponin is increased >20% above baseline. These findings suggest acute myocardial infarction.

2.   See **f3.1.**

3.   Given that myoglobin starts to rise at 2-3 hours, CKMB at 4-6 hours, and troponin at 4-6 hours after myocardial infarction, the patient's pattern suggests that the event occurred 1.5-5.5 hours before presentation.

4.   The patient has diabetes mellitus type 1 and likely has diabetic peripheral neuropathy, thereby decreasing his ability to perceive pain.

chapter 4

The laboratory diagnosis of gastrointestinal disease

4.1 Objectives

At the end of this session, the learner should be able to

➤ discuss the types of cells in the stomach

➤ discuss the process for measurement of basal, peak, and maximal gastric acid output

➤ describe differences in gastric acid output for men vs women, younger vs older people, and patients with duodenal ulcer, gastric ulcer, gastric carcinoma, pernicious anemia, and hypothyroidism vs normal people

➤ describe conditions in which achlorhydria is found

➤ discuss causes of increased serum gastrin concentrations

➤ discuss the rapid urease test, the urea breath test, and the use of serum antibody tests in suspected *Helicobacter pylori* infection

➤ discuss the causes of general malabsorption and maldigestion

➤ describe specific malabsorption and maldigestion defects

➤ discuss the nonspecific biochemical findings in malabsorption

➤ describe the disaccharidase test in the workup of malabsorption

➤ discuss the hydrogen breath test in the workup of malabsorption

➤ discuss the fecal fat measurement in the workup of malabsorption

➤ describe the use of the ^{14}C-triolein breath test in the workup of malabsorption

➤ describe the use of the IgA endomysial antibody (EMA) and the IgG and IgA tissue transglutaminase (TTG) tests in the workup of suspected celiac disease

➤ discuss the Schilling test in the workup of suspected pernicious anemia

4.2 Key terms

achlorhydria: lack of acid production by the stomach

amyloidosis: a disease in which amyloid (a misfolded protein) is deposited into vital organs (eg, heart, kidney)

blind loop syndrome: a condition caused by bypass of a portion of the intestine, leading to bacterial overgrowth and malabsorption

breath tests: tests that detect abnormalities of carbon dioxide and hydrogen elimination in breath due to defects in digestion and absorption and/or due to bacterial overgrowth

carcinoid syndrome: a group of symptoms related to carcinoid tumors in the intestine and/or lung that elaborate vasoactive substances.

celiac disease (gluten sensitive enteropathy): a disease caused by the immune mediated destructive interaction of gluten with intestinal mucosa, causing malabsorption

Crohn disease: an autoimmune chronic inflammatory bowel disease affecting any part of the gastrointestinal tract, from mouth to anus, usually with intermittent patches of healthy and diseased tissue

gastrin: a peptide hormone secreted by the antral G cells of the stomach and stimulating hydrochloric acid secretion by the parietal cells of the stomach

gluten: a protein found in wheat products

Helicobacter pylori: a bacterium that can be found in the mucous layer of the stomach and is implicated in the development of duodenal and gastric ulcers

intrinsic factor: a glycoprotein produced by the parietal cells of the stomach that is necessary for absorption of vitamin B_{12}

malabsorption: an abnormality of the small intestine causing a disorder in absorption

maldigestion: an abnormality of the digestive process due to dysfunction of the pancreas, bile acids, or small intestine

pernicious anemia: a megaloblastic anemia caused by lack of intrinsic factor production by the parietal cells of the stomach, leading to malabsorption of vitamin B_{12}

pseudo Zollinger-Ellison syndrome: hypergastrinemia caused by hyperplasia of the antral G cells of the stomach

scleroderma: an autoimmune chronic connective tissue disease resulting in sclerosis of skin and organs

steatorrhea: a condition characterized by excess fat in the feces (>7 g/day)

tropical sprue: a type of malabsorption seen in tropical areas and thought to be associated with environmental factors; its specific etiology is unknown

ulcerative colitis: a recurrent inflammatory disease of the large bowel characterized by continuous inflammation without patches of interspersed healthy tissue

Whipple disease: a rare disease caused by *Tropheryma whipplei* and leading to intestinal malabsorption

Zollinger-Ellison (ZE) syndrome: a condition resulting from a gastrin secreting tumor (gastrinoma) of the non-β pancreatic islet cells, resulting in overproduction of gastric acid and leading to fulminant ulceration of the esophagus, stomach, duodenum, and jejunum

4.3 Background/significance

Functional disorders of the gastrointestinal tract are estimated to afflict 30% of the adult population in Western countries [PMID10877233, PMID15243388]. Although endoscopy is now a "frontline" procedure in the diagnostic workup of gastrointestinal disease, it is invasive, and clinical laboratory tests are still important in establishing the diagnosis of specific disorders.

4.4 **Measurement of gastric acid output**

With the widespread use of endoscopy, the measurement of gastric acid output is performed less frequently than in the past, but is still used in certain situations (eg, determining the cause of fasting hypergastrinemia) [ISBN9780071806336].

The cell types in the stomach are the surface epithelial cells (mucus production), the antral G cells (gastrin production), the peptic (chief) cells (pepsinogen production), and the parietal cells (intrinsic factor and hydrochloric acid production).

The tests of gastric function are based on the measurement of the amount of hydrochloric acid (HCl) produced by the stomach under basal (resting, fasting) conditions and without exposure to visual, auditory, or olfactory stimuli. This is followed by testing after stimulation. Acid concentration is determined (mEq/hour) by titration with sodium hydroxide.

Basal gastric secretion is determined on a 1 hour gastric aspirate collected every 15 minutes via a nasogastric tube after at least a 12 hour overnight fast. The measured acid concentration totaled for the 1 hour aspirate represents the basal acid secretion (mEq/hour) [PMID21261669].

A synthetic analog of gastrin (eg, pentagastrin) is then injected subcutaneously, stimulating gastric acid secretion. 4 serial 15 minute specimens are collected, and the acid output in the 2 specimens with the highest output is summed to calculate the peak acid output (mEq/hour) [PMID21261669]. Maximal acid output (mEq/hour) is calculated by summing the 4 successive 15 minute results following the injection of the gastrin analog [PMID21261669].

Patients with duodenal ulcer have higher output than normal, while patients with gastric ulcer, gastric carcinoma, pernicious anemia (may have achlorhydria), and hypothyroidism have lower output than normal controls [ISBN9780803636644]. In general, younger people have higher gastric acid output than older people, and men have higher output than women [PMID13969448].

4.5 **Zollinger-Ellison syndrome**

Zollinger-Ellison syndrome is caused by a non-β islet cell gastrin producing tumor of the pancreas. The high gastrin stimulates HCl secretion by the parietal cells of the stomach. **Pseudo Zollinger-Ellison syndrome** is caused by hyperplasia of the antral G cells, and also results in elevated gastrin concentrations and excessive HCl secretion. High gastrin concentrations are also seen with pernicious anemia [PMID6732375], presumably due to attempt by the antral G cells to stimulate HCl production by the defective parietal cells.

4.6 *Helicobacter pylori*

Helicobacter pylori has been implicated in many gastrointestinal diseases, including duodenal and gastric ulcer, gastritis, and possibly gastric cancer. The organism thrives in the acidic environment of the stomach by making the enzyme urease, which breaks down urea to yield carbon dioxide and ammonia. Ammonia neutralizes the HCl in the stomach, allowing the bacterium to survive.

Tests for *Helicobacter pylori* include the rapid urease test, which involves culturing a biopsy specimen on medium containing urea and a phenol red pH indicator, which changes from yellow to red as ammonia alkalinizes the medium [PMID11996414]. Several commercial kits are available for this test. The urea breath test relies upon detection of either ^{14}C or ^{13}C labelled CO_2 in collected breath from an individual who has ingested ^{14}C or ^{13}C labelled urea [PMID11996414].

Patients who have *Helicobacter pylori* infection develop IgG, IgA, and IgM antibodies to the bacterium. Assays to detect these antibodies are available. Detection of *Helicobacter pylori* antibodies indicates that the patient was exposed to *Helicobacter pylori* at some time, but not necessarily that the infection is active, since IgG antibodies can persist for years after successful treatment with antibiotics [PMID11996414]. While most laboratories test for IgG antibodies, just a few test for all 3.

4.7 Malabsorption & maldigestion

Malabsorption is a dysfunction of the absorptive process by the gut caused by inflammation, infection, surgical resection, vitamin deficiency, and other factors. **Maldigestion** is a dysfunction of the digestive process caused by disorders of bile flow, digestive enzymes, and other factors.

4.7.1 General malabsorption

All major phases of absorption may be involved in this syndrome. It may be due to pancreatic disease (eg, chronic pancreatitis, carcinoma of the pancreas, cystic fibrosis), Zollinger-Ellison syndrome, liver disease with obstruction of bile flow, resin treatment for hyperlipidemia, and diseases or conditions that destroy the intestinal mucosa needed for absorption (eg, celiac disease, tropical sprue, Crohn disease, ulcerative colitis, Whipple disease, scleroderma, lymphoma, amyloidosis, parasitic infestations, blind loop syndrome, carcinoid syndrome, intestinal resection).

Some nonspecific biochemical abnormalities associated with general malabsorption include decreased serum/plasma concentrations of calcium, vitamin D, proteins, urea-nitrogen (reflecting decreased proteins, from which urea is derived after protein deamination), cholesterol, and vitamin A. Because the fat soluble vitamin K may also be deficient, the vitamin K dependent clotting factors (II, VII, IX, X) may be low, leading to abnormalities in coagulation resulting in an elevated prothrombin time. Serum/plasma alkaline phosphatase activity (bone) may also be elevated due to the elaboration of parathyroid hormone (PTH) in response to the low calcium and vitamin D.

4.7.1.1 Specific malabsorption defects

Some specific malabsorption defects include the disaccharidase deficiencies (eg, lactase, maltase, sucrase deficiency), celiac disease (gluten sensitive enteropathy), pernicious anemia (due to malabsorption of vitamin B_{12} from lack of intrinsic factor in the parietal cells of the stomach), and protein losing enteropathy.

4.7.1.2 Tests used in the evaluation of malabsorption

Disaccharidase deficiencies can be inferred by the oral administration of the disaccharide that appears to be malabsorbed (eg, lactose in lactase deficiency; maltose in maltase deficiency; sucrose in sucrase deficiency). Lactose is a glucose-galactose dimer; maltose is glucose-glucose; and sucrose is glucose-fructose. Following administration of 50 g of the suspected disaccharide, the serum/plasma glucose is measured every 30 minutes for a 2 hour period. Normal individuals will demonstrate an increase in serum/plasma glucose of 20-30 mg/dL over fasting glucose concentrations. If the increase is less, in order to rule out a monosaccharide absorption defect, 25 g of each monosaccharide (eg, glucose) is administered orally. Normal absorption of the monosaccharide following abnormal absorption of the disaccharide suggests the disaccharidase deficiency [ISBN9781483250793].

The hydrogen breath test is useful in the detection of bacterial fermentation of retained carbohydrates (eg, due to lactose intolerance) as well as bacterial overgrowth in the gut. Hydrogen is not produced by mammalian cells. Breath is collected into a device, and the hydrogen concentration is measured electrochemically [PMID16474100].

Steatorrhea, a consistent finding in general malabsorption, is also a frequent cause of the diarrhea seen in malabsorption. A high fecal fat concentration is the best confirmatory test for steatorrhea. Stool is collected into a large, preweighed container over a 72 hour period (to account for the great interindividual variation in frequency of bowel movements). The sample is homogenized with a known volume of water and blended to emulsify, and a measured aliquot is removed for extraction of fat using organic solvents. The solvent is evaporated, and the resulting residue (representing total fat) is weighed. Normal individuals excrete <7 g of fat per 24 hours, while individuals with general malabsorption excrete more. Less intrusive is a qualitative microscopic screen of a random stool sample. (Normal individuals average 2.5 fat droplets per high power field [PMID10761454].)

Abnormality of triglyceride absorption and metabolism can be evaluated with the ^{14}C-triolein breath test. Triolein is a triglyceride. With deficiency of pancreatic lipase, the absorption of triglyceride fat can be impaired. After administration of ^{14}C-triolein, normal individuals exhale ^{14}CO$_2$. If labelled CO$_2$ is not detected in the collected breath, triglyceride malabsorption should be expected [PMID6675178].

Celiac disease (**gluten sensitive enteropathy**) results from an immune mediated intolerance to ingestion of **gluten**, a protein found in wheat, or related proteins from barley and rye. The immunological response to gluten causes atrophy of the intestinal villi, hyperplasia of the crypts, and intraepithelial lymphocyte invasion. An endoscopic biopsy is the "gold standard" for diagnosis. However, it is invasive, and preliminary blood tests are often performed.

>95% of patients with celiac disease share the major histocompatibility complex II class human leukocyte antigen (HLA) DQ2 or DQ8 haplotype, and patients negative for both haplotypes are unlikely to suffer from celiac disease [PMID11922565]. In contrast, only 30%-35% of the normal Caucasian population has these 2 haplotypes, and of those, only 2%-5% will develop celiac disease

ISBN 978-089189-6548

[PMID6675178]. Accurate diagnosis of celiac disease requires the patient to have gluten in his or her diet at the time of testing. Serum tests that are useful in the diagnosis of the disease include IgA antitissue transglutaminase antibody (TTG; >98% specificity, >93% sensitivity) and IgA endomysial antibody (EMA; >99% specificity, >93% sensitivity) [PMID22235174]. Since IgA deficiency is more common in patients with celiac disease (3% of patients have IgA deficiency as compared with only 0.3% of the general population) [PMID10702491], the additional use of IgG antitissue transglutaminase antibody has been advocated [PMID15699419]. However, IgG TTG is less specific for celiac disease than IgA TTG and is not a "frontline" test. In addition, IgG antibodies persist long after successful treatment. The treatment of celiac disease is a lifelong gluten free diet.

Pernicious anemia is caused by the lack of elaboration of intrinsic factor by the parietal cells of the stomach, leading to vitamin B_{12} malabsorption and megaloblastic anemia, as well as by blocking antibody to intrinsic factor. Vitamin B_{12} deficiency can also result from malabsorption due to intestinal disease. Currently vitamin B_{12} deficiency is diagnosed by direct measurement of vitamin B_{12} by immunoassay as well as by monitoring concentrations of methylmalonic acid in serum and urine. Methylmalonic acid concentrations rise with vitamin B_{12} deficiency since the vitamin is required to convert methylmalonic acid to succinic acid [ISBN9781416601649]. As a biological indicator of functional vitamin B_{12}, the methylmalonic acid concentration may be the preferred test. Historically, the Schilling test has been used in the diagnosis of pernicious anemia. For this test, ^{57}Co labelled vitamin B_{12} is administered orally, and its concentration in serum and urine is measured. Normal individuals excrete >8% of the ingested dose in a 24 hour urine collection, while individuals with pernicious anemia excrete <7% of the administered dose. For patients with decreased urine concentrations of vitamin B_{12} in the Schilling test, the diagnosis is confirmed by coadministering intrinsic factor with vitamin B_{12}. Following administration of intrinsic factor with the labelled vitamin B_{12} in a patient with pernicious anemia, the abnormality is corrected [ISBN9781416601649].

4.8 References
4.8.1 Journals

PMID10702491 Prince HE, Norman GL, Binder WL [2000] Immunoglobulin A (IgA) deficiency and alternative celiac-disease associated antibodies in sera submitted to a reference laboratory for endomysial IgA testing. *Clin Diagn Lab Immunol* 7:192-6

PMID10761454 Fine KD, Ogunji F [2000] A new method of quantitative fecal fat microscopy and its correlation with chemically measured fecal fat output. *Am J Clin Pathol* 113:528-34

PMID10877233 Sandler RS, Stewart WF, Liberman JN et al [2000] Abdominal pain, bloating, and diarrhea in the United States: prevalence and impact. *Dig Dis Sci* 45:1166-71

PMID11922565 Kaukinen K, Partanen J, Maeki M et al [2002] HLA-DQ typing in the diagnosis of celiac disease. *Am J Gastroenterol* 97:695-9

PMID11996414 Meurer LN, Bower DJ [2002] Management of *Helicobacter pylori* infection. *Am Fam Phys* 65:1327-37

PMID13969448 Baron JH [1963] Studies of basal and peak acid output with an augmented histamine test. *Gut* 4:136-144

PMID15243388 Bommelaer G, Poynard T, Le Pen C et al [2004] Prevalence of irritable bowel syndrome (IBS) and variability of diagnostic criteria. *Gastroenterol Clin Biol* 28:554-61

PMID15699419 Dahlbom I, Olsson M, Forooz NK et al [2005] Immunoglobulin G (IgG) anti-tissue transglutaminase antibodies used as markers for IgA-deficient celiac disease patients. *Clin Diagn Lab Immunol* 12:254-8

PMID16474100 Simren M, Stotzer P-O [2006] Use and abuse of hydrogen breath tests. *Gut* 55:297-303

PMID21261669 Ghosh T, Lewis DI, Axon ATR et al [2011] Review article: methods of measuring gastric acid secretion. *Aliment Pharmacol Ther* 33:768-81

PMID22235174 Scanlon SA, Murray JA [2011] Update on celiac disease – etiology, differential diagnosis, drug targets, and management advances. *Clin Exp Gastroenterol* 4:297-311

PMID6675178 Einarsson K, Bjoerkhem I, Ekloef R et al [1983] ^{14}C-Triolein breath test as a rapid and convenient screening test for fat malabsorption. *Scand J Gastroenterol* 18:9-12

PMID6732375 Slingerland DW, Cardarelli JA, Burrows BA et al [1984] The utility of serum gastrin levels in assessing the significance of low serum B_{12} levels. *JAMA Intern Med* 144:1167-68

4.8.2 Books

ISBN9780071806336 McQuaid KR [2014] Gastrointestinal disorders. In: Papadakis MA, McPhee SJ, Rabow MW, ed. *Current Medical Diagnosis & Treatment*, 53e. McGraw-Hill Education, 547-640

ISBN9780803636644 Van Leeuwen AM, Poelhuis-Leth DJ, Bladh ML [2013] Gastric analysis and gastric acid stimulation test. In: Leeuwen AM, Poelhuis-Leth DJ, Bladh ML. *Davis's Comprehensive Handbook of Laboratory & Diagnostic Tests with Nursing Implications*, 5e. FA Davis, 734-35

ISBN9781416061649 Shenken A, Roberts NB [2012] Vitamins and trace elements. In: Burtis CA, Ashwood ER, Bruns DE. *Tietz Textbook of Clinical Chemistry and Molecular Diagnostics*, 5e. Elsevier Saunders, 895-984

ISBN9781483250793 Dahlqvist A, Lindquist B, Meeuwisse G [1968] Disturbances of the digestion and absorption of carbohydrates. In: Dickens F, Randle PJ, Whelan WJ, ed. *Carbohydrate Metabolism and Its Disorders*. Academic Press, 199-219

4.9 Clinical cases

4.9.1 Case 1

4.9.1.1 Question

1. List the most common symptoms (history), physical findings (signs), and laboratory abnormalities in an extreme case of malabsorption.

4.9.2 Case 2

A 48-year-old male presents with a chief complaint of chronic diarrhea and epigastric pain occurring over the past year. He states that the diarrhea is watery and without blood, pus, or mucus. He has a history of duodenal ulcer for which he took cimetidine and now takes omeprazole. He has been treated for *H pylori* without improvement of his symptoms. Over the past 6 months he has lost 25 pounds. He denies the use of laxatives.

Vital signs: oral temperature 98°F, heart rate 88 bpm, blood pressure 114/55 mmHg, respiratory rate 28 breaths/min, and weight 200 lb.

Physical examination was normal. A rectal examination was normal, and the stool was negative for occult blood.

Laboratory data: serum sodium 137 mMol/L (mEq/L), potassium 3.3 mMol/L (mEq/L), chloride 96 mMol/L (mEq/L), bicarbonate 27 mMol/L (mEq/L), urea-nitrogen 27 mg/dL, creatinine 0.8 mg/dL; stool fat 2 g/day; stool examination for ova and parasites negative; and serum gastrin 1,482 pg/mL (reference range <100).

Colonoscopy with biopsies: normal

4.9.2.1 Questions

1. What is the most likely diagnosis?

2. What is the recommended treatment?

3. What syndrome is the patient at increased risk for?

4. What are the features of that syndrome?

5. Why is the serum potassium low?

6. Why is the serum urea-nitrogen elevated?

7. Why is the blood pressure low?

4.9.3 **Case 3**

A 19-year-old male (6 ft, 165 lb) presented to a student health services physician 2 months after starting college with symptoms suggestive of an eating disorder. He reported a weight loss of 15 pounds over the last 2 weeks, diarrhea, fatigue, bloating, and vomiting after meals. An IgA endomysial antibody (EMA) test was positive.

4.9.3.1 **Questions**

1. What is the most likely diagnosis?

2. What laboratory tests should be ordered?

3. Is this a common presentation for this disease?

4. How should the patient be treated?

4.9.4 **Clinical case answers**

4.9.4.1 **Case 1 answers**

1. Common symptoms
   - ➢ abdominal distention (decreased albumin, increased gas; sign as well)
   - ➢ abdominal pain and cramping
   - ➢ diarrhea (excessive fat in stools)
   - ➢ dizziness (hypotension due to anemia)
   - ➢ easy to bleed/bruise (deficient vitamin K dependent clotting factors; sign as well)
   - ➢ easy to fracture ("brittle bones"; decreased calcium)
   - ➢ flatus (sign as well)
   - ➢ floating, malodorous stools (excessive fat in stools)
   - ➢ lethargy/weakness (anemia)
   - ➢ poor balance (vitamin B_{12} deficiency; sign as well)
   - ➢ poor night vision (vitamin A deficiency)
   - ➢ poor vibratory sensation (vitamin B_{12} deficiency; sign as well)
   - ➢ rapid heart rate (anemia; sign as well)
   - ➢ sore tongue (glossitis; vitamin B_{12} deficiency)
   - ➢ weight loss

   Physical findings
   - ➢ abdominal distention (decreased albumin, increased gas; symptom as well)
   - ➢ cachexia
   - ➢ cardiac arrhythmias (decreased potassium)
   - ➢ cheilosis (vitamin B_2 deficiency)
   - ➢ conjunctival pallor (anemia)
   - ➢ decreased blood pressure (anemia)
   - ➢ easy to bleed/bruise (deficient vitamin K dependent clotting factors; symptom as well)
   - ➢ ecchymoses (deficient vitamin K dependent clotting factors)
   - ➢ edema (decreased albumin)
   - ➢ flatus (symptom as well)
   - ➢ glossitis (vitamin B_{12} deficiency)
   - ➢ increased deep tendon reflexes (decreased calcium)
   - ➢ poor balance (vitamin B_{12} deficiency; symptom as well)
   - ➢ poor vibratory sensation (vitamin B_{12} deficiency; symptom as well)
   - ➢ rapid heart rate (anemia; symptom as well)
   - ➢ sagging skin folds (weight loss)

   Laboratory abnormalities
   - ➢ abnormal electrocardiogram (tachycardia, arrhythmias, conduction defects; low potassium, anemia, low calcium)

- decreased
  - calcium
  - carotene
  - folate
  - hematocrit
  - hemoglobin
  - red blood cells
  - potassium
  - total cholesterol
  - total proteins/albumin
  - urea-nitrogen
  - vitamin B_{12}
- increased
  - prothrombin time
  - serum alkaline phosphatase activity
  - stool fat
- pathological fractures (X rays)

4.9.4.2 Case 2 answers

1. Zollinger-Ellison syndrome is the most likely diagnosis; pseudo Zollinger-Ellison syndrome and pernicious anemia may also cause hypergastrinemia, but the gastrin concentrations are usually lower than that observed in this case

2. Surgical removal of the tumor if possible; otherwise, medical treatment for hyperacidity

3. Multiple endocrine neoplasia type I

4. Tumors of pituitary, pancreas, and parathyroid

5. Potassium has been lost in the diarrhea

6. Dehydration from diarrhea has increased the urea-nitrogen concentration. In addition it has likely caused a decreased glomerular filtration rate, leading to increased passive reabsorption of urea. This is suggested by the increased serum urea-nitrogen:creatinine ratio.

7. The blood pressure is low due to dehydration from diarrhea.

4.9.4.3 Case 3 answers

1. Celiac disease (gluten sensitive enteropathy)

2. IgG and IgA antitissue transglutaminase antibody (TTG) and colonoscopy with biopsy to look for villous atrophy, hyperplastic crypts, and intraepithelial lymphocyte infiltration

3. Yes, celiac disease often manifests itself during periods of stress (this patient had just started college)

4. The patient should be started on a gluten free diet

chapter 5

The laboratory diagnosis of renal disease

5.1 Objectives

At the end of this session, the learner should be able to

➤ identify the major nonprotein nitrogenous compounds in serum

➤ describe the influence of diet on serum urea-nitrogen

➤ discuss the passive reabsorption of urea

➤ describe the formation of creatinine

➤ discuss the use of serum urea-nitrogen, creatinine, and glomerular filtration rate in the workup of renal disease

➤ calculate the creatinine clearance as an estimate of glomerular filtration rate

➤ identify alternate methods for estimating the glomerular filtration rate

➤ describe physiological conditions in which the serum urea-nitrogen:creatinine ratio is increased and conditions in which it is decreased

➤ discuss serum cystatin C and why it may be a more sensitive indicator of changes in glomerular filtration rate than serum creatinine

➤ discuss urine osmolality, specific gravity, and renal concentrating ability as indicators of renal tubular function

➤ differentiate prerenal, renal, and postrenal azotemia

➤ discuss the most common findings in acute pyelonephritis

➤ discuss the most common findings in nephrotic syndrome

➤ discuss the most common findings in acute glomerulonephritis

➤ discuss the most common findings in chronic glomerulonephritis

5.2 Key terms

albuminuria: the presence of albumin in urine

azotemia: an excess of nitrogenous compounds in the blood

casts: imprints of renal tubules with Tamm-Horsfall protein as the matrix, often containing cells; they are excreted into the urine

creatinine: a breakdown product of creatine, mostly freely filtered into the urine and often used in estimation of glomerular filtration rate

creatinine clearance: an estimate of the glomerular filtration rate derived from measurement of serum creatinine and its rate of excretion into the urine

cystatin C: a low molecular weight protein produced by all nucleated cells that have cysteine protease inhibitor activity; since it is freely filtered into the urine at a constant rate irrespective of muscle mass, it is being used in the estimation of glomerular filtration rate

glomerular filtration rate (GFR): the rate (mL/min) that substances such as creatinine are filtered through the kidney's glomeruli; a reflection of the number of functioning nephrons; estimated by the creatinine clearance

glomerulonephritis: nephritis accompanied by inflammation of the capillary loops of the kidney's glomeruli, occurring in acute, subacute, and chronic forms

glomerulus: a tuft of blood vessels in the nephron of the kidney, involved in filtration of the blood

hematuria: blood in the urine

isosthenuria: fixed specific gravity of urine (usually 1.008-1.012)

malignant nephrosclerosis: renal disease associated with accelerated phase ("malignant") hypertension

nephrotic syndrome: a group of diseases causing increased glomerular permeability, leading to marked albuminuria and lipiduria, with varying degrees of edema, hyperlipidemia, and hypoalbuminemia

oliguria: decreased urine output

postrenal azotemia: increased concentration of nitrogenous compounds (including urea) in serum due to obstruction of urine flow (eg, prostatic hypertrophy, renal stone, tumor)

prerenal azotemia: increased concentration of nitrogenous compounds (including urea) in serum due to decreased blood flow to the kidney (eg, shock, congestive heart failure)

pyelonephritis: inflammation of the nephron due to a kidney infection

renal azotemia: increased concentration of nitrogenous compounds (including urea) in serum due to kidney damage

urea: a compound synthesized in the liver in the detoxification of ammonia and cleared into the urine

urine osmolality: a measurement of the concentration of osmotically active particles in urine

urine specific gravity: the ratio of the density of urine to that of water

5.3 Background/significance

Chronic kidney disease is an increasing public health issue, and its prevalence is estimated to be 8%-16% worldwide [PMID23727169]. While there are imaging tests and invasive procedures for evaluating renal disease, the clinical laboratory still plays a major role in the diagnosis and monitoring of this condition.

5.4 Nonprotein nitrogenous substance in serum

The kidney eliminates a vast array of nonprotein nitrogenous compounds into the urine, including urea, uric acid, creatinine, creatine, amino acids, and ammonia. Prior to the advent of measurement of specific compounds, the nonprotein nitrogen (NPN) content of serum was measured.

5.4.1 Urea-nitrogen

Ammonia, arising from catabolism of proteins, is detoxified by conversion into **urea f5.1** via the urea cycle in the liver. Urea comprises ~45% of the NPN in normal serum. The term *urea-nitrogen* is used because, instead of urea itself, the nitrogen in urea has been measured due to the purified enzyme urease's sparse availability for analytical purposes in earlier years.

f5.1 Structure of urea

Unfortunately some clinicians still refer to "blood urea-nitrogen" (BUN), although serum or plasma instead of whole blood is used for measurement of urea-nitrogen (serum urea-nitrogen [SUN]).

Urea is filtered by the glomeruli, but ~40%-50% is reabsorbed by passive diffusion into blood across the renal tubular epithelium [ISBN9780323036580]. Thus, when glomerular filtration rate is decreased, the SUN will be increased, since more time is available for passive reabsorption of urea.

In most clinical laboratories, the reference range for SUN is 8-18 mg/dL. However, it is greatly affected by the protein content of the diet as proteins are deaminated to ammonia, which is converted to urea in the liver. Thus, high protein diets yield higher SUN, while low protein diets yield lower SUN. The SUN is a less specific indicator of renal function compared to creatinine because SUN concentrations are influenced by many factors in addition to the glomerular filtration rate, which can remain essentially constant as SUN changes [ISBN9780323036580].

5.4.2 Creatinine

Creatinine, a cyclic anhydride, is derived from the spontaneous dehydration of creatine in muscle **f5.2**. Since the amount of creatine per unit of muscle mass is constant, the serum creatinine concentration remains fairly stable [ISBN9780323036580]. It follows that daily excretion is constant in normal individuals and independent of urine volume, thereby allowing the measurement of creatinine in urine to be used to evaluate the completeness of a 24 hour urine collection (1.0-1.5 g/day). Because the concentration of creatinine is a reflection of muscle mass, individuals with greater muscle mass have higher values than those with lower muscle mass [ISBN9780323036580].

The reference range for serum creatinine is 0.6-1.3 mg/dL for men; 0.5-1.1 mg/dL for women.

f5.2 Conversion of creatine to creatinine

5.4.2.1 Serum urea-nitrogen:creatinine ratio

The ratio of serum urea-nitrogen to serum creatinine (SUN:CR) can be helpful in determining the cause of altered concentrations of either analyte.

Increased ratios are noted with increased urea synthesis (eg, blood in the gastrointestinal tract, severe tissue trauma, muscle wasting diseases, and high protein diets, all of which provide a rich source of proteins, which are deaminated to yield ammonia, thereby fueling the urea cycle); increased absorption of urea (eg, intraperitoneal extravasation of urine, which is rich in urea, allowing absorption of the urea through the peritoneal membrane; urinary-enteric fistulas, which introduce urine into the intestine, allowing absorption of urine urea through intestinal mucosa); and increased tubular reabsorption of urea due to decreased glomerular filtration rate because of decreased blood flow to the kidney, allowing time for more passive reabsorption of urea to occur (eg, dehydration, congestive heart failure, shock, malignant nephrosclerosis, acute glomerulonephritis).

Decreased ratios are noted with decreased urea synthesis (eg, chronic glomerulonephritis with proteinuria leading to protein depletion, lower ammonia production, and less urea; hepatic failure with inability of liver to synthesize urea; starvation with inadequate protein intake to generate urea) and decreased urea reabsorption (eg, overhydration and rapid rehydration, both causing less renal tubular reabsorption of urea). Decreased ratios are also noted following hemodialysis because of the more efficient dialysis of urea relative to creatinine [ISBN9781416061649c].

The reference range for SUN:CR is ~12-20.

5.4.2.2 Glomerular filtration rate

The estimation of **glomerular filtration rate** (GFR) is important in evaluating renal function. It can be determined in a number of ways. Classically, the **creatinine clearance** reflects the GFR, since creatinine, for the most part, is freely filtered. The endogenous creatinine clearance is calculated by the following formula [ISBN9780683300857]:

$$C_{creat} = (U_{creat}/S_{creat}) \times V \times (1.73m^2/A)$$

where C_{creat} is the creatinine clearance (mL/min), U_{creat} is the urine creatinine concentration (mg/dL), S_{creat} is the serum creatinine concentration (mg/dL), and V is the urine flow rate in mL/min (mL volume of timed urine/min of urine collection).

Since the creatinine clearance is related to body mass, for patients whose body mass deviates substantially from normal, the result is normalized to the normal body surface area of 1.73 m^2 by multiplying the result by 1.73 m^2/A (where A is the body surface area of the patient, determined from a chart using height and weight of the patient). Thus, for individuals of small body mass (A<1.73 m^2), the result is enlarged by multiplying by a factor >1, while, for individuals of large body mass (A>1.73 m^2), the result is reduced by multiplying by a factor <1.

The reference range for creatinine clearance is 117 ± 20 mL/min for men, and 95 ± 20 mL/min for women.

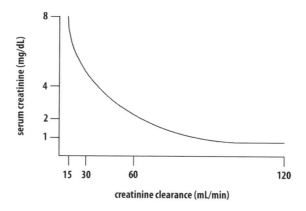

f5.3 Relationship between serum creatinine and creatinine clearance

The relationship between creatinine clearance and serum creatinine is logarithmic so that initially, small changes in serum creatinine cause significant changes in the clearance. In later stages of renal failure, small changes in the clearance are associated with significant changes in the serum creatinine **f5.3** [ISBN9780683300857].

It should be further noted that, as renal failure progresses, the small amount of tubular secretion of creatinine rises, up to as much as 60% of the total urine creatinine, resulting in a significant overestimation of the clearance in renal failure since the urine creatinine concentration appears in the numerator of the clearance calculation [ISBN9780683300857]. Thus, a low creatinine clearance in renal failure may be actually even lower than calculated.

Since collection of a timed urine specimen is unwieldy, a number of alternative methods for estimating the GFR without collecting a timed urine specimen have been developed. One is the Cockcroft-Gault formula for estimation of the creatinine clearance (mL/min) [ISBN9780323036580]:

$$C_{creat} = \frac{(140 - age) \times (weight\ in\ kg)}{72 \times (serum\ creatinine,\ mg/dL)}$$

[multiply result by 0.85 if female, due to lower muscle mass]

Yet another, more complicated formula is the Modification of Diet in Renal Disease (MDRD) formula [ISBN9781416061649c], which yields results in mL/min/1.73 m^2:

$$C_{creat} = 175 \times (serum\ creatinine)^{-1.154} \times (age)^{-0.203} \times (0.742\ if\ female;\ 1.210\ if\ African\ American)$$

The assay must be calibrated to isotope dilution mass spectrometry methods, and the age, gender, and race of the patient must be known.

More recent studies have suggested that the <u>Chronic Kidney Disease Epidemiology (CKD-EPI) formula</u> may be better for use with higher levels of GFR [PMID19414839]:

$$GFR = 141 \times \min(Scr/\kappa,1)^{\alpha} \times \max(Scr/\kappa,1)^{-1.209} \times 0.993^{age} \times (1.018, \text{ if female; } 1.159 \text{ if black})$$

where Scr is serum creatinine (mg/dL), κ is 0.7 for females and 0.9 for males, α is −0.329 for females and −0.411 for males, min indicates the minimum of Scr/κ or 1, and max indicates the maximum of Scr/κ or 1.

Fortunately, web based calculators are available for determining these parameters.

5.4.3 Cystatin C

Cystatin C is a low molecular weight (12,800) cysteine protease inhibitor that is freely filtered through the glomerular basement membrane and reabsorbed (but not secreted) with no extrarenal excretion. Its concentration is not affected by diet, muscle mass, or acute inflammation. Thus the serum concentration of cystatin C is dependent only on the GFR, making it a more sensitive indicator of changes in GFR than serum creatinine [PMID11978596, PMID7731163, ISBN9780683300857]. Furthermore, the cystatin C concentration is independent of muscle mass [ISBN9780683300857]. This marker is not yet in widespread clinical use.

5.4.4 Tests of tubular function

Tubular function can be evaluated through measuring the renal concentrating ability.

<u>Urine osmolality</u> is a measurement of the concentration of osmotically active particles in urine and expressed in mOsm/kg. Urine osmolality normally has a wide reference range, reflecting varying degrees of hydration in individuals (60-1,250 mOsm/kg). However, the failing kidney loses its capacity to concentrate urine so that the urine osmolality approaches to within 50 mOsm/kg of the serum osmolality (ie, it approaches 240-350 mOsm/kg in renal failure).

<u>Urine specific gravity</u> is the ratio of the density of urine to that of water and usually parallels the changes in urine osmolality. As a failing kidney loses the ability to concentrate urine, the specific gravity becomes fixed (1.008-1.012; **isosthenuria**). The reference range for specific gravity is 1.010-1.025.

Individuals with normal renal concentrating ability should be able to increase their urine osmolality to >850 mOsm/kg following 12 hours of fluid restriction [ISBN9781416061649b].

5.4.5 Classes of azotemia

Azotemia is the increased concentration of nitrogenous compounds (including urea) in serum. **Prerenal azotemia** is caused by a decrease in renal blood flow (eg, congestive heart failure, shock). Although the SUN is elevated, the serum creatinine is usually normal in this condition so that the SUN:CR is elevated (>20:1). **Renal azotemia** is caused by acute or chronic kidney disease (eg, glomerulonephritis, tubular necrosis), and both SUN and creatinine are usually elevated. In renal azotemia the ratio of SUN:CR varies depending on etiology.

Postrenal azotemia is due to obstruction of urine flow (eg, by prostatic hypertrophy, tumor, renal stone, renal vein thrombosis) with both SUN and creatinine being elevated. In postrenal azotemia the SUN:CR is usually elevated because the GFR is decreased, which increases passive reabsorption of urea [ISBN9781416061649c].

5.5 Laboratory findings in renal diseases

Pyelonephritis is an acute pyogenic infection of the kidney. The infection usually ascends from the lower urinary tract. Symptoms include fever, flank pain, shaking chills, and dysuria. Significant laboratory findings include a peripheral leukocytosis, bacteriuria, and white cells and white cell casts in the urine [ISBN9780071806336]. The SUN, serum creatinine, SUN:CR, and creatinine clearance are usually normal. However, if left untreated, progression to chronic pyelonephritis may lead to renal damage sufficient to produce elevation of the SUN and creatinine.

Nephrotic syndrome (nephrosis) is a group of diseases in which glomerular permeability is increased. ~75% of cases are caused by primary glomerular disease (minimal change glomerulopathy, focal segmental glomerulosclerosis, membranous glomerulonephritis, membranoproliferative glomerulonephritis) with systemic disease accounting for the remainder (eg, diabetic nephropathy, infection, neoplasms, drugs, cancer, amyloidosis, among others) [ISBN9780683300857]. The loss of albumin into the urine creates hypoalbuminemia and loss of oncotic pressure, stimulating the liver to overproduce $\alpha2$ macroglobulin [PMID9690220] and lipoproteins (very low density, low density, and intermediate density) [PMID9554862] in an attempt to preserve oncotic pressure. The elevated lipoproteins, in turn, cause an increase in serum cholesterol and triglycerides [PMID9554862]. Thus, significant laboratory findings in this condition include marked proteinuria (mostly albumin, but also binding proteins such as transferrin), hypoalbuminemia, hyperlipidemia, and occasional oval fat bodies and fat body casts in the urine [Keddis 2007]. However, the SUN, serum creatinine, and creatinine clearance can range from normal to abnormal, depending on the specific cause of the nephrotic syndrome. The loss of oncotic pressure leads to the development of edema, which, in turn, leads to secondary hyperaldosteronism due to production of renin by the juxtaglomerular cells of the kidney, causing retention of more sodium and water [ISBN9781416061649a]. Finally, patients with nephrotic syndrome are also at increased risk for thromboembolic events [PMID9554862].

Acute glomerulonephritis is an acute inflammation of the glomeruli generally resulting in oliguria, hematuria with red cells and red cell casts in the urine, increased SUN, increased serum creatinine, decreased creatinine clearance, and mild proteinuria [ISBN9780323036580]. Early in the disease process the SUN:CR may exceed 20:1.

Chronic glomerulonephritis is due to slowly progressive glomerular disease in which there is massive proteinuria. As it progresses into chronic renal failure, there is significant rise in the SUN and serum creatinine, accompanied by proteinuria, oliguria, hyponatremia, hyperkalemia, hypocalcemia, hyperphosphatemia, hyperuricemia, hypermagnesemia, and metabolic acidosis due to retention of inorganic acids [ISBN9780683300857]. Due to protein loss, the SUN:CR will often be <10:1. The decreased hydroxylation of 25-hydroxyvitamin D in the kidney, contributes to the hypocalcemia. The hypocalcemia leads to increased secretion of parathyroid hormone, which increases bone resorption and serum phosphate concentrations. Anemia is often seen due to decreased erythropoietin production by the ailing kidney [ISBN9780683300857].

5.6 References

5.6.1 Journals

PMID11978596 Laterza OF, Price CP, Scott MG [2002] Cystatin C: an improved estimator of glomerular filtration rate? *Clin Chem* 48:699-707

PMID19414839 Levey AS, Stevens LA, Schmid CH et al [2009] A new equation to estimate glomerular filtration rate. *Ann Int Med* 150:604-12

PMID23727169 Jha V, Garcia-Garcia G, Iseki K et al [2013] Chronic kidney disease: global dimension and perspectives. *Lancet* 382:260-72

PMID7731163 Newman DJ, Thakkar H, Edwards RG et al [1995] Serum cystatin C measured by automated immunoassay: a more sensitive marker of changes in GFR than creatinine. *Kidney Int* 47: 312-18 (1995).

PMID9554862 Orth SR, Ritz E [1998] The nephrotic syndrome. *N Engl J Med* 338:1202-11

PMID9690220 de Sain-van der Velden MGM, Rabelink TJ et al [1998] Plasma $\alpha 2$ macroglobulin is increased in nephrotic patients as a result of increased synthesis alone. *Kidney Int* 54:530-5

Keddis MT, Karnath BM [2007] The nephrotic syndrome. *Hosp Physician* Oct:25-30

5.6.2 Books

ISBN9780071806336 Meng MV, Walsh TJ, Stoller ML [2014] Urologic disorders. In: Papadakis MA, McPhee SJ, Rabow MW, ed. *Current Medical Diagnosis & Treatment*, 53e. McGraw Hill Education, 905-927.

ISBN9780323036580 Kaplan JM, First MR [2009] Renal function. In Kaplan LA, Pesce AJ, ed. *Clinical Chemistry: Theory, Analysis, Correlation*, 5e. Mosby, 573-8

ISBN9780683300857 Szczepiorkowski ZM, Lewandrowski K [2002] Renal function and nitrogen metabolites. In: Lewandrowski K, ed. *Clinical Chemistry: Laboratory Management and Clinical Correlations*. Lippincott Williams & Wilkins, 692-705.

ISBN9781416061649a Bertholf RF, Jialal I, Winter WE [2011] The adrenal cortex. In: Burtis CA, Ashwood ER, Bruns DE, ed. *Tietz Textbook of Clinical Chemistry and Molecular Diagnostics*, 5e. Elsevier Saunders, 1847-1904.

ISBN9781416061649b Delaney MP, Price CP, and Lamb EJ: Kidney disease. In: Burtis CA, Ashwood ER, Bruns DE, ed. *Tietz Textbook of Clinical Chemistry and Molecular Diagnostics*, 5e. Elsevier Saunders, 1523-1608.

ISBN9781416061649c Lamb EJ, Price CP [2011] Kidney function tests. In: Burtis CA, Ashwood ER, Bruns DE, ed. *Tietz Textbook of Clinical Chemistry and Molecular Diagnostics*, 5e. Elsevier Saunders, 669-708.

5.7 Clinical cases
5.7.1 Case 1

An 87-year-old male visits his primary care physician with a chief complaint of the slow onset of ankle and shin swelling, mild shortness of breath, and fatigue. Urinalysis performed in the physician's office revealed marked proteinuria (4+). Point of care testing on the patient's blood showed urea-nitrogen 35 mg/dL, creatinine 3.8 mg/dL, sodium 130 mMol/L (mEq/L), potassium 5.6 mMol/L (mEq/L), chloride 92 mMol/L (mEq/L), bicarbonate 20 mMol/L (mEq/L), total protein 4.3 g/dL, and albumin 1.4 g/dL. The patient was subsequently asked to collect a 24 hour urine specimen, in which the concentration of creatinine was 210 mg/dL, and the urine volume was 288 mL.

5.7.1.1 Questions

1. Calculate the creatinine clearance and interpret it.

2. What is the most likely diagnosis for this patient, based on the laboratory findings?

3. What additional blood tests should be ordered, and how might they be abnormal?

4. What additional studies should be performed on the urine specimen?

5.7.2 Case 2

A 5-year-old female develops swelling of her ankles and feet, along with "puffiness" in her cheeks and around her eyes. Her anxious mother brings her to her pediatrician, who has her admitted to the local children's hospital. A urinalysis shows 4+ protein. Admission blood studies show SUN 15 mg/dL, creatinine 0.5 mg/dL, sodium 135 mMol/L (mEq/L), potassium 4.6 mMol/L (mEq/L), chloride 101 mMol/L (mEq/L), bicarbonate 23 mMol/L (mEq/L), calcium 7.4 mg/dL, total cholesterol 350 mg/dL, and triglycerides 202 mg/dL. The urinalysis showed hyaline casts, oval fat bodies, and oval fat body casts.

5.7.2.1 Questions

1. What is the most likely diagnosis for this patient?

2. Describe the probable gross appearance of the patient's serum.

3. What other tests would you perform on the blood and urine?

4. Why is the calcium low?

5.7.3 Clinical cases answers
5.7.3.1 Case 1 answers

1. Creatinine clearance = (288 mL/1440 minutes) (210 mg/dL)/3.8 mg/dL = 11 mL/minutes; this is extremely low

2. The findings suggest chronic kidney disease (chronic glomerulonephritis) as demonstrated by the elevated SUN and creatinine with an SUN:CR of 9.2 (<10), hyperkalemia, hyponatremia, hypoproteinemia, proteinuria, oliguria, low bicarbonate, and elevated anion gap of 24 (suggesting metabolic acidosis)

3. Additional blood tests might include calcium (low), phosphate (elevated), uric acid (elevated), and complete blood count (anemia); arterial blood gases would likely show a decreased pH due to metabolic acidosis

4. A quantitative urine protein would be helpful to evaluate the magnitude of proteinuria; the urine specific gravity would likely be low and fixed ("isosthenuria")

5.7.3.2 Case 2 answers

1. The massive proteinuria, hyperlipidemia, edema (due to loss of oncotic pressure from albuminuria), and the presence of oval fat bodies, and oval fat body casts in the urine suggest nephrotic syndrome (nephrosis)

2. The serum would likely appear very turbid to "milky" due to the hyperlipidemia

3. Serum total proteins and albumin would be low. A quantitative urine protein would be elevated. A serum total protein electrophoresis would show decreased albumin and elevated $\alpha 2$ globulin fraction (macroglobulin, low density, very low density, and intermediate density lipoproteins). The total globulins might be reduced as well.

4. The calcium is low because of the expected low albumin due to loss of the latter into the urine

chapter 6

Urinalysis

6.1 Objectives

At the end of this session, the learner should be able to

- describe the major parts of a urinalysis, including the macroscopic, chemical, and microscopic examinations
- discuss the causes of abnormally colored urine (eg, brown-black, red, yellow-brown)
- discuss the causes of turbidity of urine
- discuss the causes of abnormal odors of urine (eg, ammoniacal, acetone)
- discuss the reference ranges for urinary pH and specific gravity
- identify nonglucose reducing substances that may appear in urine
- describe the sulfosalicylic acid test and how it is used
- identify causes of false negative glucose dipstick tests in urine
- identify causes of false negative heme dipstick tests in urine
- identify leukocytes, erythrocytes, squamous epithelial cells, renal tubular epithelial cells, and transitional epithelial cells in urine and discuss their significance
- identify hyaline, leukocyte, erythrocyte, oval fat body, granular, and waxy casts and discuss their significance
- identify calcium oxalate, sodium urate, ammonium biurate, triple phosphate, amorphous phosphate, tyrosine, leucine, cystine, and sulfonamide crystals in urine and know at what pH (alkaline or acid) they occur

6.2 Key terms

bilirubinuria: the presence of bilirubin in the urine

cast: an imprint of a renal tubule containing Tamm-Horsfall as the mucoprotein matrix and named for the predominant content of the cast (eg, red cells, white cells)

chemical examination: testing for chemical compounds in urine

dipstick test: a commercial reagent stick impregnated with test pads for the detection of protein, glucose, ketone bodies, bilirubin, heme protein, bacteria, leukocytes, urobilinogen and for estimation of pH and specific gravity in urine

hyaline cast: a transparent cast with the Tamm-Horsfall mucoprotein matrix

hydrometer: a calibrated float used for determining specific gravity of a fluid by buoyancy

ketone bodies: compounds containing a carbonyl group with hydrocarbon groups attached to the carbonyl carbon

macroscopic examination: the visual assessment of color and turbidity of a urine sample

microscopic examination: the examination of a wet unstained urine sediment at both low and high power magnification

myoglobinuria: the presence of myoglobin in the urine

refractive index: the bending of light when passing from one medium into another; in urinalysis the reference medium is water

refractometry: the measurement of the refractive index of a liquid

rhabdomyolysis: the breakdown of muscle

specific gravity: the ratio of the density of a substance to that of a reference substance; in urinalysis, the reference is water

Tamm-Horsfall protein: the mucoprotein matrix of casts

urinalysis: analysis of urine including macroscopic, chemical, and microscopic examination

urobilinogen: a compound formed by the action of bacteria on conjugated bilirubin in the gut

6.3 Background/significance

Urinalysis is one of the oldest biological fluid examinations in human history. For many years, the procedure was performed manually. Now most clinical laboratories use high throughput automated systems that are equipped with a spectrophotometer to read the color of the dipstick and with either a video camera that photographs the formed elements (using digital imaging software to classify them for verification by the operator) or a flow cytometer to classify them [PMID18623125]. Nonetheless, manual urinalysis is still performed in many instances, particularly in office laboratories, and an understanding of the procedure and its interpretation is important.

6.4 Examination
6.4.1 Macroscopic examination

The **macroscopic examination** of urine is performed visually. Normal urine color ranges from straw to pale yellow. Other colors suggest various conditions: yellow-brown (**bilirubinuria**), red (beets, porphyrins, hemoglobin, myoglobin), and brown-black (melanin, alkapton bodies resulting from oxidized homogentisic acid). Turbidity is caused by diffraction of light by formed elements in the urine (eg, cells, crystals, casts, mucus). Normal urine should be clear. While not reported, odor can suggest a variety of conditions: ammoniacal (breakdown of urea by urease containing bacteria such as *Proteus* species), acetone (diabetic ketoacidosis), rotten (tyrosinuria), mousy (phenylketonuria), and food odors (asparagus).

6.4.2 Chemical examination (dipstick)

The **chemical examination** of urine is performed for the most part with commercial dipsticks, which are compartmentalized strips containing separate reagents for each test. Automated instruments detect the color change of each compartment spectrophotometrically, while manual urinalysis relies on the operator visually detecting color using a color chart for comparison. The interpretation of the specific tests below is described in the individual chapters of this book.

6.4.2.1 Specific gravity

Since **specific gravity** of urine is directly proportional to the **refractive index**, it is measured by **refractometry** in many automated urinalysis instruments. It can also be measured manually with a handheld refractometer, by dipstick (pK_a change of pretreated electrolytes in relation to the ionic concentration of the sample, creating a color change), and with a **hydrometer** (a calibrated float detecting buoyancy). Refractometry and the **dipstick test** require only a few drops of urine, while the hydrometer requires at least 10 mL of urine. A little used method (the "falling drop" method) measures the rate of fall of a drop of urine through a synthetic liquid, with higher specific gravity urine falling faster. Specific gravity reference range is 1.010-1.025 [ISBN9780683300857].

6.4.2.2 pH

The maximum physiological range for urine pH is 4.5-8.0, but most patients have urine pH in the range of 5.0-7.0. Urinary pH <4.5 or higher than 8.0 suggests contamination and/or adulteration. The dipstick uses a combination of colorimetric indicators to cover the urine pH range [ISBN9780683300857].

6.4.2.3 Protein

The dipstick is most sensitive to albumin and relatively insensitive to globulins. It does not detect light chains. The test is based on the protein error of pH indicators with the strip test area buffered to a constant low pH (usually <3) so that any color change reflects the amount of protein present [ISBN9780683300857].

The sulfosalicylic acid test (3% aqueous sulfosalicylic acid) is a supplementary, nonspecific test that causes precipitation of albumin, globulins, light chains, iodinated radiographic contrast media, penicillin, cephalosporins, and sulfonamides. The test is semiquantified visually by the turbidity produced when equal volumes of urine and reagent are mixed. Thus a negative dipstick protein and a positive sulfosalicylic acid test together suggest the presence of nonalbumin substances. The sulfosalicylic acid test is often included in the workup of multiple myeloma.

6.4.2.4 Glucose

Glucose is detected using a glucose oxidase reaction, in which glucose is converted to gluconic acid and hydrogen peroxide. The hydrogen peroxide is then converted to oxygen by peroxidase (also present in the strip). The oxygen oxidizes a chromogen, causing color development [ISBN9780683300857].

In addition to glucose, other reducing substances such as galactose, lactose, fructose, pentose, ascorbic acid (vitamin C), aspirin, and homogentisic acid may be present in urine [ISBN9780683300857]. Until recently, reducing substances were detected with a copper reduction test (Clinitest, Bayer, Pittsburgh, PA). The reagent tablet contained copper sulfate, sodium hydroxide, sodium bicarbonate, and citric acid. When added to diluted urine that contained a reducing substance, the copper sulfate was reduced to cuprous oxide, producing a brick red color [ISBN9780683300857]. Thus the presence of a positive copper reduction test together with a negative dipstick for glucose suggested the presence of a nonglucose reducing substance (eg, lactose), which can be particularly important in the neonatal population. However, this test has now been discontinued due to improved and widespread newborn screening for nonglucose reducing sugars. In addition, other tests are available if carbohydrate malabsorption is suspected (see chapter 4).

High urine concentrations of reducing substances such as ascorbic acid can quench the glucose oxidase-peroxidase coupled reaction, leading to a false negative reaction for glucose.

6.4.2.5 Ketone bodies

Ketone bodies are intermediates of fat metabolism and found in carbohydrate deficient states such as starvation and when carbohydrates cannot be effectively used as an energy source (eg, type 1 diabetes mellitus). They include acetone and acetoacetic acid. The reaction utilizes nitroprusside to form a color. Since acetone does not react well with the dipstick, detection of ketone bodies for the most part suggests acetoacetic acid. It should be noted that β-hydroxybutyric acid is not a ketone and does not react with the dipstick [ISBN9780683300857].

6.4.2.6 Heme proteins

The heme proteins that can be found in urine include hemoglobin and myoglobin. The latter can be seen with **rhabdomyolysis**. **Myoglobinuria** can also occur following acute myocardial infarction, but in that condition the concentrations of myoglobin are generally too low to be detected by dipstick. It should be noted that intact erythrocytes must be lysed by the lysing agent on the dipstick before the reaction occurs. Thus intact red cells seen in a freshly voided urine will usually cause a speckled pattern on the dipstick strip, while free hemoglobin in urine causes an even color. If the urine is allowed to sit for a prolonged period prior to testing, the red cells will lyse so that the liberated hemoglobin will produce an even color. The dipstick reaction is based on the pseudoperoxidase activity of heme proteins, which act upon the organic peroxide in the strip, liberating oxygen, oxidizing the substrate, and generating color. As with the glucose test, large amounts of reducing substances such as ascorbic acid can quench the oxidation reaction [ISBN9780683300857].

6.4.2.7 Bilirubin

Conjugated (water soluble) bilirubin is detected by dipstick with the "diazo" reaction, producing a color change. If urine containing bilirubin is allowed to sit for a prolonged period of time before testing, it can be deconjugated to bilirubin and then photo-oxidized to biliverdin, causing a false negative test [ISBN9780683300857].

6.4.2.8 Urobilinogen

Urobilinogen is produced by intestinal bacteria acting upon conjugated bilirubin in the intestine, followed by urobilinogen reabsorption from the intestine via the enterohepatic circulation and subsequent filtration into the urine by the kidneys. The urobilinogen reagent present on the dipstick utilizes the Ehrlich reaction [ISBN9780683300857]. If urine containing urobilinogen is allowed to sit for a prolonged period of time before testing, it can be oxidized to urobilin, causing a false negative test.

6.4.2.9 Nitrite

The detection of nitrite in urine suggests the reduction of urinary nitrate to nitrite by enteric Gram– rods such as *Escherichia coli*. The reaction depends on diazotization of nitrite [ISBN9780683300857].

6.4.2.10 Leukocyte esterase

The presence of leukocyte esterase suggests the presence of neutrophils in the urine. It is detected through conversion of an ester into a chromogen on the dipstick [ISBN9780683300857].

6.4.3 Microscopic examination

The **microscopic examination** should be performed soon after specimen collection to avoid deterioration of formed elements. ~10 mL of well mixed urine should be centrifuged for ~5 minutes (1,200-2,000 rpm). The supernatant urine should be carefully decanted, and the resulting sediment should be suspended in the few drops of urine remaining in the tube. The sediment should be examined wet, without stain, and under both low power and high dry power. Because the images are often pale, low microscope light should be used. The number of larger formed elements (eg, casts, crystals) per low power field (LPF) and the number of smaller formed elements (eg, cells, bacteria) per high power field (HPF) should be estimated in ~10 different fields and reported as #/LPF and #/HPF.

6.4.3.1 Cells

Cell types noted in urine sediment may include erythrocytes, leukocytes, squamous epithelial cells (urethra, vagina), transitional epithelial cells (bladder), and renal tubular epithelial cells (renal tubules).

6.4.3.2 Casts

Casts are imprints of renal tubules formed by precipitation of **Tamm-Horsfall protein** in tubular fluid. The classification of casts is largely based on the type of cellular contents they contain. Since they are formed in the renal tubules, they are usually elongated. Cast production is enhanced by decreased glomerular filtration rate.

Types of casts include **hyaline casts** (consisting only of the Tamm-Horsfall protein and excreted by the normal kidneys in small amounts); leukocyte casts (associated with diseases that involve inflammation and infection, such as pyelonephritis); erythrocyte casts (associated with injury to the glomerular basement membrane, such as acute glomerulonephritis, Goodpasture syndrome, lupus nephritis, and subacute bacterial endocarditis); renal tubular epithelial cells (reflecting renal tubular damage); and fatty casts (from leakage of lipoproteins through the glomerulus as may occur in nephrotic syndrome, diabetes mellitus, and renal tubular cell damage). Mixed casts can also be seen. Cellular casts deteriorate over time, first becoming coarsely granular casts, then finely granular casts, and then waxy casts.

6.4.3.3 Crystals

Crystals occur when urine becomes so supersaturated with compounds that their solubility is exceeded. Since solubility is pH dependent, certain crystals are found only in acid urine, while others are found only in alkaline urine. Crystals are usually symmetrical.

Crystals found in <u>acid</u> urine along with descriptors about their appearance include the following: calcium oxalate ("envelopes"; seen following ingestion of food with high oxalate content, such as beets, spinach, nuts, wheat bran, rhubarb; after massive ingestion of vitamin C; after poisoning with ethylene glycol, which is metabolized to oxalic acid), sodium urates ("whetstones"; seen with high serum uric acid concentrations, as in gout), and sulfonamides ("sheaves"; seen following administration of sulfonamide medications). Amino acid crystals can also be found in acidic urine when their concentrations are high (eg, as in end stage liver disease, when the liver cannot make proteins): tyrosine ("needles in rosettes"), leucine ("spheres"), and cystine ("hexagons"). Cystine crystals can also be found in cystinosis. Crystals found in <u>alkaline</u> urine include the following: triple phosphates ("coffin lids"), ammonium biurates ("thorn apples"; seen with high serum uric acid concentrations, as in gout), and amorphous phosphates ("amorphous debris").

6.5 References
6.5.1 Journal

PMID18623125 Mayo S, Acevedo D, Quinones-Torrelo C et al [2008] Clinical laboratory automated microscopy, flow cytometry, 2 test strips analyzers, and manual microscopic examination of the urine sediments. *J Clin Lab Anal* 22:262-70

6.5.2 Book

ISBN9780683300857 Clarke W, Palmer-Toy DE [2002] Clinical chemistry of urine, pleural effusions, and ascites. In: Lewandrowski K, ed. *Clinical Chemistry: Laboratory Management and Clinical Correlations*. Lippincott Williams & Wilkins, 850-61

6.6 Clinical cases

6.6.1 Case 1

A 65-year-old male notes progressive swelling of his lower extremities as well as the onset of severe back pain. A urinalysis performed in his physician's office reveals the following: appearance (clear, light yellow), specific gravity 1.030, pH 6.3, glucose negative, ketones negative, bilirubin negative, protein negative, heme protein negative, erythrocytes 0-1/HPF, leukocytes 0-1/HPF, and hyaline casts 0-1/HPF. A sulfosalicylic acid test was 4+.

6.6.1.1 Questions

1. Interpret the positive sulfosalicylic acid test with the negative dipstick protein test.

2. What additional tests should be performed?

3. Why is the specific gravity high?

6.6.2 Case 2

A 26-year-old diabetic woman has an elevated fingerstick glucose. She decides to check her urine and is surprised to find that her urine dipstick test for glucose is negative. She is having her menses and is also surprised to note that her blood tinged urine is dipstick negative for heme protein.

6.6.2.1 Question

What is the likely explanation for these findings?

6.6.3 **Clinical case answers**

6.6.3.1 **Case 1 answers**

1. The positive sulfosalicylic acid test with negative dipstick protein test suggests the presence of a radiographic contrast medium (perhaps given during an imaging study in the workup of the patient's back pain), light chains, or antibiotics. Light chains would suggest multiple myeloma, which could be a cause of the patient's back pain.

2. Serum total protein and albumin, quantitative light chain analysis, serum protein and immunofixation electrophoresis, serum free light chain analysis, and urine immunofixation electrophoresis would be helpful in pursuing the diagnosis of multiple myeloma. The urinalysis should also be repeated in a clinical laboratory. Imaging studies of the back would be helpful as well.

3. The specific gravity reflects the substance(s) detected with the sulfosalicylic acid test (eg, light chains, contrast medium).

6.6.3.2 **Case 2 answers**

Dipstick glucose and heme detection depend on oxidation reactions. Thus they may be quenched by strong reducing substances in the urine. It is probable that the patient has a large concentration of a reducing substance in her urine, the most likely one being ascorbic acid (vitamin C).

chapter 7

The laboratory examination of body fluids

7.1 **Objectives**

At the end of the session, the learner should be able to

➤ describe the formation of cerebrospinal fluid and its distribution in the various compartments

➤ describe the characteristics of normal cerebrospinal fluid

➤ discuss causes of increased cerebrospinal fluid pressure

➤ describe the collection of cerebrospinal fluid for chemistry tests, microbiology studies, and cell counts

➤ define Froin syndrome

➤ discuss oligoclonal banding in the diagnosis of multiple sclerosis

➤ discuss myelin basic protein in monitoring active demyelination

➤ discuss the IgG index in monitoring demyelinating diseases

➤ discuss the IgG synthesis rate in monitoring demyelinating diseases

➤ describe the cerebrospinal fluid protein, glucose, and cell count in acute bacterial meningitis, tuberculous meningitis, and aseptic meningitis

➤ discuss the physicochemical differences between an exudate and a transudate

➤ describe the causes of a transudate

➤ describe the causes of an exudate

➤ discuss the serum-ascites albumin gradient (SAAG) and its use

➤ Differentiate chylous from pseudochylous effusions

➤ describe the characteristics of normal synovial fluid

➤ describe the mucin clot (ROPES) test and how it is used

➤ discuss the glucose difference (serum/plasma vs synovial fluid) in normal, inflamed, and septic joints

7.2 **Key terms**

ascitic fluid: an abnormal collection of fluid in the peritoneum, often due to portal hypertension accompanied by decreased oncotic pressure due to hypoalbuminemia

blood-brain barrier: the barrier between the brain and blood that allows the brain to maintain a cerebrospinal fluid composition different from that of blood

cerebral venous sinus thrombosis: a clot in the dural venous sinuses that drain blood

cerebrospinal fluid: an ultrafiltrate of blood produced by the cells that line the choroid plexus and the cells that line the cerebral ventricles

choroid plexus: a venous plexus contained within the cerebral ventricles

chylous effusion: an abnormal collection of fluid (usually in the thoracic cavity) that contains chyle (lymphatic drainage)

effusion: fluid in a body cavity that is produced by a pathologic process

exudate: a fluid rich in protein and cells that leak out of blood vessels

Froin syndrome: the finding of xanthochromia and high protein, leading to coagulation, and caused by meningeal irritation and blockage of cerebrospinal fluid flow by tumor or abscess

gout: a condition in which joints are inflamed due to deposition of urate crystals because of elevated serum uric acid

hyaluronic acid: a viscous glycosaminoglycan present in synovial fluid and in ocular vitreous humor

IgG index: the ratio of the concentration of CSF IgG to that of serum IgG

IgG synthesis rate: the calculation of the production of IgG (mg/day) in the central nervous system

intrathecal: of the area within the spinal cord

lacrimation: production of tears

lumbar puncture: the procedure by which cerebrospinal fluid is obtained

meninges: the 3 membranes covering the brain and spinal cord (dura, arachnoid, and pia)

meningitis: inflammation of the meninges, often caused by viral or bacterial infections

mucin clot (ROPES) test: the formation of a clot by addition of glacial acetic acid to synovial fluid

myelin basic protein: a myelin sheath component that rises in response to neuronal damage and central nervous system inflammation

oligoclonal banding: the finding of multiple immunoglobulin bands, which, if present in cerebrospinal fluid but absent in serum, suggests active central nervous system demyelination

otorrhea: the flow of fluid from the ears

paracentesis: a procedure for removal of fluid from the peritoneal cavity

pseudochylous effusion: an effusion similar in appearance to a chylous effusion except the white color and turbidity are due to leukocytes or tumor cells

pseudogout: a condition in which joints are inflamed due to deposition of calcium pyrophosphate crystals

rhinorrhea: the flow of fluid from the nose

serum ascites albumin gradient (SAAG): the difference between serum albumin concentration and ascitic fluid albumin concentration in a patient

subarachnoid cistern: the space between the arachnoid and pia mater

subarachnoid hemorrhage: intracranial bleeding into the subarachnoid cistern

synovial fluid: a thick fluid that serves as a lubricant in joints, tendon sheaths, and bursa

thoracentesis: a procedure for removal of fluid from the thoracic cavity

transferrin: a β globulin present in serum and in CSF

transudate: an extravascular fluid with low protein concentration and low specific gravity

traumatic tap: a lumbar puncture in which there is contamination from peripheral blood during the procedure

ventricles: the 4 cavities within the brain that are filled with cerebrospinal fluid

xanthochromia: a yellow coloring of the cerebrospinal fluid caused by degradation products of hemoglobin

7.3 Background/significance

The study of body fluids other than blood and urine (eg, cerebrospinal fluid, transudates, exudates, chylous effusions, pseudochylous effusions, synovial fluid) requires invasive procedures to obtain the fluid; therefore such collections are performed only in specific instances in order to confirm a diagnosis. Since the collection of such fluids is often time sensitive and repeat collection is often impossible, an understanding of the information provided by analysis of the fluids is important.

7.4 Cerebrospinal fluid
7.4.1 Characteristics

Cerebrospinal fluid (CSF) is an ultrafiltrate of blood produced by the cells that line the **choroid plexus** as well as those that line the surfaces of the cerebral **ventricles**. The total volume of CSF in normal adults is 125-150 mL, with ~20% in the ventricles, ~30% in the **subarachnoid cisterns**, and ~50% in the spinal column. ~500 mL of fluid is produced per day, so the volume turnover is ~3-4× per day [PMID22278331, ISBN9780683300857].

The **blood-brain barrier** allows the brain to maintain a CSF composition that is different from that in blood while remaining in osmotic equilibrium with blood. The rate of entry of compounds that diffuse into the brain is dependent on their lipid solubility, molecular size, and charge state. Compounds such as ethanol are completely extracted from blood during a single passage through the brain, while more polar molecules enter the brain slowly. Compounds that are tightly bound to serum proteins also enter the brain at a rate slower than that predicted by their lipid solubility. Gases diffuse rapidly into the brain [ISBN9780397518203].

7.4.1.1 Lumbar puncture

The CSF is usually collected by performing a **lumbar puncture** at the area of L3-L4 or L4-L5 using a 22-24 gauge needle after cleaning the area with antiseptic agents and anesthetizing the area with a topical anesthetic. The patient lies flat in the lateral decubitus position with legs extended. Immediately after achieving lumbar puncture, the opening pressure is measured by a manometer into which is affixed a 3 way stopcock to direct the flow of CSF into the manometer and to the collection vessels. A total of 10-20 mL of fluid is usually distributed among 3-4 tubes [ISBN9780683300857].

7.4.1.2 Appearance

Normal CSF is clear and colorless. In bacterial **meningitis**, the fluid is turbid, while with a **traumatic tap**, it is bloody [ISBN9780683300857]. With **subarachnoid hemorrhage**, the fluid is also bloody, but after centrifugation, the supernatant fluid shows **xanthochromia** [ISBN9780683300857]. With **Froin syndrome** the CSF is also xanthochromic due to the high protein concentration, which may even lead to clotting [ISBN9780071794794].

7.4.1.3 Pressure

Normal opening pressure in adults is 100-200 mm water [PMID22278331]. Causes of increased CSF pressure include intracranial space occupying lesions, meningitis (bacterial, viral, fungal, tuberculous), subarachnoid hemorrhage, and **cerebral venous sinus thrombosis** [PMID22278331, ISBN9780683300857]. Decreased CSF pressure may be caused by a CSF leak or diuretic drugs [PMID22278331].

7.4.1.4 Glucose & protein

The CSF collected into tube 1 is submitted for measurement of glucose and protein. The concentration of glucose in the CSF is usually 1/3-2/3 that of simultaneously measured plasma/serum glucose, and the protein concentration is normally 15-45 mg/dL [ISBN9780683300857]. Decreased glucose concentration can be seen with bacterial, fungal, and tuberculous meningitis, due to glucose utilization by the microorganisms and neutrophils, while a normal glucose concentration is seen with viral meningitis and neurosyphilis [ISBN9780683300857]. Increased protein concentration is seen with bacterial, fungal, viral, and tuberculous meningitis, as well as neurosyphilis, subarachnoid hemorrhage, and Froin syndrome [ISBN9780071794794, ISBN9780683300857], all due to increased permeability of the meninges. Obviously, traumatic taps also lead to elevations of the glucose and protein, since their concentrations are higher in peripheral blood than in CSF. For every 1,000 erythrocytes, ~1 mg of protein is added to the CSF [ISBN9780071794794]. Fluid obtained from cisternal puncture has a lower protein concentration that than obtained from lumbar puncture [ISBN9780071794794], presumably due to more reabsorption of water in the lumbar region.

7.4.2 Microbiology studies

CSF collected into tube 2 should be submitted for microbiology studies, since it is analogous to a "clean catch midstream" collection (due to reduced contact with skin flora). If meningitis is suspected, a culture and sensitivity should be ordered. Additional studies (eg, India ink preparation for cryptococcal infection, special antigen studies, smears) may be performed depending on the clinical impression.

7.4.3 Cell count

CSF collected into tube 3 should be submitted for manual microscopic cell count, since usually by tube 3, contaminating cells from a traumatic tap should have cleared. With a subarachnoid hemorrhage, red cells remain. The examination should be performed soon after collection, since cells may deteriorate upon standing. Normal CSF contains no neutrophils or erythrocytes but may contain up to 5 lymphocytes/mm^3 [ISBN9780683300857]. In bacterial meningitis, neutrophils predominate, while in viral, fungal, and tuberculous meningitis, and neurosyphilis, lymphocytes predominate [ISBN9780683300857]. If a traumatic tap has occurred, for every 1,000 erythrocytes, the leukocyte count is elevated by 1 [PMID22278331].

7.4.4 Specialized studies

Many clinicians obtain a fourth tube of fluid in order to allow performance of specialized studies as may be indicated from the initial laboratory findings.

Electrophoresis of concentrated CSF to look for **oligoclonal banding** of immunoglobulins (chiefly IgG and IgM) may be useful in the workup of suspected demyelinating diseases such as multiple sclerosis. To rule out the possibility that the CSF proteins may be due to systemic production (eg, as with multiple myeloma), a serum protein electrophoresis should be performed simultaneously. Bands present only in the CSF suggest an abnormal B cell central nervous system immune response, although other conditions such as paraneoplastic disorders, systemic lupus erythematosus, neurosarcoidosis, cerebral angiitis and cerebral infections have been reported to produce isolated bands in the CSF [PMID22278331].

The **IgG index** is the ratio of the concentration of CSF IgG to that of serum IgG ($IgG_{csf}:IgG_{serum}$) and, when increased >0.003, is consistent with an increased intrathecal synthesis of IgG by the infiltrating B lymphocytes. However, this ratio does not take into account any leakage across the blood-brain barrier. To account for this, albumin concentrations are included in the following measurement:

$$IgG\ index = \frac{[IgG_{CSF}\ (mg/dL)/IgG_{serum}\ (g/dL)]}{[Albumin_{CSF}\ (mg/dL)/Albumin_{serum}\ (g/dL)]}$$

Since the units cancel out, the index is dimensionless. The reference range for this calculation is 0.3-0.7, with results >0.7 suggesting increased intrathecal synthesis of immunoglobulins [ISBN9780683300857].

The **IgG synthesis rate** is also increased in demyelinating diseases due to production by B cells that infiltrate the areas of demyelination. It can be calculated as follows:

$$\begin{aligned}
IgG\ synthesis\ rate\ (mg/day) = &[(IgG_{CSF} - IgG_{serum}/369) \\
&- (Albumin_{CSF} - Albumin_{serum}/230) \\
&\times (IgG_{serum}/Albumin_{serum}) \times 0.43] \times 0.5
\end{aligned}$$

where concentrations are in mg/L, 369 is the average normal serum:CSF mass ratio for IgG, 230 is the average normal serum:CSF mass ratio for albumin, 0.43 is the molecular mass ratio of albumin:IgG, and 0.5 is the daily production of CSF in liters. Rates >8 mg/day suggest increased intrathecal synthesis rates [PMID3802456].

Myelin basic protein is an important component of the myelin sheath and accounts for ~1/3 of the total central nervous system myelin protein [PMID22904139]. Its concentrations rise in response to neuronal damage, and thus it is a nonspecific marker of central nervous system inflammation. However, some believe that it does not enhance the sensitivity and specificity for diagnosis of multiple sclerosis above and beyond the use of CSF electrophoretic analysis for oligoclonal banding, and the use of the IgG index and the IgG synthesis rate [PMID22904139].

Occasionally, when clear, colorless fluid leaks from the nose (**rhinorrhea**), ear (**otorrhea**), or eyes (**lacrimation**), one may question whether or not the fluid is CSF. In those instances, measurement of β2 **transferrin** (desialated transferrin) may be helpful, since it is present in CSF and inner ear perilymph but not normally found in nasal secretions, tears, sweat, or saliva [ISBN9780683300857]. Serum transferrin is β1 transferrin. Another differentiator is glucose, since it is present in CSF at concentrations >30 mg/dL, while its concentrations are negligible in secretions [PMID1449183, ISBN9780683300857].

7.5 Effusions

Fluid in the mesothelium lined body cavities is an ultrafiltrate of plasma, and is usually watery and colorless to slight yellow. If the fluid accumulates due to a pathologic process, then it is classified as either an **exudate** or a **transudate**, largely based on its protein content [PMID1449183]. Depending upon the clinical history, **effusions** may be submitted for cell count, chemistry studies (see below), and culture and sensitivity.

7.5.1 Exudates

Exudates are usually produced by inflammation from chemical injury or infection, both of which cause increased capillary permeability. As a result, their removal is usually beneficial. Exudates are usually cloudy, and may contain leukocytes and bacteria. Pleural fluids are considered to be exudates if the total protein concentration is ≥3 g/dL or if the specific gravity is ≥1.015. Also, if the ratio of pleural fluid protein to that of serum protein is ≥0.5, and the glucose concentration is less than that in plasma/serum, then the fluid is considered to be an exudate. Due to the high protein concentrations (including fibrinogen), exudates may clot [ISBN9780323036580].

Peritoneal fluid (**ascitic fluid**) is considered to be an exudate if the protein concentration exceeds 2.5 g/dL. The difference between the serum albumin concentration and that of ascitic fluid (the so called **serum ascites albumin gradient** [**SAAG**]) is usually <1.1 g/dL if the ascitic fluid is an exudate [ISBN9780323036580].

7.5.2 Transudates

Transudates are usually produced by disturbances in hydrostatic or colloid osmotic pressure (eg, congestive heart failure, nephrotic syndrome, hepatic cirrhosis). As a result, they usually recur after removal. Transudates are usually clear and colorless to light yellow. Their glucose concentration is about the same as that of plasma/serum. The total protein concentration is less than that of exudates. Pleural fluids are considered to be transudates if the total protein concentration is <3 g/dL or if the specific gravity is <1.015. Also, if the ratio of pleural fluid protein to that of serum protein is <0.5, then the pleural fluid is considered to be a transudate. Peritoneal fluid is considered to be a transudate if the SAAG is >1.1 g/dL [ISBN9780323036580].

7.5.3 Special effusions

Chylous effusions are white because they contain fatty lymph fluid that is rich in chylomicrons and originates from the intestinal lymphatics. These effusions result from blockage of the thoracic duct due to tumor, granulomatous lesions, or parasitic infestation. They can also occur due to trauma to the thoracic duct (eg, stab injury). Such effusions contain high concentrations of triglycerides (usually >110 mg/dL) [ISBN9780323036580]. The ratio of a chylous pleural effusion cholesterol concentration to that of the concentration in serum is typically <1, while the ratio of a chylous pleural effusion triglyceride concentration to that of the serum triglyceride is usually >1 [Karkhanis 2012].

Pseudochylous effusions look like chylous effusions, but the white color is due to leukocytes or tumor cells instead of lymph fluid. These effusions are rich in cholesterol (usually >200 mg/dL) and, in fact, are sometimes called cholesterol effusions. They do not have elevated triglyceride concentrations or contain chylomicrons. Exceedingly high cholesterol concentrations may result in the so called "gold paint" effusion due to the intense opaque yellowish-orange color imparted by cholesterol. Since ether extracts the cholesterol, shaking a pseudochylous effusion with it will cause the effusion to clear, while shaking a chylous effusion with cholesterol will not cause it to clear [Karkhanis 2012].

7.5.4 Synovial fluid

Synovial fluid is colorless to light yellow and highly viscous due to high concentrations of **hyaluronic acid**. It functions as a lubricant for joints. The volume of fluid in the largest joints is <4 mL; thus, it is very difficult to sample. It is an ultrafiltrate of plasma, and the protein concentration is insufficient (no fibrinogen) to cause clotting. Analysis of synovial fluid may include chemistry, culture and sensitivity, and cell count. In the case of **gout**, monosodium urate crystals can be seen in the fluid, while in **pseudogout**, calcium pyrophosphate crystals are noted [ISBN9780683307511].

The **mucin clot (ROPES) test** is performed by adding glacial acetic acid to synovial fluid. Normal fluid forms a firm clot (complex of protein and hyaluronic acid) that is not broken when the tube is shaken. With inflammatory joints, hyaluronidase (present in the infiltrating neutrophils) destroys hyaluronic acid so that the fluid loses it viscosity, and a clot does not form with the addition of acid [ISBN9780323036580, ISBN9780683307511].

In noninflammatory joints, the synovial fluid glucose is about the same as that of the plasma/serum. In inflammatory joints, it is ~25 mg/dL lower than that of the plasma/serum (due to glucose utilization by infiltrating leukocytes), while in septic joints it is >40 mg/dL lower (due to utilization of glucose by bacteria and leukocytes) [ISBN9780323036580].

The range of leukocyte count in normal synovial fluid is 200-2,000 cells/mm^3. In inflammatory joints, it ranges from 2,000-100,000, and in septic joints it ranges from 10,000 to >100,000 [ISBN9780323036580].

7.6 **References**

7.6.1 **Journals**

PMID1449183 Bassiouny M, Hirsch B, Kelly RF et al [1992] Beta$_2$-transferrin application in otology. *Am J Otol* 13:552-55

PMID22278331 Wright BLC, Lai JTF, Sinclair AJ [2012] Cerebrospinal fluid and lumbar puncture: a practical review. *J Neurol* 259:1530-45

PMID22904139 Greene DN, Schmidt RL, Wilson AR et al [2012] Cerebrospinal fluid myelin basic protein is frequently ordered but has little value – a test utilization study. *Am J Clin Pathol* 138:262-72

PMID3802456 Hische EAH, van der Helm HJ [1987] Rate of synthesis of IgG within the blood-brain barrier and the IgG index compared in the diagnosis of multiple sclerosis. *Clin Chem* 31:113-14

Karkhanis VS, Joshi JM [2012] Pleural effusion: diagnosis, treatment, and management. *Open Access Emerg Med* 4:31-52

7.6.2 **Books**

ISBN9780071794794 Ropper AH, Samuels MA, Klein JP [2014] Imaging, electrophysiologic, and laboratory techniques for neurologic diagnosis. *Adams and Victor's Principles of Neurology*, 10e. McGraw-Hill Education, 13-44

ISBN9780323036580 Glasser L [2009] Extravascular biological fluids. In: Kaplan LA, Pesce AJ, ed. *Clinical Chemistry: Theory, Analysis, Correlation*, 5e. Mosby, 896-903

ISBN9780397518203 Laterra J, Keep R, Betz LA, Goldstein GW [1998] Blood-brain barrier. In: Siegel GJ, Agranoff BW, Albers RW et al, ed. *Basic Neurochemistry: Molecular, Cellular and Medical Aspects*, 6e. Lippincott-Raven

ISBN9780683300857 Boyer PJ, Simmons Z, Nifong TP [2002] Cerebrospinal fluid. In: Lewandrowski K, ed. *Clinical Chemistry: Laboratory Management & Clinical Correlations*. Lippincott Williams & Wilkins, 877-82

ISBN9780683307511 Curry JL, Amin HM, Theil KS [2002] Synovial, pleural, and peritoneal fluids. In: McClatchey KD, ed. *Clinical Laboratory Medicine*, 2e. Lippincott Williams & Wilkins, 501-16

7.7 **Clinical cases**

7.7.1 **Case 1**

A 64-year-old alcoholic man is hospitalized with lethargy, mental confusion, and abdominal pain. Physical examination suggests the presence of a large amount of fluid in the abdominal cavity, and a paracentesis is performed. ~150 mL of fluid is obtained. Because of respiratory difficulty, a second paracentesis is performed, and ~500 mL of fluid is removed. The albumin concentration of the fluid is 1.1 g/dL, and the serum albumin concentration is 2.5 g/dL.

7.7.1.1 **Questions**

1. What is the most likely diagnosis?

2. What laboratory studies should be performed on the peritoneal fluid?

3. Calculate the serum ascites albumin gradient (SAAG).

4. Calculate the peritoneal fluid albumin to serum albumin ratio.

5. Is the peritoneal fluid a transudate or an exudate?

6. What dangers, if any, to the patient might additional paracentesis present?

7. Why might the patient be confused?

7.7.2 **Case 2**

A 23-year-old male presents to the emergency department with a temperature of 101°F and a painful swollen metatarsal-phalangeal joint of the right great toe. The rheumatologist on call taps the joint and withdraws 0.5 mL of serosanguineous fluid.

7.7.2.1 **Questions**

1. What laboratory studies should be performed on the fluid?

2. What do you expect the leukocyte count to be (high, normal, or low)?

3. What do you expect the glucose concentration to be, relative to the plasma/serum (high, normal, or low)?

4. What do you expect the result of a mucin clot test to be?

5. Knowing that the serum uric acid is 13.2 mg/dL (reference range 3.6-7.5 mg/dL), what might you expect to see on microscopic examination of the fluid?

7.7.3 Clinical case answers

7.7.3.1 Case 1 answers

1. The most likely diagnosis is hepatic cirrhosis caused by chronic alcoholism. The liver can no longer make albumin, thus decreasing the oncotic pressure, and the cirrhosis causes portal hypertension. This combination yields ascites.

2. Culture and sensitivity (if infection is suspected), cell count, cytology (if malignancy is suspected), protein, and glucose; for comparison, serum/plasma protein and glucose concentrations should also be measured

3. 1.4 g/dL

4. 0.4

5. It is a transudate

6. Additional massive paracentesis could deplete the albumin stores, thereby further diminishing the oncotic pressure; it could also cause dehydration and shock, leading to secondary hyperaldosteronism

7. The patient likely has hepatic encephalopathy due to inability of the cirrhotic liver to convert ammonia into urea

7.7.3.2 Case 2 answers

1. Glucose, cell count, microscopic examination, culture and sensitivity, and mucin clot test

2. High due to inflammation

3. Low due to glycolysis by leukocytes

4. There would be no clot due to the presence of hyaluronidase in the infiltrating neutrophils, destroying the hyaluronic acid needed to make the clot

5. Monosodium urate crystals might be seen

chapter 8

The laboratory diagnosis of electrolyte & acid-base disturbances

8.1 **Objectives**

At the end of this session, the learner should be able to

- ➢ describe proper specimen collection for electrolyte analysis
- ➢ describe the effect of clotting on serum potassium
- ➢ discuss the effect of refrigeration of intact blood samples on serum/plasma potassium
- ➢ describe the effect of antidiuretic hormone and aldosterone on electrolytes
- ➢ discuss the renin-angiotensin system and its role in maintaining electrolyte balance
- ➢ describe the calculation of an anion gap
- ➢ discuss causes of increased and decreased anion gap
- ➢ describe the calculation of serum/plasma osmolality
- ➢ discuss causes of increased and decreased serum/plasma osmolality
- ➢ describe the calculation of the osmolal gap
- ➢ apply the Henderson-Hasselbalch equation to acid-base disorders
- ➢ discuss renal compensatory mechanisms in respiratory acidosis and respiratory alkalosis
- ➢ discuss pulmonary compensatory mechanisms in metabolic acidosis and metabolic alkalosis
- ➢ describe the criteria for determining whether or not there is maximum pulmonary compensation in metabolic acidosis and metabolic alkalosis
- ➢ describe the criteria for determining whether or not there is maximum renal compensation in chronic respiratory acidosis and in chronic respiratory alkalosis
- ➢ discuss the major causes for increased and decreased serum/plasma bicarbonate
- ➢ discuss the major causes for increased and decreased serum/plasma potassium
- ➢ discuss the major causes for increased and decreased serum/plasma sodium
- ➢ discuss the major causes for increased and decreased serum/plasma chloride

8.2 **Key terms**

acidosis: a pathological condition resulting from accumulation of acid in the blood or from loss of base from the blood

aldosterone: a mineralocorticoid hormone produced by the adrenal cortex that induces renal excretion of potassium and hydrogen ion, renal retention of sodium and water, and reclamation of bicarbonate; it is released through the action of angiotensin II

aldosteronism: a pathological condition resulting in increased concentration of aldosterone; it can be either primary (autonomous production of aldosterone) or secondary (resulting from another condition)

alkalosis: a pathological condition resulting from accumulation of base in the blood or from loss of acid from the blood

angiotensin: a vasoconstrictive polypeptide produced by the action of renin on angiotensinogen, forming the biologically inactive angiotensin I; angiotensin converting enzyme in the lung converts angiotensin I to the biologically active angiotensin II

angiotensinogen: a precursor of angiotensin I

anion: a negatively charged ion

anion gap: the difference between unmeasured anions and unmeasured cations in a serum or plasma specimen

antidiuretic hormone (ADH, vasopressin): a hormone produced by the hypothalamus and stored in the pituitary gland; it causes water to be reabsorbed by the renal collecting ducts and the ascending loop of Henle, and its release is regulated by serum osmolality

cation: a positively charged ion

cirrhosis: progressive disease of the liver leading to scarring and failure of hepatic parenchymal cells

diabetes insipidus: a pathological condition caused either by insufficient production of antidiuretic hormone by the hypothalamus and/or secretion by the pituitary (central diabetes insipidus), or by the lack of hormone effect on the kidney (nephrogenic diabetes insipidus), resulting in excretion of voluminous amounts of hypoosmolar urine and causing hyperosmolality of the serum/plasma

familial hypokalemic periodic paralysis: a congenital condition in which extracellular potassium enters the muscle, leading to transient paralysis

hemoconcentration: the decrease of the fluid content of blood, causing increased concentration of analytes

Henderson-Hasselbalch equation: a formula describing the relationship among pH and pK_a of a buffer system, and the ratio of the conjugate base to its corresponding weak acid

hypercortisolism: an increase in the serum/plasma concentration of cortisol

hypocortisolism: a decrease in the serum/plasma concentration of cortisol

hypovolemia: an abnormally low blood volume

juxtaglomerular cells: smooth muscle cells that synthesize and store renin, and release it in response to decreased renal perfusion pressure (decreased renal blood flow; hypovolemia) and/or decreased sodium concentration

metabolic acidosis: pathological accumulation of acid or loss of base from the body

metabolic alkalosis: pathological accumulation of base or loss of acid from the body.

osmolal gap: the difference between measured osmolality and calculated osmolality

osmolality: the concentration of osmotically active substances, expressed as mOSm in a kilogram of water

polydypsia: excessive thirst causing ingestion of large amounts of water

polycythemia vera: a disorder of the bone marrow resulting in overproduction of red blood cells, white blood cells, and platelets

polyuria: excessive urine output

pseudohyperkalemia: artifactually high serum or plasma potassium in the absence of a true elevation of potassium in a patient

renin: an enzyme produced, stored, and excreted by the juxtaglomerular cells of the kidney; responsible for converting angiotensinogen to angiotensin I

respiratory acidosis: pathological retention of carbon dioxide caused by low respiration rates

respiratory alkalosis: pathological decrease of carbon dioxide caused by increased respiration rates

rhabdomyolysis: breakdown of muscle

sodium-potassium ATPase pump: the mechanism residing in the red cell membrane that exchanges 2 potassium ions (into the red cell) for 3 sodium ions (out of the red cell) per molecule of ATP utilized

spurious hyponatremia: artifactually low serum or plasma sodium in the absence of a true depression of sodium in a patient

syndrome of inappropriate antidiuretic hormone (SIADH): a pathological condition that can be caused by tumor, granulomatous diseases, and drugs, and is characterized by excessive production of antidiuretic hormone, resulting in serum hypoosmolality and urine hyperosmolality

8.3 Background/significance

Electrolyte and acid-base balance disturbances are among the most commonly encountered disorders in medicine. They can be either primary causes of disease themselves or reflections of other pathology.

8.4 Sample collection for electrolyte analysis

Samples for electrolyte analysis can be serum (no anticoagulant) or plasma. If the latter, the anticoagulant must be heparin, since other anticoagulants (eg, citrate, oxalate, ethylenediaminetetraacetate) contribute electrolytes, thereby contaminating the sample. Some anticoagulants also bind calcium and magnesium.

Since, by definition, serum is plasma that has been allowed to clot so that it is devoid of clotting factors, the serum potassium is higher than the plasma potassium due to release of potassium from platelets during clotting (on average 0.4 mEq/L higher) [PMID23724399]. With substantial elevations of the platelet count (eg, **polycythemia vera**), this **pseudohyperkalemia** may be even more pronounced. With the advent of gel separator blood collection tubes, which facilitate the analysis of plasma without contamination by the underlying cell mass, many laboratories prefer to use heparinized plasma as the specimen of choice because the sample does not need to sit to permit clotting before analysis. Use of plasma also eliminates pseudohyperkalemia due to potassium release from platelets. Unfortunately, however, pseudohyperkalemia can still result from prolonged application of the tourniquet during blood drawing by causing **hemoconcentration**. It can also be caused by the forearm muscle releasing potassium if the fist is pumped during blood drawing [PMID23724399]. Yet another cause of pseudohyperkalemia can be refrigeration of the intact blood sample because refrigeration inhibits the sodium-potassium ATPase pump, thereby reducing the amount of potassium transported into the erythrocyte [PMID23724399]. Finally, although less profound, allowing samples to sit intact for long periods of time before processing them for analysis can also result in pseudohyperkalemia due to failure of the sodium-potassium ATPase pump as the supply of available glucose to generate ATP is exhausted [PMID23724399]. Since these conditions do not cause hemolysis, if the clinical laboratory staff then analyzes the specimen, they will be unaware of the artifact. Of particular concern, pseudohyperkalemia can mask hypokalemia by driving the potassium into the reference range. Samples for potassium analysis ideally should be centrifuged prior to delivery to the laboratory in order to separate the serum or plasma from the erythrocytes, especially if delivery time to the laboratory will be prolonged.

As noted in Chapter 2, hemolysis increases potassium concentrations in serum and plasma due to its release from the erythrocyte. In fact, it has been reported that 1 g of liberated hemoglobin will contribute 3.3 mEq/L of potassium to plasma or serum [PMID14422258]. In order to identify hemolysis, most clinical laboratories check serum indices (ie, measurements that detect hemolysis, lipemia, and icterus). Using computer algorithms, the laboratory evaluates the potential for any of these to interfere with the analysis prior to reporting the result. If there is a possible interferent, no result is reported.

8.5 Hormones important in electrolyte & acid-base balance

Antidiuretic hormone (**ADH, vasopressin**) is produced in the hypothalamus and stored in the pituitary. It causes water to be reabsorbed by the renal collecting ducts and the ascending loop of Henle. Its release is stimulated by increases in serum/plasma **osmolality**. Defects of ADH production or release (central **diabetes insipidus**) or kidney response (nephrogenic diabetes insipidus) lead to **polyuria** and **polydipsia** with increased serum/plasma osmolality and decreased urine osmolality. In contrast, excessive production of ADH (**syndrome of inappropriate ADH [SIADH]**) can be due to central nervous system disorders, pulmonary lesions, malignancies, and drugs, and causes decreased serum/plasma osmolality and increased urine osmolality [ISBN9780071824866].

Renin is an enzyme produced, stored, and secreted by the juxtaglomerular cells of the kidney in response to low sodium concentration and decreased renal perfusion (as may occur with edematous conditions). Renin causes conversion of **angiotensinogen** to **angiotensin** I, which is converted to angiotensin II by angiotensin converting enzyme in the lung. Angiotensin II causes release of aldosterone.

Aldosterone, produced by the zona glomerulosa of the adrenal cortex, induces the urinary excretion of potassium and hydrogen ion, and the renal retention of sodium and water. Thus, hyperaldosteronism causes a hypokalemic metabolic alkalosis. Aldosterone is released in response to angiotensin II. In adrenal insufficiency, the amount of aldosterone and cortisol (which has mineralocorticoid effects in high concentration) is deficient. In contrast, in primary **aldosteronism** (caused by bilateral hypertrophy of the zona glomerulosa, adrenal adenoma, adrenal carcinoma), excessive production of aldosterone reduces renin production (high serum aldosterone and low renin). In secondary aldosteronism (caused by congestive heart failure, hepatic cirrhosis, nephrotic syndrome), the **juxtaglomerular cells** secrete renin in response to **hypovolemia**, thus prompting the release of aldosterone with retention of more sodium and water so that the total body sodium is increased while the serum or plasma sodium is low due to concomitant retention of water and release of ADH (high serum renin and high aldosterone).

8.6 Anion gap

The so called Gamblegram **f8.1**, named for James L Gamble [1954], provides a simple way of understanding the **anion gap**, which is the difference between the unmeasured **anions** (ions with negative charge; *an-* = without) and the unmeasured **cations** (ions with positive charge). It should be emphasized that *unmeasured* does not mean *unmeasurable*, since all of the analytes can be measured. Rather, *unmeasured* refers to analytes that are not normally measured when one orders a set of electrolytes. Such orders usually include only sodium, potassium, chloride, and bicarbonate.

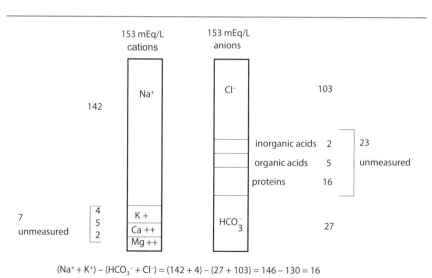

$$(Na^+ + K^+) - (HCO_3^- + Cl^-) = (142 + 4) - (27 + 103) = 146 - 130 = 16$$

(the anion gap reflects the fact that there are more unmeasured anions than there are unmeasured cations: 23 − 7 = 16)

f8.1 Balance of cations & anions with a gap between unmeasured anions & unmeasured cations

Since more anions than cations are unmeasured, normal individuals have a gap **f8.1**. The anion gap can be calculated as follows:

$$(Na^+ + K^+) - (HCO_3^- + Cl^-)$$

The reference range is 12-20 mEq/L. An alternate formula does not use K^+ because its numerical contribution to the anion gap is small, in which case the reference range is 8-16 mEq/L [ISBN9781594251023]. It should be noted that **f8.1** uses mean normal values for each of the 4 measured electrolytes and for the major categories of unmeasured cations (magnesium and calcium) and unmeasured anions (proteins; organic acids such as lactic acid, pyruvic acid; inorganic acids such as phosphate and sulfate—all of which are negatively charged at physiological pH). In this particular example, the sum of measured and unmeasured anions and the sum of measured and unmeasured cations are each 153 mEq/L. Obviously, in other individuals with different analyte concentrations, the sum is different. Nevertheless, in each instance, the sum of the anions must equal the sum of the cations in order to preserve electroneutrality.

The anion gap is diagnostically useful, and for that reason, it should be calculated whenever a set of electrolytes is obtained. Increased and decreased anion gaps can suggest certain abnormalities.

An increased anion gap can be due to increases in any of the unmeasured anions shown in the Gamblegram, since increases in the unmeasured anions cause proportionate decreases in the measured anions in order to preserve electroneutrality. The measured anions that decrease in concentration do so by being cleared from the extracellular space. Common causes of an increased anion gap are the following: increases of organic acids, including ketoacids (eg, acetoacetic acid and β hydroxybutyric acid in diabetic ketoacidosis), lactic acidosis, treatment with substances that are unmeasured anions at physiological pH (eg, salicylates, citrate in transfused blood), poisoning with agents that are metabolized to organic acids (eg, methanol, ethylene glycol); and increases of inorganic acids, including retention of phosphate, sulfate (increased in renal failure). Obviously hypocalcemia and hypomagnesemia will also cause some increase in the anion gap by causing a proportionate increase in sodium and potassium.

Common causes of a decreased anion gap are the following: decreases of unmeasured anions, as in hypoalbuminemia (eg, nephrotic syndrome, hepatic failure, burns), causing an increase in the measured anions; and increases of unmeasured cations, such as paraproteins (monoclonal proteins that are positively charged at physiological pH), hypercalcemia, and hypermagnesemia, all of which diminish the concentration of measured cations, thereby decreasing the anion gap. Finally, hemodilution also decreases the anion gap because more anions than cations are unmeasured. For example, a 20% dilution would reduce the concentrations of measured analytes to 80% of their baseline values:

$$0.8(Na^+ + K^+) - 0.8(HCO_3^- + Cl^-)$$

$$= 0.8\,(142 + 4) - 0.8\,(27 + 103)$$

$$= 0.8[16] = 12.8$$

8.7 Osmolality

Osmolality is the concentration of osmotically active substances in mOsm per kg of water (serum/plasma is mostly water). Compounds must be water soluble in order to contribute to serum/plasma and urine osmolality. For <u>nondissociable</u> water soluble compounds (eg, glucose, urea, ethanol), 1 osmole = 1 mole, and 1 mOSm = 1 mMol. Thus, using glucose as an example, 1 mole (180 g) = 1 osmole, and 1 mMol (180 mg) = 1 mOsm. Thus, for glucose, 1 mOsm/kg = 180 mg/kg. Since serum/plasma is mostly water, and since 1 kg of water yields 1 L, then, for glucose, 1 mOsm/kg = 180 mg/kg = 180 mg/L = 18 mg/dL. Therefore, for every 18 mg/dL of serum or plasma glucose, there is a contribution of 1 mOsm/kg to the osmolality. Similarly, since urea has 2 nitrogens (each atomic weight 14 for a total of 28), then for every 2.8 mg/dL of serum/plasma urea nitrogen (SUN), there is a contribution of 1 mOsm/kg to the osmolality. By a similar derivation, if ethanol (molecular weight 46) were present, then for every 4.6 mg/dL of ethanol, there would be a contribution of 1 mOsm/kg to the osmolality. For <u>dissociable</u> water soluble compounds, the number of particles yielded per mole must be considered (eg, 1 mole of NaCl theoretically yields 2 moles of solute, but due to shielding by molecules of water, the osmotic coefficient is <1 and the yield is thus somewhat <2; however, for ease of calculation, the number 2 is used) [ISBN9781416061649b]. Thus, the osmotic contribution of sodium to serum/plasma osmolality is estimated by 2(Na).

Although various formulas have been developed for calculation of serum osmolality, using the parameters described above, the formula of Worthly et al [PMID16006260, Worthly 1987] has been recommended due to its simplicity [ISBN9781416061649b]:

$$2(Na) + (glucose/18) + (SUN/2.8)$$

Using normal values, this would yield

$$2(Na) + (glucose/18) + (SUN/2.8) = 2(142) + (100/90) + (14/2.8)$$
$$= 294 \text{ (reference range 275-300 mOsm/kg)}$$

Most measurements of osmolality are based on the principle of freezing point depression by solutes in solution. 1 mole of solute depresses the freezing point of water by 1.86°C [ISBN9781416061649b]. This is the principle behind using salt to treat ice on highways as it lowers the freezing point of water <0°C (32°F). Thus an osmotically active substance will lower the freezing point by a multiple of this amount depending on the molar concentration of osmolutes. The osmometer is designed to detect the heat of fusion released when the slowly cooled, supersaturated sample freezes. The heat of fusion liberated is directly proportional to the osmolality of the sample.

It should be emphasized that osmolality must be measured in either serum or heparinized plasma because other anticoagulants are themselves osmotically active and will contribute to the osmolality.

Some common causes of serum <u>hyperosmolality</u> include hyperglycemia, uremia, and hypernatremia, since glucose, urea, and sodium are osmotically active. Thus, any conditions causing them (eg, dehydration, diabetes insipidus, uncontrolled diabetes mellitus, renal failure) will increase the serum osmolality. Obviously, ingestion of other osmotically active substances (eg, ethanol) will also increase the osmolality.

Some common causes of serum hypo-osmolality include overhydration, compulsive water drinking, and SIADH because they each cause dilution of the osmotically active compounds.

The **osmal gap** is the difference between measured osmolality and calculated osmolality and, if positive, suggests the presence of other osmotically active compounds that may not have been measured. Some of these (eg, ethanol) may not affect the anion gap.

8.8 Henderson-Hasselbalch equation

An appreciation of the **Henderson-Hasselbalch equation** is essential to understanding acid-base balance. This equation describes the establishment and maintenance of the pH of a buffer solution based on the concentrations of the weak acid and its conjugate base:

$$pH = pK_a + \log([base]/[acid])$$

The pK_a is a physical constant of the buffer system and is the pH at which the concentration of the base (ionized) equals that of the acid (unionized) so that [base]/[acid] = 1, and the log(1) = 0, leaving $pH = pK_a$. The bicarbonate/carbonic acid buffer system is the most important buffer system for maintenance of the physiological pH. Applying the Henderson-Hasselbalch equation to this system and using average concentrations for bicarbonate and carbonic acid:

$$pH = pK_a + \log([base]/[acid]) = 6.1 + \log([HCO_3^-]/[H_2CO_3])$$
$$= 6.1 + \log([24 \text{ mMol/L}]/[1.2 \text{ mMol/L}])$$
$$= 6.1 + \log(20) = 6.1 + 1.3 = 7.4$$

Since pK_a is fixed, the maintenance of physiological pH depends on the preservation of the 20:1 ratio between $[HCO_3^-]$ and $[H_2CO_3]$. Since the concentration of carbonic acid is equal to pCO_2 (the partial pressure of carbon dioxide in the blood, mm/Hg) × 0.03, this means that maintenance of the ratio can occur by regulation of carbon dioxide through rapid or slower breathing and/or by retention or loss of hydrogen ion by the kidney:

$$pH = pK_a + \log([base]/[acid]) = 6.1 + \log([HCO_3^-]/[H_2CO_3])$$
$$= 6.1 + \log([HCO_3^-]/[pCO_2 \times 0.03])$$

Obviously, if 2 of the 3 variables (ie, pCO_2, pH, HCO_3^-) are known, the third can be calculated.

8.9 Respiratory acidosis & alkalosis & renal compensation

Acute **respiratory acidosis** is caused by retention of carbon dioxide through suppressed breathing (eg, partial airway obstruction). The immediate effect, by law of mass action, is to shift the following equilibrium to the left as the expiration of carbon dioxide is suppressed:

$$H^+ + HCO_3^- \Leftrightarrow H_2CO_3 \rightarrow H_2O + CO_2 \uparrow$$

For every 10 mmHg increase in pCO_2 above the normal level of 40, the HCO_3^- increases by 1 mMol/L (mEq/L), and the H^+ concentration increases (pH falls) [ISBN9781416061649a].

Chronic respiratory acidosis is caused by retention of carbon dioxide through suppressed breathing for longer periods of time (eg, chronic obstructive pulmonary disease). Due to the chronicity of the disorder, the kidneys have time to compensate by clearing H^+ through its elimination as hydrogen phosphate, elimination as ammonium ion, reclamation of filtered HCO_3^-, and tubular exchange of sodium for H^+ [ISBN9781416061649a]. The loss of H^+ in this manner causes elevation of HCO_3^- since there is less hydrogen to convert HCO_3^- to H_2CO_3. Thus, in compensated chronic respiratory acidosis, for every increase in pCO_2 above the normal level of 40, the HCO_3^- increases by 3.5 mMol/L (mEq/L) [ISBN9781416061649a].

Acute **respiratory alkalosis** is caused by loss of carbon dioxide through sudden hyperventilation (eg, hysteria). The immediate effect, by law of mass action, is to shift the following equilibrium to the right as carbon dioxide is removed:

$$H^+ + HCO_3^- \Leftrightarrow H_2CO_3 \rightarrow H_2O + CO_2\uparrow$$

For every 10 mmHg decrease in pCO_2 below the normal level of 40, the HCO_3^- decreases by 2 mMol/L (mEq/L), and the H^+ concentration decreases (pH rises) [ISBN9781416061649a].

Chronic respiratory alkalosis is caused by loss of carbon dioxide through hyperventilation on a prolonged basis (eg, living at high altitudes, which necessitates rapid breathing to maintain adequate oxygenation; ascites with inability to inspire fully due to elevated diaphragms). Due to the chronicity of this disorder, the kidneys have time to compensate by exchanging sodium for H^+, by excreting less hydrogen phosphate, reclaiming less bicarbonate, and generating less ammonium ion [Worthly 1987]. The retention of H^+ causes further reduction of the HCO_3^- as the H^+ converts it to H_2CO_3. Thus, in compensated chronic respiratory alkalosis, for every reduction in pCO_2 of 10 mmHg below the normal level of 40, the HCO_3^- decreases by 5 mMol/L (mEq/L) [ISBN9781416061649a].

8.10 Metabolic acidosis & alkalosis & pulmonary compensation

By their very nature, **metabolic acidosis** and **metabolic alkalosis** occur only chronically because their etiology requires disturbances over a period of time. Metabolic acidosis is caused by either production or retention of acid (eg, diabetic ketoacidosis, lactic acidosis, renal failure, hypocortisolism) or by loss of bicarbonate (eg, massive diarrhea). In contrast, metabolic alkalosis is caused by excess bicarbonate (eg, overadministration of bicarbonate; massive blood transfusion with hepatic metabolism of the citrate to bicarbonate) or by loss of acid (eg, profound vomiting, nasogastric suction, hypercortisolism and hyperaldosteronism with loss of H^+ into the urine).

Compensation of metabolic acidosis and alkalosis occurs via the lungs. Metabolic acidosis stimulates hyperventilation (in attempt to correct the acidosis). Pulmonary compensation is evidenced when $pCO_2 = 1.5(HCO_3^-) + 8$ (±2) [ISBN9781416061649a].

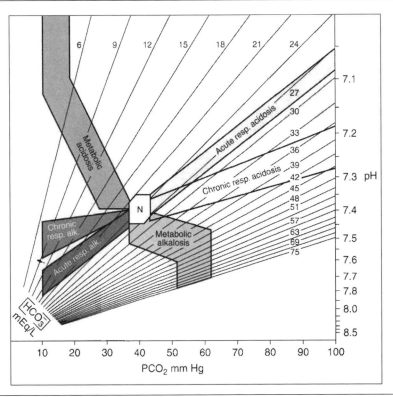

f8.2 Acid-base map [modified from Goldberg 1973]

In contrast, metabolic alkalosis stimulates hypoventilation. Pulmonary compensation is evidenced when the pCO_2 is increased by 6 mmHg for every 10 mMol/L (mEq/L) increase in HCO_3^- above the normal 24 mMol/L (mEq/L) [ISBN9781416061649a].

The relationships of each of these conditions with the pH, HCO_3^-, and pCO_2 is depicted in the classical "acid-base map" of Goldberg et al **f8.2** [1973].

f8.3 illustrates how to determine if an acid-base disorder is a respiratory or a metabolic problem.

8.11 Causes of electrolyte abnormalities
8.11.1 Bicarbonate
Bicarbonate (reference range 22-28 mMol/L, mEq/L) is <u>increased</u> as a compensatory mechanism in respiratory acidosis, which can be caused by prolonged hypoventilation, central nervous system depression (eg, opiate usage), chronic obstructive pulmonary disease, paralysis of the respiratory musculature, diseases of the airway, sleep apnea, and cardiac disease [ISBN9781416061649a]. It is also <u>increased</u> as a primary cause of metabolic alkalosis (which can be caused by loss of acid from the stomach through vomiting or excessive drainage of the

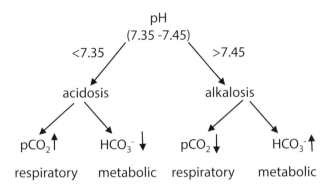

f8.3 Interpretation of acid-base disorders

stomach), hypercortisolism and hyperaldosteronism (loss of hydrogen ion into the urine along with potassium), administration of excess base (eg, massive blood transfusion), and use of diuretics (loss of hydrogen ion into the urine along with potassium) [ISBN9781416061649a].

Bicarbonate is <u>decreased</u> as a compensatory mechanism in respiratory alkalosis, which can be caused by hyperventilation due to fever, hysteria, extreme obesity (with inability to mobilize the diaphragms), and living at high altitudes [Worthly 1987]. It is also <u>decreased</u> as a primary cause of metabolic acidosis, which can be caused by overproduction of acids (eg, lactic acidosis, diabetic ketoacidosis), retention of acid (eg, renal failure), and loss of base (eg, diarrhea) [ISBN9781416061649a].

8.11.2 Chloride

Chloride (reference range 98-107 mMol/L, mEq/L) is <u>increased</u> in dehydration (eg, due to water loss, diabetes insipidus), with most decreases in bicarbonate (compensatory increase to preserve electroneutrality; an exception is diabetic ketoacidosis, in which both the bicarbonate and chloride are decreased due to the expansion of ketoacids), hyperventilation (compensatory increase to preserve electroneutrality as the bicarbonate decreases; eg, hysteria, living at high altitudes, massive ascites with inability to mobilize the diaphragms), and overtreatment with normal saline solutions [ISBN9781416061649a].

Chloride is <u>decreased</u> in overhydration, hypoventilation (compensatory decrease to preserve electroneutrality due to the increased bicarbonate; eg, chronic obstructive pulmonary disease), SIADH, central nervous system depression (compensatory decrease to preserve electroneutrality as the bicarbonate increases; eg, opiate usage), chronic renal disease (urinary loss of chloride with sodium), adrenal insufficiency (urinary loss of chloride with sodium), hypercortisolism (urinary loss of chloride with potassium), metabolic alkalosis (compensatory decrease to preserve electroneutrality due to the increased bicarbonate; eg, massive blood transfusion, loss of H^+ through vomiting), and loss of chloride with vomiting [ISBN9781416061649a].

8.11.3 **Sodium**

Sodium (reference range 136-145 mMol/L, mEq/L) is increased in dehydration, hypercortisolism (retention of sodium), hyperaldosteronism (retention of sodium), and diarrhea (with water loss).

Sodium is decreased in overhydration, hypoadrenalism (urinary loss), renal disease (urinary loss), diabetic ketoacidosis (urinary loss with the ketoacids), SIADH, prolonged use of potassium sparing diuretic agents (eg, spironolactone), compulsive water drinking, and hypothyroidism (impairment of free water excretion). Dilutional hyponatremia can be caused by hyperglycemia, which exerts an osmotic effect, resulting in an extracellular shift of water or an intracellular shift of sodium to maintain the osmotic balance between the extracellular and intracellular compartments. For every increase in glucose >100 mg/dL, the plasma or serum sodium is decreased by 1.6-2.4 mMol/L (mEq/L) [ISBN9781416061649a]. Secondary hyperaldosteronism (which can be caused by nephrotic syndrome, congestive heart failure, and hepatic cirrhosis) stimulates the juxtaglomerular cells to secrete renin in response to the decreased renal blood flow, resulting in production of aldosterone, which causes retention of sodium and water so that the total body sodium is increased while the serum/plasma sodium is decreased due to water retention and the secretion of ADH. This produces a vicious cycle. Finally, if serum/plasma sodium is measured by indirect ion selective electrode potentiometry (ie, using a dilution of sample prior to analysis), hyperlipidemia will cause **spurious hyponatremia** due to a sampling artifact caused by volume displacement of sodium by the lipid content of the sample [ISBN9781416061649a].

8.11.4 **Potassium**

Potassium (reference range 3.5-5.1 mMol/L, mEq/L) is increased by hemolysis, hemoconcentration, fist pumping during phlebotomy, refrigeration of an intact whole blood sample (due to inhibition of the sodium-potassium ATPase pump), and letting intact whole blood samples sit for prolonged periods before processing for analysis, as previously noted. It is also increased by dehydration, hypoadrenalism (potassium retention), metabolic acidosis (shift of potassium from erythrocyte into the plasma/serum as the blood pH decreases; eg, diabetic ketoacidosis), polycythemia vera (if a serum sample is used, due to release of potassium from the increased number of platelets during clotting), tumor lysis (potassium release), **rhabdomyolysis** (potassium release), and renal failure (potassium retention) [ISBN9781416061649a].

Potassium is decreased in malnutrition (inadequate potassium intake), diarrhea (potassium loss), vomiting (potassium loss), hypercortisolism (urinary potassium loss), hyperaldosteronism (urinary potassium loss), diuretic use (urinary potassium loss), and **familial hypokalemic periodic paralysis** (a condition in which extracellular potassium leaks into the myocytes) [ISBN9781416061649a].

8.12 **References**
8.12.1 **Journals**

PMID14422258 Mather A, Mackie NR [1960] Effects of hemolysis on serum electrolyte values. *Clin Chem* 6:223-7

PMID16006260 Rasouli M, Kalantari KR [2005] Comparison of methods for calculating serum osmolality: multivariate linear regression analysis. *Clin Chem Lab Med* 43:635-40

PMID23724399 Asirvatham JR, Moses V, Bjornson L [2013] Errors in potassium measurement: a laboratory perspective for the clinician. *N Am J Med Sci* 5:255-9

Goldberg M, Green SB, Moss ML et al [1973] Computer-based instruction and diagnosis of acid-base disorders: a systematic approach. 223:269-75

Worthly LI, Guerin M, Pain RW [1987] For calculating osmolality, the simplest formula is the best. *Anesthaesia and Intensive Care* 15:199-202

8.12.2 **Books**

ISBN9780071824866 Cho, K [2014] Electrolytes & acid-base disorders. In: Papadakis MA, McPhee SJ, Rabow MW, ed. *Current Medical Diagnosis & Treatment*, 53e. McGraw Hill Education, 837-64

ISBN9781416061649a Hood JL, Scott MG [2012] Physiology and disorders of water, electrolyte, and acid-base metabolism. In: Burtis CA, Ashwood ER, Bruns DE, ed. *Tietz Textbook of Clinical Chemistry and Molecular Diagnostics*, 5e. Elsevier Saunders, 1609-636.

ISBN9781416061649b Scott MG, LeGrys VA, Hood JL [2013] Electrolytes and blood gases In: Burtis CA, Ashwood ER, Bruns DE, ed. *Tietz Textbook of Clinical Chemistry and Molecular Diagnostics*, 5e. Elsevier Saunders, 807-836.

ISBN9781594251023 Toffaletti JG [2011] Blood gas and critical care testing. In: Clarke W, ed. *Contemporary Practice in Clinical Chemistry*, 2e. A Press, 372.

Gamble J [1954] *Chemical Anatomy Physiology and Pathology of Extracellular Fluid: A Lecture Syllabus*, 6e. Harvard University Press, chart 4

8.13 **Clinical cases**
8.13.1 **Case 1**

A febrile 84-year-old female is brought from a nursing home to the emergency department. She is severely cachectic and confused, and has sagging skin folds and extremely dry skin. Admission serum laboratory results are as follows: sodium 168 mMol/L (mEq/L), potassium 6.2 mMol/L (mEq/L), chloride 130 mMol/L (mEq/L), bicarbonate 26 mMol/L (mEq/L), osmolality 360 mOsm/kg, and urea-N 38 mg/dL. Her hematocrit was 58%.

8.13.1.1 **Questions**

1. Explain the elevated sodium, potassium, chloride, urea-N, osmolality, and hematocrit.

2. Why was the bicarbonate not increased?

3. What other laboratory studies should be obtained?

4. How might this situation have occurred?

8.13.2 **Case 2**

A 25-year-old female with a history of surgical removal of an adenoma of the pituitary gland returns to her endocrinologist with complaints of unquenchable thirst and excretion of voluminous amounts of urine daily. Laboratory tests performed on her serum reveal the following: sodium 160 mMol/L (mEq/L), potassium 4.8 mMol/L (mEq/L), chloride 125 mMol/L (mEq/L), bicarbonate 24 mMol/L (mEq/L), and osmolality 345 mOsm/kg.

8.13.2.1 **Questions**

1. What is the most likely diagnosis?

2. What additional laboratory tests should be performed?

8.13.3 **Case 3**

A 40-year-old male is brought to the emergency department; he is confused and has the odor of alcohol on his breath. Laboratory tests performed on serum show the following: sodium 137 mMol/L (mEq/L), potassium 4.2 mMol/L (mEq/L), chloride 100 mMol/L (mEq/L), bicarbonate 26 mMol/L (mEq/L), urea-N 14 mg/dL, glucose 90 mg/dL, and osmolality 360 mOsm/kg.

8.13.3.1 **Questions**

1. What is the most likely explanation for the elevated serum osmolality?

2. How would you confirm the explanation?

3. Calculate the osmolal gap.

4. If the osmolal gap were entirely due to ethanol, what would the ethanol concentration (mg/dL) be?

8.13.4 **Case 4**

A 14-year-old male was severely injured in an automobile accident. He was hospitalized and required the use of a ventilator during the acute phase of his illness. When he appeared to be recovering, he was weaned off the ventilator with no apparent ill effects. Analysis of his blood at that time showed the following: arterial pH 7.32, arterial pO_2 52 mmHg, arterial pCO_2 70 mmHg, serum bicarbonate 35 mMol/L (mEq/L), serum chloride 90 mMol/L (mEq/L), serum sodium 136 mMol/L (mEq/L), and serum potassium 4.5 mMol/L (mEq/L).

8.13.4.1 **Questions**

1. What is the type of acid-base balance disorder?

2. What is its cause in this case?

3. Is there evidence for compensation in this case?

4. Why is the serum chloride decreased?

8.13.5 **Case 5**

An 8-year-old female is hospitalized following 1 week of uncontrollable diarrhea. She is listless and responds incoherently to questions. Her skin turgor is poor, and her eyes are soft and sunken. Her pulse is 114 beats per minute, blood pressure 98/66 mmHg, temperature 100°F, and respirations 26/min (deep). The following laboratory results were obtained: arterial pH 7.13, arterial pO_2 96 mmHg, arterial pCO_2 18 mmHg, serum bicarbonate 6 mMol/L (mEq/L), serum chloride 115 mMol/L (mEq/L), serum sodium 133 mMol/L (mEq/L), and serum potassium 3.1 mMol/L (mEq/L).

8.13.5.1 Questions

1. What is the type of acid-base balance disorder?

2. What is its cause in this case?

3. Is there evidence for compensation in this case?

4. Why does the patient have low blood pressure and a high pulse rate?

5. Why is the serum potassium low?

6. Why is serum potassium not a good indicator of total body potassium in this case?

7. Why is the serum chloride increased?

8.13.6 **Case 6**

A 21-year-old female with a 12 year history of diabetes mellitus type I was hospitalized in a coma. On admission she had a blood pressure of 92/40 mmHg, a pulse of 122 beats per minute, and deep respirations of 32/min. Her laboratory results were as follows: arterial pH 7.10, arterial pO_2 90 mmHg, arterial pCO_2 15 mmHg, serum bicarbonate 4 mMol/L (mEq/L), serum chloride 95 mMol/L (mEq/L), serum sodium 121 mMol/L (mEq/L), serum potassium 6.4 mMol/L (mEq/L), serum urea-N 74 mg/dL, serum creatinine 2.3 mg/dL, and serum glucose 1,200 mg/dL. Her serum was strongly positive for ketones.

8.13.6.1 Questions

1. What is the type of acid-base balance disorder?

2. What is its cause in this case?

3. Is there evidence for compensation in this case?

4. Why is the serum potassium elevated?

5. Why is the serum sodium low?

6. Calculate the anion gap and explain the value.

7. Why are the blood pressure low and the pulse rate high?

8. Why are the serum urea-N and creatinine elevated?

9. Why is the SUN:CR elevated?

8.13.7 Case 7

A 40-year-old alcoholic male with massive ascites is brought to the emergency department after being found wandering in a confused state. His blood pressure is 158/92 mmHg, temperature 101°F, respirations 26/min (shallow), and pulse rate 75 beats per minute. His laboratory results are as follows: arterial pH 7.58, arterial pO_2 90 mmHg, arterial pCO_2 10 mmHg, serum bicarbonate 9 mMol/L (mEq/L), serum chloride 103 mMol/L (mEq/L), serum sodium 131 mMol/L (mEq/L), serum potassium 3.1 mMol/L (mEq/L), serum calcium 8.2 mg/dL, and serum albumin 2.2 g/dL.

8.13.7.1 Questions

1. What is the type of acid-base balance disorder?

2. What is its cause in this case?

3. Is there evidence for compensation in this case?

4. Why is the serum calcium low?

5. Why is the serum albumin low?

6. Why is the serum potassium low?

7. Why is the serum sodium low?

8. Why is the blood pressure high?

8.13.8 Case 8

A 58-year-old female is hospitalized after 3 days of intractable vomiting. Her blood pressure is 100/50 mmHg, respirations 8/min (shallow), pulse rate 101 beats per minute, and temperature 100°F. Laboratory results were as follows: arterial pH 7.55, arterial pO_2 95 mmHg, arterial pCO_2 52 mmHg, serum bicarbonate 44 mMol/L (mEq/L), serum chloride 82 mMol/L (mEq/L), serum sodium 135 mMol/L (mEq/L), and serum potassium 3.2 mMol/L (mEq/L).

8.13.8.1 Questions

1. What is the type of acid-base balance disorder?

2. What is its cause in this case?

3. Is there evidence for compensation in this case?

4. Why is the serum potassium low?

5. Why is the blood pressure low?

6. Why is the serum chloride low?

8.13.9 Clinical case answers

8.13.9.1 Case 1 answers

1. The sodium, potassium, chloride, urea-N, osmolality, and hematocrit are increased due to dehydration; this also causes decreased glomerular filtration rate, which allows for more passive reabsorption of urea-N (prerenal azotemia)

2. A bicarbonate increase would be compensated by respiratory and renal mechanisms

3. Urine, if obtainable, should be submitted for urinalysis and for measurement of osmolality. Dehydration should cause a urine high specific gravity and osmolality. Serum creatinine should be obtained as well. The creatinine should also be elevated due to decreased glomerular filtration rate, and the SUN:CR should be elevated (prerenal azotemia). Laboratory studies should be repeated after hydration of the patient.

4. The patient had dementia and could not ask for water; the nursing home staff was inattentive to her care

8.13.9.2 Case 2 answers

1. With the history of pituitary surgery, it is likely that the patient has central diabetes insipidus, since antidiuretic hormone (vasopressin) is produced by the hypothalamus and stored in the pituitary. Either the adenoma has recurred (if there was only a partial hypophysectomy), or the patient has stopped taking her replacement vasopressin (if there was a complete hypophysectomy)

2. A urine osmolality and specific gravity should be ordered. Both would be low if the patient has central diabetes insipidus. Vasopressin should be administered, and the serum and urine tests should be repeated. They should return to normal with vasopressin.

8.13.9.3 Case 3 answers

1. Given the odor of alcohol on the breath, the osmolality elevation is likely due to ethanol ingestion

2. A serum or plasma ethanol should be ordered

3. Osmolal gap = measured osmolality – calculated osmolality = measured osmolality – 2(Na$^+$) + (glucose/18) + (urea-N/2.8) = 360-2(137) + (90/18) + (14/2.8) = 360-284 = 76

4. Ethanol is an osmotically active compound; every 4.6 mg/dL of ethanol contributes 1 mOsm/kg; thus the expected serum ethanol concentration would be (4.6 mg/dL) × 76 = 350 mg/dL

8.13.9.4 Case 4 answers

1. As the pH is slightly low, this is acidosis; since the patient has been on a ventilator and thus breathing has been impaired, this is respiratory acidosis (chronic), which is further evidenced by the increased pCO_2 and the decreased pO_2

2. The likely cause is damage to the central nervous system and spinal cord; alternatively, he may have been placed into induced coma

3. For chronic respiratory acidosis, compensation is achieved by the kidneys. For every 10 mmHg increase in pCO_2 above the normal level of 40, the HCO_3^- increases by 3.5 mMol/L (mEq/L) as the kidneys eliminate H^+ by exchanging it for Na^+, forming hydrogen phosphate, forming ammonium ion, and reclaiming bicarbonate. Since there are 3 increments of 10 mmHg increase in the pCO_2, there would be an increase of 3×3.5, or 10.5 mMol/L (mEq/L) in HCO_3^- above the normal of 24, yielding $24 + 10.5 = 34.5$ mMol/L (mEq/L) HCO_3^-. Since the measured HCO_3^- is 35 mMol/L (mEq/L), full renal compensation has occurred.

4. The serum chloride is decreased in order to preserve electroneutrality

8.13.9.5 Case 5 answers

1. As the pH is low, this is acidosis; since her primary imbalance is a low bicarbonate, this is metabolic acidosis

2. Massive diarrhea with loss of bicarbonate

3. For metabolic acidosis, compensation is achieved by the lungs (hyperventilation). With full compensation, $pCO_2 = 1.5 (HCO_3^-) + 8 (\pm 2) = 1.5 (6) + 8 (\pm 2) = 17 \pm 2 = 15\text{-}19$. The observed pCO_2 is 18 mmHg, demonstrating full compensation. This is also consistent with the patient's rapid and deep respirations.

4. Due to the profound diarrhea, the patient is dehydrated, leading to increased pulse rate and low blood pressure; the dehydration is further evidenced by the poor skin turgor and soft and sunken eyes

5. Potassium has been lost in the diarrhea; also, due to the decreased renal blood flow from the dehydration, the juxtaglomerular cells secrete renin, stimulating aldosterone secretion and leading to urinary potassium loss

6. In metabolic acidosis, potassium is shifted from the red cell into the serum/plasma

7. The serum chloride is increased in order to preserve electroneutrality

8.13.9.6 Case 6 answers

1. As the pH is low, this is acidosis; since the primary imbalance is a low bicarbonate, this is metabolic acidosis

2. Diabetic ketoacidosis resulting from oxidation of free fatty acids due to insulin deficiency

3. For metabolic acidosis, compensation is achieved by the lungs (hyperventilation). With full compensation, $pCO_2 = 1.5 (HCO_3^-) + 8 (\pm2) = 1.5 (4) + 8 (\pm2) = 14\pm2 = 12\text{-}16$. The observed pCO_2 is 15 mmHg, demonstrating full compensation. This is also consistent with the patient's rapid and deep respirations.

4. The potassium is elevated due to shift from the red cells in acidosis; also, in diabetic ketoacidosis, potassium urinary excretion may be decreased

5. The sodium is decreased due to dilutional hyponatremia caused by the osmotic effect of glucose. For every 100 mg/dL increase in glucose >100 mg/dL, there is a 1.6-2.4 mMol/L (mEq/L) decrease in sodium as the extracellular fluid is diluted. In this case, 1,200/100 = 12 (11 increments of 100 mg/dL >100); 11 × (1.6-2.4) = 17.6-26.4. Thus the corrected sodium would be in the range 138-147 mMol/L (mEq/L).

6. Anion gap = $(Na^+ + K^+) - (HCO_3^- + Cl^-) = (121 + 6.4) - (4 + 95) = 26$ (elevated due to the presence of ketoacids)

7. The patient is dehydrated due to the osmotic diuresis stimulated by the hyperglycemia, resulting in decreased blood pressure and increased pulse rate

8. The serum urea-N and serum creatinine are increased due to dehydration, causing decreased glomerular filtration rate

9. The SUN:CR is elevated due to decreased glomerular filtration rate from dehydration, allowing for more passive reabsorption of urea-N (prerenal azotemia)

8.13.9.7 Case 7 answers

1. As the pH is high, this is alkalosis; since the pCO_2 is low, this imbalance is respiratory alkalosis

2. The massive ascites prevents the patient from mobilizing his diaphragms, thereby causing hyperventilation, as evidenced by the rapid, shallow respirations

3. For chronic respiratory alkalosis, compensation is achieved by the kidneys. With full compensation, for every decrease in pCO_2 of 10 mmHg <40, the HCO_3^- decreases by 5 mMol/L (mEq/L) as the kidneys retain H^+ by reducing exchange of Na^+ for H^+, forming less hydrogen phosphate, forming less ammonium ion, and reclaiming less bicarbonate. In this case, the pCO_2 is 30 mmHg <40 (3 increments of 10) so that (3 × 5) = a 15 mMol/L (mEq/L) reduction in bicarbonate below the normal of 24 = 24 −15 = 9 mMol/L (mEq/L). Since the observed bicarbonate is 9, there is full compensation.

4. The serum calcium is low because serum albumin (to which it is bound) is low

5. The serum albumin is low due to hepatic cirrhosis, as evidenced by the massive ascites

6. The serum potassium is low due to malnutrition (commonly seen in alcoholics) plus secondary hyperaldosteronism due to the ascites (low albumin results in decreased oncotic pressure, which, when coupled with portal hypertension from the cirrhosis, leads to ascites). The juxtaglomerular cells respond to decreased renal blood flow and secrete renin, leading to stimulation of aldosterone secretion. Aldosterone results in loss of potassium into the urine and retention of sodium and water.

7. The serum sodium is low due to dilutional hyponatremia from secondary hyperaldosteronism (see answer to previous question) as well as secretion of ADH, although the total body sodium is high

8. The blood pressure is high due to retention of water with sodium (secondary hyperaldosteronism)

8.13.9.8 Case 8 answers

1. As the pH is high, this is alkalosis; since the bicarbonate is high, this is metabolic alkalosis

2. Intractable vomiting causing loss of acid

3. In metabolic alkalosis compensation is via hypoventilation. For every increase in bicarbonate of 10 mMol/L (mEq/L) above the normal of 24, the pCO_2 increases by 6 mmHg. In this case the bicarbonate is 44 (2 increments of increase of 10 mMol/L each). Thus $(2 \times 6) = 12$ mmHg increase in pCO_2 above the normal level of 40 = 52 mmHg (matching the observed value). Thus, compensation has been achieved. This is consistent with the observed decreased rate and depth of respirations.

4. The serum potassium is low due to loss with vomiting; also, due to dehydration, the juxtaglomerular cells respond to decreased renal blood flow by secreting renin, stimulating aldosterone which causes urinary loss of potassium

5. The blood pressure is low due to dehydration

6. The chloride is decreased due to loss in the vomitus; also, it is decreased in order to preserve electroneutrality

chapter 9

The laboratory diagnosis of calcium, phosphorus & magnesium disorders

9.1 **Objectives**

At the end of this session, the learner should be able to

➤ discuss the percentage of calcium present in bone and the serum fractions of calcium that are free, bound, and complexed with anions

➤ describe the correction of serum calcium concentration for abnormal serum albumin concentrations

➤ discuss the interaction between parathyroid hormone (PTH) and calcium

➤ discuss the interaction between PTH and phosphate

➤ describe the forms of vitamin D

➤ describe the conversion of vitamin D to its hormonally active form

➤ describe the role of 1,25-dihydroxyvitamin D in calcium homeostasis

➤ discuss the assessment of vitamin D stores

➤ describe causes of hypocalcemia

➤ discuss primary hypoparathyroidism and its associated laboratory findings

➤ describe pseudohypoparathyroidism and pseudohypohyperparathyroidism, and their associated laboratory findings

➤ list etiologies of calcium deficiency as a cause of hypocalcemia

➤ describe causes of hypercalcemia

➤ discuss primary, secondary, and tertiary hyperparathyroidism, and their associated laboratory findings

➤ describe mechanisms for the hypercalcemia of malignancy

➤ describe the mechanism for hypercalcemia in hypothyroidism and in hyperthyroidism

➤ describe the mechanism for hypercalcemia in granulomatous diseases

➤ discuss the percentage of phosphorus present in bone and the serum fractions of phosphate that are free, bound, and complexed with cations

➤ discuss causes of hypophosphatemia

➤ discuss causes of hyperphosphatemia

➤ discuss the percentage of magnesium present in bone and the serum fractions of magnesium that are free, bound, and complexed with anions

➤ discuss causes of hypomagnesemia

➤ discuss causes of hypermagnesemia

9.2 **Key terms**

calcidiol: 25-hydroxyvitamin D_3, inactive prehormone produced by the monohydroxylation of vitamin D_3 in the liver

calcitonin: a hormone synthesized by the C cells of the thyroid gland in response to an inceased ionized calcium concentration

calcitriol: 1,25-dihydroxyvitamin D_3, the active hormone produced by a second hydroxylation of calcidiol in the kidney

eclampsia: a potentially life threatening disorder of pregnancy in which there is profound hypertension, proteinuria, and seizures

familial hypocalciuric hypercalcemia: an autosomal dominant cause of mild hypercalcemia resulting from a loss of function mutation in the calcium receptors on the parathyroid gland chief cells and on the renal tubular cells

Fanconi syndrome: a congenital defect involving the kidney tubules, characterized by loss of phosphate, amino acids, uric acid, glucose, and bicarbonate into the urine

fibroblast growth factor 23 (FGF23): a key modulator of phosphate homeostasis, increasing the fractional excretion of phosphate by the kidney and inhibiting the production of 1,25-dihydroxyvitamin D

hypoparathyroidism: a disorder in which the parathyroid glands do not produce enough parathyroid hormone, resulting in elevated serum phosphate and decreased serum calcium

milk alkali syndrome: an acquired condition in which there is hypercalcemia with associated metabolic alkalosis, caused by ingestion of excess calcium and base (eg, milk and antacids)

multiple endocrine neoplasia (MEN) 1 & 2: syndromes featuring 2 or more tumors of the endocrine glands (eg, pancreas, pituitary, parathyroid: MEN1; thyroid and pheochromocytoma: MEN2)

nephrolithiasis: the formation of kidney stones

osteoclasts: cells that resorb bone

parathyroid hormone (PTH): the hormone (parathormone) secreted by the chief cells of the parathyroid glands, stimulating renal tubular reabsorption of calcium and renal excretion of phosphate, calcium resorption from bone, and intestinal absorption of calcium and phosphate

pre-eclampsia: a potentially life threatening disorder of pregnancy characterized by hypertension and proteinuria, but not seizures (which occur in eclampsia)

primary hyperaldosteronism: a condition caused by elaboration of aldosterone by an adrenal tumor, an adrenal adenoma, or bilateral adrenal hyperplasia

primary hyperparathyroidism: the overproduction of parathyroid hormone due to an adenoma, carcinoma, or hyperplasia of the parathyroid glands, causing increased serum calcium and decreased serum phosphate

primary hypoparathyroidism: the underproduction of parathyroid hormone due to autoimmune destruction of the glands, congenital defect of the glands, irradiation, or surgical removal

pseudohypoparathyroidism: a genetic disorder in which there is resistance to the effects of parathyroid hormone, resulting in low serum calcium, high serum phosphate, and high parathyroid hormone

pseudohypohyperparathyroidism: a genetic disorder in which there is renal resistance but not bone resistance to the effects of parathyroid hormone

PTH related protein (PTHrP): protein produced by certain malignancies and having an effect similar to that of parathyroid hormone

rhabdomyolysis: the breakdown of muscle

secondary hyperparathyroidism: a condition characterized by excessive production of parathyroid hormone in response to hypocalcemia, leading to stimulation of the parathyroid glands

tertiary hyperparathyroidism: a condition characterized by autonomous production of parathyroid hormone by hypertrophic parathyroid glands after prolonged secondary hyperparathyroidism

vitamin D_2: ergocalciferol, present in food and plants

vitamin D_3: cholecalciferol, synthesized by the skin in response to ultraviolet B light; this is the predominant form of endogenous vitamin D in humans

9.3 Background/significance

Disorders of mineral metabolism (calcium, phosphorus, and magnesium) are common. Normal homeostatic regulatory mechanisms target 3 organ systems (intestines, kidneys, and bone) in the maintenance of serum, intracellular, and bone mineral content. **Parathyroid hormone** (PTH), 1,25-dihydroxyvitamin D_3 (**calcitriol**), and **calcitonin** are important in maintaining homeostasis.

9.4 Calcium
9.4.1 Calcium homeostasis

Calcium plays the major role in formation of bone. It is also important in blood coagulation, neuromuscular function, and intracellular signaling. Most calcium (99%) is contained in bone. The serum calcium is ~50% ionized ("free" or "active"), 40% bound to albumin, and 10% complexed to other anions. The "total" calcium is the sum of these 3. Total serum calcium is affected by the serum albumin concentration. For every 1 g/dL of serum albumin, 0.8 mg/dL of calcium is bound. Thus, when there are abnormalities of the serum albumin concentration, either ionized calcium should be measured or total calcium should be adjusted as follows:

Corrected total calcium = measured total calcium (mg/dL) + 0.8 (4.0 – X)

where X = measured serum albumin concentration (g/dL) and 4.0 is a normal serum albumin concentration. It should be noted that this corrected calcium is an estimate and direct measurements of ionized calcium are more precise. Calcium is bound to the negatively charged sites on albumin. Since alkalosis increases the negative charge (and thus increases binding of calcium), it follows that alkalosis will decrease the ionized calcium. Conversely, acidosis decreases the negative charge (and thus decreases binding of calcium) so that the ionized calcium is increased. For every 0.1 unit change in systemic pH, the ionized calcium changes by 0.2 mg/dL (0.1 mEq/L) [ISBN9781416061649].

The 4 parathyroid glands respond to ionized calcium through their calcium sensing receptors. A decrease in ionized calcium stimulates PTH secretion by the chief cells of the glands, while an increase in ionized calcium suppresses PTH secretion. The PTH stimulates the renal tubular cells to increase calcium absorption and decrease phosphate reabsorption (ie, to increase phosphate excretion), and it also stimulates the **osteoclasts** to release calcium from bone. Additionally, it induces the renal conversion of 25-hydroxyvitamin D_2 and D_3 (**calcidiol**) to their active 1,25-dihydroxyvitamin D_2 and D_3 (**calcitriol**) forms, which then stimulate the intestinal reabsorption of calcium and phosphate (as well as their release from bone), and the renal tubular reabsorption of calcium. However, the phosphaturic effect of PTH predominates over the phosphate resorption from bone. Thus, PTH causes an increase in serum calcium and a decrease in serum phosphate. Because the intact (84 amino acid) PTH molecule is metabolized shortly after secretion, many fragments are in the blood, and many immunoassays exist for the different forms (eg, intact PTH, N terminal PTH, C terminal PTH). The intact PTH is one of the most widely used, however [ISBN9780683300857, ISBN9781416061649, ISBN9781594251023].

Vitamin D is important in calcium and phosphorus homeostasis. There are 2 forms of vitamin D: **vitamin D$_2$** (ergocalciferol), found in the diet (a relatively minor component of total vitamin D), and **vitamin D$_3$** (cholecalciferol), produced in the skin after ultraviolet B exposure (major component). Both vitamins D_2 and D_3 are hydroxylated in the liver to produce their respective inactive 25-hydroxyvitamin D analogs (calcidiol). As noted above, PTH then stimulates the renal hydroxylation of the 25-hydroxyvitamin D analogs to form the respective biologically active 1,25-dihydroxyvitamin D analogs. Also as noted above, the 1,25-dihydroxyvitamin D stimulates calcium and phosphate absorption in the intestine as well as renal tubular reabsorption of calcium, and it enhances PTH induced bone resorption of calcium and phosphate [ISBN9780683300857].

The assessment of vitamin D stores is based on measurement of total 25-hydroxyvitamin D. This generally includes the sum of the concentrations of 25-hydroxyvitamin D_2 and 25-hydroxyvitamin D_3. Not all assays for total 25-hydroxyvitamin D are equivalent, since immunoassays do not always have the same cross reactivity to 25-hydroxyvitamin D_2 and 25-hydroxyvitamin D_3. Properly validated mass spectrometry based methods do not suffer from this problem. Measurement of 1,25-dihydroxyvitamin D (calcitriol) is inappropriate for assessing vitamin D stores because its formation is regulated by PTH and phosphate [ISBN9780683300857, ISBN9781594251023]. In addition, the serum half-life of 25-hydroxyvitamin D is much longer than that of 1,25-dihydroxyvitamin D; thus, 25-hydroxyvitamin D provides a better indication of vitamin D status than does 1,25-dihydroxyvitamin D. Due to the rapid fluctuation of 1,25-dihydroxyvitamin D, patients can have a low 1,25-dihydroxyvitamin D concentration but be vitamin D sufficient. Assessment of 1,25-dihydroxyvitamin D is only indicated in the setting of renal disease, some malignancies, and unexplained hypercalcemia.

With large increases (>10%) in serum ionized calcium, **calcitonin**, which is a hormone synthesized and secreted by the C cells of the thyroid gland, reduces calcium by inhibiting osteoclastic activity as well as the effects of both PTH and vitamin D [ISBN9780683300857].

9.4.1.1 Reference ranges

Serum total calcium: 8.6-10.4 mg/dL (4.3-5.2 mEq/L)
Serum ionized calcium: 4.5-5.3 mg/dL (2.25-2.65 mEq/L)
Serum intact PTH: 15-65 pg/mL
Serum 25-hydroxyvitamin D (calcidiol): 30-80 ng/mL (measured by mass spectrometry)
    (It should be noted that there is an active debate on what constitutes an adequate amount of 25-hydroxyvitamin D.)

9.4.2 **Hypocalcemia**

Hypocalcemia lowers the threshold for depolarization of the sodium channel. This leads to hyperreflexia, seizures, cramps, tetany, paresthesias, and cardiac conduction defects [ISBN9781594251023].

Chronic renal failure causes retention of phosphate by the kidney, loss of albumin into the urine, decreased conversion of 25-hydroxyvitamin D to 1,25-dihydroxyvitamin D in the kidney, and skeletal resistance to PTH, all leading to hypocalcemia [ISBN9781416061649]. In this disorder, serum calcium is low, serum phosphate is elevated, and serum PTH is high.

Primary hypoparathyroidism is caused by neck surgery (eg, parathyroid gland destruction during thyroidectomy), autoimmune destruction of the parathyroid glands, irradiation of the neck, and genetic disorders (eg, DiGeorge syndrome, idiopathic hypoparathyroidism) [ISBN9781594251023]. The serum calcium is low, the serum phosphate is elevated, and the serum PTH is low in this disorder.

In **pseudohypoparathyroidism**, there is inherited resistance to the effects of PTH. This disorder has several variants. The serum calcium is low, the serum phosphate is elevated, and the PTH is elevated as the parathyroid gland attempts to overcome resistance [ISBN9781594251023].

In **pseudohypohyperparathyroidism**, there is renal resistance to the effects of PTH but no bone resistance. This causes a low serum calcium, an elevated serum phosphate, and an increased serum PTH. Because of bone sensitivity to PTH, bone resorption occurs [ISBN9781594251023].

Vitamin D deficiency can be caused by lack of the vitamin in diet, lack of adequate exposure to sunlight, malabsorption (eg, due to pancreatic or intestinal disease), and/or deficient conversion of 25-hydroxyvitamin D to 1,25-hydroxyvitamin D due to an autosomal recessive defect. Deficient vitamin D activity results in decreased intestinal absorption of both calcium and phosphate, decreased bone resorption of calcium and phosphate, and decreased renal tubular reabsorption of calcium. The serum calcium is normal to low, the serum phosphate is low, and the PTH is elevated [ISBN9780683300857, ISBN9781594251023].

Secondary hyperparathyroidism is a consequence of longstanding hypocalcemia, often due to chronic renal failure, in which there is phosphate retention leading to deposition of calcium phosphate in tissues. The hyperphosphatemia impairs the renal enzymatic conversion of 25-hydroxyvitamin D to 1,25-dihydroxyvitamin D. The serum calcium is low, phosphate high, and PTH high [ISBN9781594251023].

Calcium deficiency is yet another cause of hypocalcemia. It can be caused by the rapid removal of calcium by healing bone (the so called "hungry bone" syndrome), certain drugs (eg, bisphosphonates used in treatment of osteoporosis because they inhibit osteoclastic activity), intestinal malabsorption (may be related to malabsorption of vitamin D and calcium), hemorrhagic pancreatitis (due to calcium binding by released free fatty acids), and dietary deficiency of calcium (rare). These conditions cause a low serum calcium and an elevated serum PTH [PMID10818080, ISBN9780683300857, ISBN9781594251023]. It appears that the serum phosphate can be variable depending on the magnitude of the calcium deficiency and its effect on PTH secretion.

Massive blood transfusion can cause acute depression of the serum calcium due to binding of calcium by citrate in the blood product [ISBN9781416061649].

 ISBN 978-089189-6548

9.4.3 Hypercalcemia

Hypercalcemia can cause **nephrolithiasis**, corneal calcification, constipation, polyuria, nausea, vomiting, lethargy, and calcification of blood vessels [ISBN9780071824866]. The most common causes of hypercalcemia are described below.

Primary hyperparathyroidism is the most common cause of hypercalcemia. Patients with primary hyperparathyroidism often present with "moans" (central nervous system complaints of depression, weakness, apathy), "bones" (bone pain), "groans" (gastrointestinal tract disturbances), and "stones" (kidney stones). The condition is caused by a solitary parathyroid adenoma (80%-85% of cases), hyperplasia of all 4 parathyroid glands (15%), and parathyroid carcinoma (<1% of cases). In this condition the serum calcium is elevated, the serum phosphate is low, and the serum PTH is increased [ISBN9781416061649].

Tertiary hyperparathyroidism results from longstanding secondary hyperparathyroidism, which causes the parathyroid glands to be sufficiently chronically stimulated to become hyperplastic and secrete PTH autonomously [ISBN9781594251023]. The serum calcium is elevated, the serum phosphate is low, and the PTH is elevated.

Malignancy is the second most common cause of persistent hypercalcemia. One mechanism is the secretion of **PTH related proteins (PTHrPs)** that have action similar to PTH. These proteins are not detected by the PTH assay, so they require a separate assay. The second mechanism is local bone destruction by tumor metastases. Finally, certain lymphomas can stimulate conversion of 25-hydroxyvitamin D to 1,25-dihydroxyvitamin D, thereby increasing intestinal calcium absorption and bone resorption [ISBN9781594251023]. The serum phosphate and the serum PTH are normal to low due to the PTHrP.

Hypothyroidism decreases the metabolism of 1,25-dihydroxyvitamin D, thereby prolonging its half-life and causing hypercalcemia. Hyperthyroidism causes increased bone turnover, with bone loss leading to hypercalcemia [ISBN9781594251023].

In most granulomatous diseases (eg, sarcoidosis, histoplasmosis, leprosy, cryptococcosis), the macrophages acquire the ability to convert 25-hydroxyvitamin D to 1,25-dihydroxyvitamin D, thereby leading to hypercalcemia [ISBN9781594251023].

Obviously, vitamin D ingestion in excess can lead to hypercalcemia through mechanisms described previously. Vitamin A in high doses causes bone resorption. Thiazide diuretics increase tubular reabsorption of calcium. The ingestion of large amounts of calcium together with alkali (**milk alkali syndrome**) leads to increased calcium absorption and metabolic alkalosis, while chronic lithium therapy raises the parathyroid gland set point for negative feedback by calcium, thereby causing hypercalcemia [ISBN9781594251023].

Prolonged immobilization (especially in growing teenagers) increases the calcium as it is released from bone [ISBN9781594251023].

Familial causes of hypercalcemia include **familial hypocalciuric hypercalcemia**, an autosomal dominant form of mild chronic hypercalcemia resulting from a loss of function mutation in the calcium receptors of the parathyroid gland chief cells and the renal tubular cells. This causes mild hypersecretion of PTH relative to the calcium concentration. The serum phosphate concentration is usually normal, and the urine calcium concentration is not increased because the renal tubules perceive a state of calcium deficiency in this condition. **Multiple**

endocrine neoplasia (MEN) 1 and 2 usually involves 2 or more tumors of the endocrine glands. MEN1 usually involves tumors of pituitary, parathyroid, and pancreas, while MEN2 often involves medullary carcinoma of the thyroid gland and pheochromocytoma [ISBN9781594251023].

9.5 Phosphorus
9.5.1 Phosphorus homeostasis

Phosphorus (P), which exists primarily as phosphate (PO_4) at physiological pH, is important in energy metabolism, cell signaling, bone formation, and maintenance of acid-base balance. While blood contains both organic and inorganic phosphate, only the inorganic phosphate is measured. Most of the phosphate resides in bone (85%). Of the total serum phosphate, 55% is ionized ("free" or "active" phosphate), 10% is protein bound, and 35% is complexed with sodium, calcium, and magnesium [ISBN9781416061649].

Phosphate is considered to be the "servant" of calcium in that the body primarily regulates calcium, with phosphate responding to that. As noted above, PTH decreases the renal tubular reabsorption of phosphate (ie, increases phosphate excretion) while 1,25-dihydroxyvitamin D increases the gastrointestinal absorption of phosphate.

Fibroblast growth factor 23 (FGF23) is a key modulator of phosphate homeostasis. It increases the fractional excretion of phosphate by the kidney and inhibits the enzymatic production of 1,25-dihydroxyvitamin D, both of which decrease the serum phosphate concentration. It is secreted by bone cells in response to increased serum phosphate and increased 1,25-dihydroxyvitamin D [ISBN9781416061649].

9.5.1.1 Reference range
Serum phosphate: 2.7-4.5 mg/dL (adults) and 4.0-7.0 mg/dL (children; higher due to increased growth hormone activity)

9.5.2 Hypophosphatemia

The symptoms of hypophosphatemia can include muscle pain, paresthesias, cardiac arrhythmias, diaphragmatic weakness, and hemolytic anemia (increased red cell fragility) [ISBN9780071824866]. Hypophosphatemia can be caused by inadequate dietary intake of phosphorus, vitamin D deficiency (leading to inadequate intestinal reabsorption of phosphate), phosphate redistribution into cells (eg, acute respiratory alkalosis, insulin administration, healing bone), renal loss (eg, hyperparathyroidism, renal tubular defects such as **Fanconi syndrome**), and gastrointestinal loss (eg, vomiting, diarrhea, use of phosphate binding antacids, intestinal malabsorption) [ISBN9781416061649, ISBN9781594251023].

9.5.3 Hyperphosphatemia

The symptoms of hyperphosphatemia are largely those of the underlying cause [ISBN9780071824866]. Hyperphosphatemia can be caused by increased phosphate intake (eg, ingestion of phosphate salts, transfusion of outdated blood), excessive vitamin D ingestion, milk alkali syndrome (see above), decreased renal clearance of phosphate (eg, renal failure, hypoparathyroidism, pseudohypo-parathyroidism), acromegaly (growth hormone increases tubular reabsorption of phosphate), prolonged immobilization (release of phosphate from bone), thyrotoxicosis (release from bone), and increased cellular release of phosphate (eg, tumor lysis, metabolic acidosis, **rhabdomyolysis**, infection, hemolysis) [ISBN9781594251023].

9.6 Magnesium
9.6.1 Magnesium homeostasis
Magnesium is a cofactor for >300 enzymes in the body. Unlike calcium and phosphate, however, no primary hormone regulates serum magnesium. Of the total magnesium, 55% resides in bone. Of the serum magnesium, 55% is ionized ("free" or "active"), 30% is protein bound (mostly albumin), and 15% is complexed with phosphate, citrate, and other anions [ISBN9781416061649, ISBN9781594251023].

9.6.1.1 Reference range
Serum magnesium: 1.6-2.6 mg/dL

9.6.2 Hypomagnesemia
Hypomagnesemia can be characterized by hypertension, tachycardia, ventricular arrhythmias, muscle weakness, and cramps [ISBN9780071824866]. Hypomagnesemia can result from malabsorption, malnutrition, vomiting, nasogastric suction, diarrhea, renal magnesium wasting from drugs (eg, thiazide diuretics), endocrine disorders (eg, **primary hyperaldosteronism**, which causes volume expansion with decreased renal tubular reabsorption of magnesium; hyperthyroidism, which causes increased renal excretion of magnesium), alcohol use (due to poor nutrition and alcohol induced impairment of magnesium renal tubular reabsorption), use of proton pump inhibitors (presumably due to intestinal losses), and osmotic diuresis [PMID18235082, PMID22762246, ISBN9781416061649, ISBN9781594251023].

9.6.3 Hypermagnesemia
The symptoms of hypermagnesemia can include mental obtundation, muscle weakness, decreased deep tendon reflexes, hypotension, and urinary retention [ISBN9780071824866]. The most common cause is iatrogenic (administration of magnesium sulfate in the treatment of **pre-eclampsia** and **eclampsia**). Other causes include excessive intake (usually in the presence of chronic renal failure), milk alkali syndrome, rhabdomyolysis, and tumor lysis [ISBN9781594251023].

9.7 References
9.7.1 Journals
PMID10818080 Jorde R, Sundsfjord J, Haug E et al [2000] Relation between low calcium intake, parathyroid hormone, and blood pressure. *Hypertension* 35:1154-59

PMID18235082 Martin KJ, Gonzalez EA, Slatopolsky E [2009] Clinical consequences and management of hypomagnesemia. *J Am Soc Nephrol* 20:2291-95

PMID22762246 Hess MW, Hoenderop JGJ, Bindels RJM et al [2012] Systematic review: hypomagnesaemia induced by proton pump inhibition. *Aliment Pharmacol Ther* 36:405-13

9.7.2 Books

ISBN9780071824866 Cho KC [2014] Electrolyte & acid-base disorders. In: Papadakis MA, McPhee SJ, Rabow MW, ed. *Current Medical Diagnosis & Treatment*, 53e. McGraw Hill Education, 837-864.

ISBN9780683300857 Toffaletti JG [2002] Calcium, magnesium, and phosphate. In: Lewandrowski K, ed. *Clinical Chemistry: Laboratory Management & Clinical Correlations*. Lippincott Williams & Wilkins, 710-724.

ISBN9781416061649 Risteli J, Winter WE, Kleerekoper M et al [2013] Bone and mineral metabolism. In: Burtis CA, Ashwood ER, Bruns DE, ed. *Tietz Textbook of Clinical Chemistry and Molecular Diagnostics*, 5e. Elsevier Saunders, 1733-1802.

ISBN9781594251023 Winter WE, Harris NS [2011] Calcium biology and disorders. In: Clarke W, ed. *Contemporary Practice in Clinical Chemistry*, 2e. A Press, 505-24

9.8 Clinical Cases

9.8.1 Case 1

A 47-year-old female visits her primary care physician with the chief complaints of numbness, "tingling," and occasional cramps in her extremities. The neuromuscular examination reveals profound hyperreflexia. The astute clinician orders a series of clinical chemistry tests and notes a serum total calcium of 7.2 mg/dL with an ionized calcium of 3.6 mg/dL and a serum phosphate of 6.2 mg/dL. He orders subsequent testing.

9.8.1.1 Questions

1. What is the likely etiology if the serum intact PTH is very low?

2. What is the likely etiology if the serum intact PTH is very high, and what additional tests might be helpful in establishing the diagnosis?

3. What is the likely etiology if the serum phosphate is 1.0 mg/dL?

9.8.2 Case 2

A 72-year-old female visits her primary care physician with complaints of a lump in her right breast that she has had for 4 months. She also complains of severe back pain. Laboratory studies obtained by the physician show a serum total calcium of 12.8 mg/dL with an ionized calcium of 6.5 mg/dL and a serum phosphate of 1.7 mg/dL.

9.8.2.1 Questions

1. What is the most likely explanation for these findings?

2. What additional studies should be ordered?

9.8.3 Clinical case answers

9.8.3.1 Case 1 answers

1. A low serum intact PTH would suggest primary hypoparathyroidism

2. An elevated serum intact PTH would suggest pseudohypoparathyroidism (renal and bone resistance to PTH effects) or pseudohypohyperparathyroidism (renal resistance but not bone resistance to PTH effects), and could also suggest chronic renal failure with retention of phosphate, decreased conversion of 25-hydroxyvitamin D to 1,25-dihydroxyvitamin D, and skeletal resistance to the effects of PTH; thus a serum urea-N, serum creatinine, urine protein, and urinalysis should be obtained

3. A low serum phosphate with a low serum calcium would suggest severe vitamin D deficiency; the serum PTH would be elevated

9.8.3.2 Case 2 answers

1. The patient may have metastatic breast carcinoma with elaboration of PTH related proteins

2. Additional studies should include testing for PTHrP and serum intact PTH. The former would be positive, and the latter would be normal to low. Imaging studies should be performed to look for metastases, especially to bone. A biopsy of the breast lesion is essential to establish the diagnosis.

chapter 10

The laboratory diagnosis of iron disorders

10.1 Objectives

By the end of this session, the learner should be able to

➤ describe the distribution of iron in the body

➤ discuss the role of hepcidin and ferroportin in iron homeostasis

➤ discuss the mechanisms for "anemia of chronic disease," "anemia of inflammation," and anemia secondary to bacterial infection

➤ discuss the causes of hereditary hemochromatosis

➤ discuss the transport of iron in blood

➤ discuss the causes of a decreased and an increased serum iron

➤ discuss the causes of a decreased and an increased serum total iron binding capacity

➤ discuss the causes of a decreased and an increased percent saturation of transferrin

➤ discuss the causes of a decreased and an increased serum ferritin

10.2 Key terms

apotransferrin: a β globulin that has 2 unoccupied iron binding sites per molecule

apoferritin: an analog of ferritin that complexes with iron, forming ferritin

ferritin: the iron-apoferritin complex, one of the chief storage forms of iron in the body

ferroportin: the hepcidin receptor, a cellular iron exporter

hemochromatosis: a disorder caused by the deposition of hemosiderin in the parenchymal cells, causing tissue damage and dysfunction of liver, pancreas, pituitary, and heart

hemosiderin: an intracellular storage form of iron, consisting of ferritin, denatured ferritin, and other materials

hepcidin: the iron regulatory protein produced in the liver

transferrin: a β globulin that transports iron in the blood; it is the apotransferrin-iron complex

10.3 Background/significance

Iron deficiency anemia is prevalent in 2% of adult men, 9%-12% of non-Hispanic white women, and nearly 20% of black and Mexican-American women [PMID17375513]. In fact, iron deficiency is considered to be the leading single nutritional deficiency in the world [PMID19242589]. In adults it is most usually caused by chronic blood loss, while in children it is mostly due to dietary deficiency. Coupled with the fact that hereditary iron overload is the most common autosomal recessive disorder in Caucasians, affecting 1 in every 200-400 people [PMID16493621], an understanding of iron disorders is important.

10.4 Iron homeostasis

Of the total body iron, 67% (2 g) resides in hemoglobin. The liver stores 0.5-1.0 g of iron, and every 1 mL of blood contains 1 mg of iron. In the US, the average daily diet contains ~10-15 mg of iron, mostly in the form of hemoglobin and myoglobin ingested in meat. Given its importance and the fact that there is no regulated pathway for iron excretion, it is tightly conserved in the body, with only ~0.1% of total body iron being lost per day. Iron normally leaves the body through menstruation in women, and through sloughing of epithelial cells from skin and from gastrointestinal, biliary, and urinary tract mucosa [PMID11252750, ISBN9781416061649].

Hepcidin, a 25 amino acid peptide hormone produced in the liver, is the major regulatory hormone in iron metabolism [PMID12663437]. Its receptor is **ferroportin**, which is present on the surfaces of cells responsible for gathering and recycling iron (ie, hepatocytes, macrophages, placenta, intestine). When hepcidin is bound to ferroportin, the ferroportin is internalized and degraded, leading to decreased extracellular export of cellular iron. Iron regulates the secretion of hepcidin, which in turn controls the concentration of ferroportin on the cell surfaces [PMID15514116]. Hepcidin is feedback regulated by iron concentrations in the serum and the liver, and by the erythropoietic demand for iron [PMID21346250]. Thus, increased serum iron causes increased hepcidin, leading to decreased export of iron from cells, while decreased serum iron causes decreased hepcidin, leading to increased export of iron from cells.

Apotransferrin is a β globulin that transports iron in the blood. When iron is bound, the complex is known as **transferrin**. Iron is stored as **ferritin**, which is present in nearly all cells and acts as a reservoir of iron for formation of heme proteins [ISBN9781416061649].

10.4.1 Disorders of iron homeostasis

In the so called "anemia of chronic disease" and "anemia of inflammation," hepcidin is increased, leading to decreased export of iron from cells. Similarly, in anemia secondary to bacterial infection, the release of liposaccharides and cytokines stimulates hepcidin, leading to decreased iron export from cells [PMID21346250].

Hereditary hemochromatosis can be caused by 1) a mutation leading to decreased hepcidin and/or 2) by a mutation in ferroportin leading to resistance to hepcidin [PMID21346250]. Both lead to increased export of iron from the cell. Nonhereditary hemochromatosis can be caused by excessive administration of iron orally or massive blood transfusion.

10.4.1.1 Evaluation of iron disorders
10.4.1.1.1 Serum iron

Serum iron is the iron bound to transferrin. Thus it is decreased in iron deficiency, leading to iron deficiency anemia (eg, blood loss, celiac disease, increased demand for iron as in pregnancy), acute inflammation (since transferrin is a negative acute phase reactant), malignancies (presumably due to decreased transferrin synthesis), and chronic inflammation (due to stimulation of hepcidin production by cytokine release as well as decreased transferrin synthesis). It may also be low in the early stages of treatment for anemias because rapid synthesis of hemoglobin draws iron from serum and iron stores [ISBN9781416061649].

Serum iron is increased with use of oral contraceptives (presumably due to stimulation of transferrin synthesis), and in iron overload (eg, excessive iron ingestion, hereditary hemochromatosis) and hepatitis (due to increase in ferritin from hepatocyte injury) [ISBN9781416061649].

10.4.1.1.1.1 Reference range
Women: 37-145 µg/dL (bound to transferrin)
Men: 59-158 µg/dL (bound to transferrin)

10.4.1.1.2 Serum total iron binding capacity (TIBC)

The serum total iron binding capacity (TIBC) is a measurement of the maximum amount of iron that serum proteins (mainly transferrin) can bind. It represents the sum of the unsaturated iron binding capacity (UIBC; apotransferrin, which is transferrin able to bind iron) and the iron that is bound: TIBC = UIBC + iron (bound). Thus, UIBC = TIBC – iron (bound). The UIBC and iron (bound) can be measured directly while the TIBC is usually calculated [ISBN9781416061649].

The TIBC is decreased in acute inflammation (due to decreased transferrin concentration), iron overload (eg, excessive iron ingestion, hereditary hemochromatosis; due to transferrin iron binding sites already being saturated and due to decreased synthesis of transferrin), and chronic inflammation and malignancies (both presumably due to decreased synthesis of transferrin) [ISBN9781416061649].

The TIBC is increased in iron deficiency (due to unfilled iron binding sites) and with use of oral contraceptives (presumably due to increased transferrin synthesis) [ISBN9781416061649].

10.4.1.1.2.1 Reference range
TIBC (women & men) : 148-506 µg/dL
Transferrin (women & men) : 200-360 mg/dL

10.4.1.1.3 Percent saturation of transferrin

The percent saturation of transferrin is the amount of transferrin that has iron bound relative to the total amount of transferrin. It is decreased in iron deficiency (due to low amounts of iron bound). It is increased in iron overload (due to high amounts of iron bound) [ISBN9781416061649]. The percent saturation of transferrin is simply calculated as serum iron (µg/dL) divided by TIBC (µg/dL) multiplied by 100%.

10.4.1.1.3.1 Reference range
Women and men: 15%-50% of TIBC

10.4.1.1.4 Serum ferritin

Ferritin, the chief storage form of iron in the body, consists of an **apoferritin** protein shell around a core of iron and is present in nearly all cells. It provides a reserve of iron that can be used for heme protein production. The release of iron from ferritin is believed to be nonenzymatic [ISBN9781416061649].

Only a small amount of ferritin is present in serum, mostly as apoferritin. Serum ferritin is decreased in iron deficiency, with such decreases manifesting themselves even before decline of the serum iron. Serum ferritin is increased in iron overload, and it may be the first indicator of this condition, long before symptoms appear. Other conditions in which serum ferritin is increased include hepatitis (release from the inflamed liver), acute inflammation (ferritin is an acute phase reactant), and chronic inflammation and malignancies (both presumably due to decreased synthesis of transferrin, resulting in increases of free iron) [ISBN9780323036580].

10.4.1.1.4.1 Reference range
Women: 20-200 ng/mL
Men: 20-250 ng/mL

10.4.1.1.5 Tissue iron
Cytochemical staining of hemosiderin in bone marrow aspirates is a qualitative but definitive test of iron status. Quantitative measurement of iron in liver biopsies can also be helpful in the diagnosis of hemochromatosis.

10.5 References
10.5.1 Journals

PMID11252750 Andrews NC [2000] Iron homeostasis: insights from genetics and animal models. *Nat Rev Genet* 1:208-17

PMID12663437 Ganz T [2003] Hepcidin, a key regulator of iron metabolism and mediator of anemia of inflammation. *Blood* 102:783-8

PMID15514116 Nemeth E, Tuttle MS, Powelson J et al [2004] Hepcidin regulates cellular iron efflux by binding to ferroportin and inducing its internalization. *Science* 306:2090-3

PMID16493621 Franchini M [2006] Hereditary iron overload: update on pathophysiology, diagnosis, and treatment. *Am J Hematol* 81:202-9

PMID17375513 Killip S, Bennett JM, Chambers MD [2007] Iron deficiency anemia. *Am Fam Phys* 75:671-8

PMID19242589 Gautam CS, Saha L, Sekhri K et al [2008] Iron deficiency in pregnancy and the rationality of iron supplements prescribed during pregnancy. *Medscape J Med* 10:283

PMID21346250 Ganz T [2011] Hepcidin and iron regulation, 10 years later. *Blood* 117:4425-33

10.5.2 Books

ISBN9780323036580 Schreiber WE [2010] Iron and porphyrin metabolism. In: Kaplan LA, Pesce AJ, ed. *Clinical Chemistry: Theory, Analysis, Correlation*, 5e. Mosby, 761

ISBN9781416061649 Higgins T, Eckfeldt JH, Barton JC et al [2013] Hemoglobin, iron, and bilirubin. In: Burtis CA, Ashwood ER, Bruns DE, ed. *Tietz Textbook of Clinical Chemistry and Molecular Diagnostics*, 5e. Elsevier Saunders, 985-1030.

10.6 Clinical Cases

10.6.1 Case 1

A 56-year-old Caucasian male presented to his primary care physician with the chief complaint of increasing abdominal swelling of several months' duration. He denied ethanol usage. He looked tan, even though it was winter. His vital signs were normal. Physical examination revealed massive ascites with a fluid wave. The liver edge could not be palpated.

Laboratory studies showed a normal complete blood count and electrolytes, a marginally elevated serum bilirubin, and elevated alanine aminotransferase (ALT) and aspartate aminotransferase (AST). The serum iron was 316 µg/dL, transferrin 218 mg/dL, transferrin saturation 95%, and ferritin 2,542 ng/mL.

10.6.1.1 Questions

1. What is the likely diagnosis?

2. Why does the patient have ascites?

3. Why does the patient appear tan?

4. What would you expect the total iron binding capacity to be?

10.6.2 **Clinical case answers**

10.6.2.1 **Case 1 answers**

1. The patient likely has hemochromatosis (probably hereditary since he has no history of other causes of iron overload)

2. Iron deposition in the liver causes fibrosis and cirrhosis, leading to portal hypertension and decreased synthesis of albumin; the 2 together cause ascites

3. The hemosiderin produces a slate gray color, and bronzing results from increased melanin production; one theory is that iron deposition in the pituitary stimulates production of melanocyte stimulating hormone

4. Percent saturation of transferrin = 95% or 0.95 = iron/TIBC = 316/TIBC so that TIBC = 316/0.95 = 332 µg/dL (normal), which is consistent with the normal transferrin observed (218 mg/dL), suggesting that the iron overload has not yet suppressed transferrin synthesis

chapter 11

The laboratory diagnosis of pancreatic disease

11.1 Objectives

At the end of this session, the learner should be able to

➤ describe the nonspecific biochemical findings in serum from a patient with acute pancreatitis

➤ discuss the use of serum amylase in the workup of acute pancreatitis

➤ discuss the use of serum lipase in the workup of acute pancreatitis

➤ identify nonpancreatic conditions in which serum amylase may be elevated

➤ discuss the concept of macroamylasemia

➤ identify nonpancreatic conditions in which serum lipase may be elevated

➤ calculate and interpret the amylase:creatinine clearance ratio

11.2 Key terms

acute pancreatitis: inflammation of the pancreas causing diffuse enzymatic destruction

amylase: an enzyme that hydrolyzes polysaccharides into simple sugars

chronic pancreatitis: chronic inflammation of the pancreas, often irreversible

glucagon: a pancreatic hormone produced by the α cells of the islet of Langerhans that stimulates gluconeogenesis and glycogenolysis

insulin: a pancreatic hormone produced by the β cells of the islet of Langerhans that stimulates lowering of glucose

islet of Langerhans: clusters of α, β, and δ cells that provide the endocrine functions of the pancreas

lipase: a pancreatic enzyme that cleaves triglycerides sequentially into a monoglyceride and 2 fatty acids, and then into glycerol and an additional fatty acid

macroamylasemia: a benign condition characterized by hyperamylasemia due to amylase being complexed with immunoglobulins

saponification: the formation of insoluble soaps by reaction of a free fatty acid with a metal such as calcium

triglycerides: glycerol esters of long chain fatty acids

11.3 **Background/significance**

Symptoms of pancreatic insufficiency usually manifest only when 90% or more of the glandular function is lost. However, when pancreatic disorders occur, they can be extremely serious, with pancreatic cancer and **acute pancreatitis** having a high mortality, and **chronic pancreatitis** causing much suffering and morbidity. The financial cost for pancreatic disease has been estimated to be almost 10% of the total cost of diagnosing and treating common digestive diseases [PMID15802095]. Thus, understanding the laboratory workup of pancreatic disorders is important.

11.4 **Acute pancreatitis**

Acute pancreatitis is characterized by sudden onset of severe, steady pain that radiates into the back and is accompanied by nausea and vomiting. The abdomen may be distended, and bowel sounds may be absent. Most cases are related to biliary tract disease or heavy alcohol usage (alcohol is thought to be toxic to the pancreas), although other conditions (eg, hyperlipidemia and hypercalcemia) have been associated with it [ISBN9780071824866].

11.5 **Amylase**

Amylase is present in several organs and tissues. The greatest concentration is in the salivary glands, which secrete S type amylase to initiate the hydrolysis of starches in the mouth and esophagus. The P type amylase is produced by the pancreatic acinar cells and then secreted into the intestinal tract. Amylase activity is also found in semen, testes, ovaries, fallopian tubes, striated muscle, lungs, and adipose tissue. However, the enzyme normally found in serum and urine is of pancreatic and salivary origin [ISBN9781594251023].

When serum amylase activity rises to ≥3× the upper reference limit, it suggests acute pancreatitis. However, the degree of elevation does not correlate with the severity of the pancreatitis. Increase in serum amylase typically starts within a few hours after the onset of acute pancreatitis, and after 3-7 days the serum amylase decreases toward normal [ISBN9780071802154]. Being a relatively small molecule (molecular weight 45,000), amylase is readily cleared into the urine and into pleural and peritoneal effusions that may accompany pancreatitis. Thus, increases of amylase activity in serum are usually accompanied by increases in urine amylase activity when renal function is normal, and urine amylase activity can remain elevated for 7-10 days after the serum amylase has returned to normal [PMID13410166].

Extrapancreatic causes of elevated serum amylase activity include salivary gland lesions (eg, mumps, parotitis), perforated peptic ulcer (release of amylase containing gastric secretions into the peritoneum), intestinal obstruction, cholecystitis, ruptured ectopic pregnancy (fallopian tube amylase), mesenteric infarction, acute appendicitis, renal failure (impaired amylase clearance), ectopic production by tumors (rare), and diabetic ketoacidosis (salivary gland amylase due to carbohydrate metabolic derangement) [ISBN9781451118698]. In addition, while highly variable, there is evidence that administration of opiates such as morphine may increase serum amylase activity (presumably due to causing spasm of the sphincter of Oddi) [PMID13009210]. However, these conditions typically do not produce serum amylase elevations of 3 fold or greater.

Macroamylasemia is a benign condition in which amylase (usually salivary amylase) complexes with immunoglobulins (usually IgG or IgA). Because of the high molecular weight of the complex (>200,000), macroamylase cannot be cleared by the kidney, resulting in a persistent elevated serum amylase activity [ISBN9781594251023]. It is estimated that 1%-2% of the population manifests this condition [ISBN9781451118698]. Urine amylase activity is low in this condition.

11.5.1 Amylase reference range
Serum: 28-100 U/L
Urine, random: men 16-491 U/L; women 21-447 U/L

11.6 Lipase
Lipase catalyzes the hydrolysis of **triglycerides**. Measurement of serum lipase activity is primarily used to investigate pancreatic disorders. In acute pancreatitis the activity increases within 4-6 hours, peaks near 24 hours, and decreases toward normal by 8-14 days [ISBN9780683300857]. Elevation of serum lipase activity >3× the upper reference limit, in the absence of renal failure, is a more specific diagnostic finding for acute pancreatitis than an increase in serum amylase activity [ISBN9781594251023]. In fact, an increase of serum amylase with a normal lipase usually suggests an extrapancreatic cause of hyperamylasemia.

Extrapancreatic causes of elevated serum lipase activity include cholecystitis, perforated peptic ulcer, intestinal obstruction, peritonitis, trauma to the pancreas, renal insufficiency, and spasm of the sphincter of Oddi [ISBN9781594251023]. Urine lipase measurements are not clinically useful.

11.6.1 Lipase reference range
Serum: 13-60 U/L

11.7 Amylase:creatinine clearance ratio
The renal clearance of amylase in normal individuals is <5% of the creatinine clearance. However, in acute pancreatitis, it rises to ≥10% due to increased renal permeability to amylase in that condition [PMID1117961]. It is believed that in acute pancreatitis, the tubular reabsorption of amylase is reduced (probably secondary to competition from other lower molecular weight proteins that may be released from the inflamed pancreas) [PMID1117961, ISBN9780721686349]. Elevations of the ratio have also been reported in burns, myeloma, march hemoglobinuria (hemoglobinuria seen following heavy exercise), and light chain proteinuria, all of which might cause elaboration of small molecular weight proteins that could compete with amylase for tubular reabsorption. Because of the low urine amylase activity, in macroamylasemia, the amylase:creatinine clearance ratio is <2% [ISBN9780721686349].

$$\frac{\text{amylase clearance}}{\text{creatinine clearance}} \% = \frac{\dfrac{\text{urine amylase}}{\text{serum amylase}} \times \dfrac{\text{urine volume}}{\text{unit time}}}{\dfrac{\text{urine creatinine}}{\text{serum creatinine}} \times \dfrac{\text{urine volume}}{\text{unit time}}} \times 100$$

$$= \frac{\text{urine amylase}}{\text{serum amylase}} \times \frac{\text{serum creatinine}}{\text{urine creatinine}} \times 100$$

f11.1 Calculation of amylase: creatinine clearance ratio

Note that the urine volume and time cancel out in the calculation of the clearance ratio **f11.1** so that timed urine and blood collections are not required. The test can thus be conducted on simultaneously collected random samples of blood and urine.

11.7.1 Amylase:creatinine clearance ratio reference ranges
Normal: <5%
Acute pancreatitis: >10%
Macroamylasemia: <2%

11.8 Nonspecific biochemical changes
Acute pancreatitis is frequently accompanied by relatively nonspecific changes in clinical chemistry tests. Hypocalcemia occurs in ~25% of patients and is thought to be due to intraperitoneal **saponification** of calcium by free fatty acids released in pancreatitis. Hyperbilirubinemia occurs in ~10% of patients due to the release of hemoglobin in hemorrhagic pancreatitis and subsequent conversion of the hemoglobin to bilirubin. Hypertriglyceridemia is noted in ~5%-10% of patients, and hypertriglyceridemia is thought to be a cause of acute pancreatitis due to release of toxic free fatty acids from the triglycerides. Hyperglycemia is common and is due to decreased release of **insulin** from the damaged pancreas; increased release of **glucagon** from the inflamed pancreas; and an increased output of adrenal glucocorticoids and catecholamines [ISBN9780071802154].

11.9 **References**
11.9.1 **Journals**

PMID1117961 Warshaw AL, Fuller AF [1975] Specificity of increased renal clearance of amylase in diagnosis of acute pancreatitis. *N Engl J Med* 292:325-8

PMID13009210 Wapshaw H [1953] The pancreatic side-effects of morphine. *Br Med J* 1:373-5

PMID13410166 Saxon EI, Hinkley WC, Vogel WC et al [1957] Comparative value of serum and urinary amylase in the diagnosis of acute pancreatitis. *AMA Arch Intern Med* 99:607-21

PMID15802095 Lowenfels AB, Sullivan T, Fiorianti J et al [2005] The epidemiology and impact of pancreatic diseases in the United States. *Curr Gastroenterol Rep* 7:90-5

11.9.2 **Books**

ISBN9780071802154 Conwell DL, Banks P, Greenberger, NJ [2015] Acute and chronic pancreatitis. In: Kasper D, Fauci A, Hauser S et al, ed. *Harrison's Principles of Internal Medicine*, 19e. McGraw Hill Education, 2090-2102

ISBN9780071824866 Friedman LS [2014] Liver, biliary tract, & pancreas disorders. In: Papadakis MA, McPhee SJ, Rabow MW, ed. *Current Medical Diagnosis & Treatment*, 53e. McGraw Hill Education, 641-697.

ISBN9780683300857 Chun KY [2002] Clinical enzymology. In: Lewandrowski K, ed. *Clinical Chemistry: Laboratory Management & Clinical Correlations*. Lippincott Williams & Wilkins, 517-518.

ISBN9780721686349 Henderson AR, Moss DW [2001] Enzymes. In: Burtis CA, Ashwood ER, ed. *Tietz Fundamentals of Clinical Chemistry*, 5e. WB Saunders Company, 374

ISBN9781451118698 Johnson-Davis KL [2013] Enzymes. In: Bishop ML, Fody EP, Schoeff LE. *Clinical Chemistry: Principles, Techniques, and Correlation*, 7e. Lippincott Williams & Wilkins, 262-91

ISBN9781594251023 Panteghini M [2011] Laboratory evaluation of the pancreas. In: Clarke W, ed. *Contemporary Practice in Clinical Chemistry*, 2e. A Press, 333-41

11.10 **Clinical cases**
11.10.1 **Case 1**

A 29-year-old female is seen in the emergency department with a chief complaint of diffuse abdominal pain. She also has swollen, painful salivary glands. Her serum amylase is 250 U/L.

11.10.1.1 **Questions**

1. What clinical conditions may explain the hyperamylasemia?

2. What laboratory tests should be conducted to evaluate each of them?

11.10.2 **Case 2**

A 38-year-old alcoholic male with a history of hepatobiliary disease presents to the emergency department with an 8 hour history of acute abdominal pain. He was noted to be lying on the gurney with his knees drawn up to reduce the pain. He described the pain as very intense and radiating to his back. He also complained of nausea. His blood pressure was 148/90 mmHg, pulse 85/minute, and temperature 101.5°F. There was tenderness and rigidity in the left upper quadrant. On admission to the hospital, laboratory tests on plasma showed the following: glucose 186 mg/dL, calcium 7.8 mg/dL, cholesterol 187 mg/dL, triglycerides 453 mg/dL, amylase 870 U/L, and lipase 1,205 U/L. The serum amylase activity returned toward normal after 5 days, and the serum lipase activity returned toward normal after 10 days.

11.10.2.1 **Questions**

1. What is the most likely diagnosis, and what evidence supports this?
2. What additional studies should be ordered?

11.10.3 **Case 3**

A 43-year-old male who is 3 years postpneumonectomy for pulmonary adeno-carcinoma is distressed to learn on routine evaluation that his serum amylase is 450 U/L. He has no new chief complaints other than chronic pain, which is alleviated by use of Vicodin (hydrocodone with acetaminophen).

11.10.3.1 **Questions**

1. What clinical conditions might explain the hyperamylasemia?
2. What laboratory tests should be ordered to evaluate them?

11.10.4 Clinical case answers

11.10.4.1 Case 1 answers

In addition to basic clinical chemistry and hematology tests as well as any imaging studies that may be indicated, the following tests (denoted in parentheses) may be performed for each condition listed:

➢ acute pancreatitis; though the serum amylase is <3× the upper reference range, it could be on the increase (serum lipase should be elevated >3× the upper reference range; amylase:creatinine clearance ratio should be 10% or greater)

➢ mesenteric infarction (serum lipase and amylase:creatinine clearance ratio should be normal)

➢ appendicitis (serum lipase and amylase:creatinine clearance ratio should be normal)

➢ cholecystitis (serum lipase should be elevated but amylase:creatinine clearance ratio should be normal)

➢ ruptured ectopic pregnancy (serum lipase and amylase:creatinine clearance ratio should be normal); urine pregnancy test should be positive

➢ intestinal obstruction (serum lipase should be elevated but amylase:creatinine clearance ratio should be normal)

➢ perforated peptic ulcer (serum lipase should be elevated but amylase:creatinine clearance ratio should be normal)

➢ amylase producing tumor (serum lipase and amylase:creatinine clearance ratio should be normal)

➢ renal failure, though it does not explain the abdominal pain (serum lipase should be elevated but amylase:creatinine clearance ratio should be normal)

➢ sialitis, though it does not explain the abdominal pain (serum lipase and amylase:creatinine clearance ratio should be normal)

➢ macroamylasemia, though it does not explain the abdominal pain (serum lipase should be normal but amylase:creatinine clearance ratio should be low)

➢ diabetic ketoacidosis, though it does not explain the abdominal pain (serum lipase and amylase:creatinine clearance ratio should be normal)

11.10.4.2 **Case 2 answers**

1. The most likely diagnosis is acute pancreatitis, based on the findings of acute abdominal pain radiating to the back, nausea, the history of hepatobiliary disease and alcoholism, the elevated serum amylase and lipase activities with the lipase remaining elevated longer than the amylase, hypocalcemia, hypertriglyceridemia, and hyperglycemia

2. Additional studies should include an amylase:creatinine clearance ratio (should be elevated), serum bilirubin (may be elevated), and imaging studies of the abdomen (may show pancreatic calcifications, peritoneal effusion)

11.10.4.3 **Case 3 answers**

Since the patient has no new chief complaints other than chronic pain, the following should be considered:

➤ occult tumor producing amylase (urine amylase would be high; serum lipase would be normal; amylase:creatinine clearance ratio would be normal); imaging studies should be ordered

➤ macroamylasemia (urine amylase would be low; serum lipase would be normal; amylase:creatinine clearance ratio would be low).

➤ spasm of the sphincter of Oddi due to use of opiates for pain (urine amylase would be high; serum lipase would be high; amylase:creatinine clearance ratio would be normal)

chapter 12

The laboratory diagnosis of liver disease

12.1 Objectives

At the end of this session, the learner should be able to

➢ describe the general functions of the liver

➢ discuss the use of serum bilirubin, alanine aminotransferase, and aspartate aminotransferase in evaluating hepatic parenchymal function

➢ discuss the use of serum alkaline phosphatase, γ glutamyl transferase, and bilirubin in evaluating biliary tract function

➢ describe conditions in which the serum unconjugated (indirect) bilirubin is elevated without significant elevation of the conjugated (direct) bilirubin

➢ describe conditions in which both serum unconjugated and conjugated bilirubin are elevated

➢ discuss δ bilirubin (biliprotein) and its significance

➢ discuss alteration of serum proteins in liver disease

➢ discuss alteration of blood coagulation in liver disease

➢ discuss causes of hyperammonemia

➢ discuss the causes of De Ritis ratio >1 and <1

➢ discuss alkaline phosphatase isoenzymes

12.2 Key terms

alkaline phosphatase (ALP): enzymes found in a variety of tissues and that catalyze the phosphorylation of proteins; useful in diagnosing bone and hepatic diseases

alanine aminotransferase (ALT): an enzyme catalyzing the transfer of an amino group from alanine to α ketoglutarate; useful in evaluating hepatocellular disease

Arias syndrome: a congenital condition in which there is reduced uridine 5'-phosphate glucuronyl transferase activity, leading to elevation of the unconjugated bilirubin; also referred to as type II Crigler Najjar syndrome

aspartate aminotransferase (AST): an enzyme catalyzing the transfer of an amino group from aspartic acid to α ketoglutarate; useful in evaluating hepatocellular disease

bilirubin: the end product of heme catabolism, conjugated in the liver

cholestasis: decreased bile flow due to either intrahepatic or extrahepatic obstruction

cirrhosis: liver disease characterized by diffuse interlacing bands of fibrous tissue dividing the hepatic parenchyma into micronodular or macronodular patterns

conjugated bilirubin: bilirubin that is conjugated with glucuronic acid to form the water soluble bilirubin monoglucuronide and bilirubin diglucuronide

Crigler Najjar syndrome: a congenital condition in which uridine 5'-phosphate glucuronyl transferase is absent (type I) or markedly reduced (type II, Arias syndrome), leading to inability or markedly reduced ability to conjugate bilirubin

De Ritis ratio: the ratio of AST to ALT activities

direct bilirubin: an approximation of the sum of the conjugated forms of bilirubin (bilirubin monoglucuronide, bilirubin diglucuronide, δ bilirubin) plus some unconjugated bilirubin

Dubin-Johnson syndrome: a congenital condition in which there is a defect in the ability of hepatocytes to excrete bilirubin; liver tissue is often black on gross examination

γ glutamyl transferase: an enzyme present in liver, kidney, and pancreas and that catalyzes the transfer of γ glutamyl functional groups; useful in determining if alkaline phosphatase elevations are due to bone or liver; also very sensitive to ethanol ingestion; elevated in cholestasis

Gilbert syndrome: a benign congenital condition in which there is impaired bilirubin uptake by the liver and decreased conjugating ability of the liver, resulting in mildly elevated unconjugated bilirubin

hemolytic disease of the newborn: hemolysis in the newborn due to Rh incompatibility between maternal and fetal antigens

hepatic encephalopathy: a neuropsychiatric condition due to advanced liver disease and hyperammonemia; often progresses to coma

hepatitis: inflammation of the liver, usually due to viruses or drugs

indirect bilirubin: an approximation of the unconjugated bilirubin calculated as the difference between total bilirubin and direct bilirubin

Paget disease of bone: a disorder characterized by excessive breakdown and formation of bone followed by disorganized bone remodeling

Reye syndrome: a rare condition causing swelling of the brain and liver and associated with elevated blood ammonia, usually in children

Rotor syndrome: a congenital condition in which there is a defect in the ability of hepatocytes to excrete bilirubin; normal liver histology

thrombocytopenia: a deficiency of platelets

total bilirubin: the sum of all forms of bilirubin (bilirubin monoglucuronide, bilirubin diglucuronide, δ bilirubin, and unconjugated bilirubin)

unconjugated bilirubin: bilirubin that has not been conjugated with glucuronic acid

varices: dilated blood vessels in the stomach or esophagus

δ bilirubin: conjugated bilirubin covalently bound to albumin

12.3 **Background/significance**

The liver has more varied functions than perhaps any other organ in the body. The hepatic parenchymal cells are involved in protein synthesis (almost all plasma/serum proteins including blood coagulation factors; immunoglobulins are not made in the liver but are made by plasma cells in the bone marrow), lipid metabolism (fat, cholesterol, phospholipids, lipoproteins), carbohydrate metabolism (gluconeogenesis, glycogenolysis), storage functions (most vitamins, iron, copper, trace metals), excretory functions (**bilirubin**, bile salts), and detoxification (ammonia, steroids, drugs, poisons).

Liver disease may be confined to the organ itself (eg, **cirrhosis,** infection, neoplasms) or can be secondary to systemic disease (eg, congestive heart failure, hemochromatosis).

A basic understanding of laboratory testing of liver function is important in the diagnostic workup of liver disease.

12.4 **Bilirubin**

Bilirubin is the end product of heme catabolism. It is transported from sites of production (mostly spleen) to the liver to be conjugated with glucuronic acid as the monoglucuronide and the diglucuronide, which are then excreted via the bile. δ bilirubin (aka "biliprotein") is an additional form of conjugated bilirubin that is covalently bound to albumin. In healthy subjects, **unconjugated bilirubin** is noncovalently bound to albumin. Clinical laboratories typically measure **direct bilirubin** (all conjugated forms of bilirubin, including the monoglucuronide, bilirubin diglucuronide, and δ bilirubin, plus a small amount of unconjugated bilirubin). The total bilirubin is measured separately, and the concentration of **indirect bilirubin** (an estimate of unconjugated bilirubin, since some unconjugated bilirubin is also measured in the direct fraction) is calculated by subtraction of the two. δ bilirubin is not available as a routine measurement in the clinical laboratory, but since it reacts in measurements of direct bilirubin (see above), it can account for a prolonged direct hyperbilirubinemia following disappearance of bilirubinuria. Jaundice is usually detectable when the serum total bilirubin exceeds 2-3 mg/dL. Bilirubin is photosensitive, and exposure to light causes lowering of the concentration [ISBN9781416061649]. Measurement of bilirubin is an evaluation of both the synthetic and excretory functions of the liver.

Elevations of unconjugated (indirect) bilirubin without significant elevation of conjugated (direct) bilirubin are seen with hemolysis (due to the amount of unconjugated bilirubin overwhelming the conjugation capacity of the liver), end stage cirrhosis (due to loss of the liver's conjugating ability), congenital defects in the liver's conjugating ability (due to reduced uridine 5'-phosphate glucuronyl transferase activity, as in **Crigler Najjar syndrome** type I and type II, the latter known as **Arias syndrome** and milder), and hepatic immaturity of the newborn (occurring at 2-4 days after birth of a full term infant) [ISBN9780683300857, ISBN9781416061649, ISBN9781594251023]. **Gilbert syndrome** is a benign asymptomatic condition in which there is impaired bilirubin uptake by the liver and decreased amount of uridine 5'-phosphate glucuronyl transferase activity in the hepatocytes. The syndrome is seen in 2%-3% of the population and is characterized by elevated unconjugated bilirubin concentrations but total bilirubin <3 mg/dL [ISBN9780683300857, ISBN9781594251023].

Elevations of the conjugated (direct) plus unconjugated (indirect) bilirubin are seen in mechanical or functional impairment of bilirubin excretion. Such conditions include nonendstage cirrhosis, acute **hepatitis,** cholestasis (due to hepatocellular injury, drug induced **cholestasis**, intrahepatic biliary tree obstruction), posthepatic obstruction (eg, gallstones, tumors, strictures), and congenital excretory defects (eg, **Dubin-Johnson syndrome** and **Rotor syndrome**, in which the ability of the hepatocytes to excrete bilirubin is defective) [ISBN9780683300857, ISBN9781416061649].

12.4.1 Plasma/serum bilirubin reference range

Total bilirubin: <1.2 mg/dL
Direct bilirubin: <0.2 mg/dL

12.5 Plasma/serum proteins

The serum albumin concentration decreases with liver injury (eg, cirrhosis, autoimmune hepatitis, alcoholic hepatitis) due to loss of synthetic ability of the hepatocytes. However, the total protein frequently is near normal since the globulin fraction increases concurrently. Accordingly, the ratio of albumin to globulin (the so called A:G ratio) declines in liver disease (normal 1.5-2.5:1.0). The A:G ratio also declines in inflammation since cytokines inhibit albumin synthesis while immunoglobulin synthesis is stimulated [ISBN9780683300857]. Furthermore, in liver disease the catabolism of IgA is compromised, leading to an increase in that immunoglobulin.

The loss of albumin compromises the ability to retain oncotic pressure so that edema and ascites occur (commonly seen in chronic alcoholics).

Serum albumin and total proteins are measured directly, while the globulin concentration is calculated as the difference between the two.

12.5.1 Plasma/serum protein reference range

Total proteins: 6.0-8.0 g/dL
Albumin: 3.5-5.2 g/dL

12.6 Blood coagulation

The liver synthesizes almost all of the proteins in the coagulation cascade with factor VIII and von Willebrand factor also being made in endothelial cells. In addition the liver produces antithrombin III and protein C. Thus, end stage liver disease is usually associated with coagulopathies (eg, elevated prothrombin time and partial thromboplastin time). In liver disease most of the clotting factors are deficient except for factor VIII, which may even be elevated since it is a positive acute phase reactant. Similarly, fibrinogen (factor I) may be decreased in advanced liver disease (decreased synthesis) or elevated in hepatitis (since fibrinogen is a positive acute phase reactant). If there is malabsorption of vitamin K (eg, as in general malabsorption, cholestasis, biliary obstruction), synthesis of clotting factors II, VII, IX, and X may be impaired [ISBN9780683300857]. These coagulopathies are of particular concern since patients with end stage liver disease often have portal hypertension, **varices**, and **thrombocytopenia**, and are thus at risk for hemorrhage.

12.7 Ammonia

The liver is the site of the urea cycle, which detoxifies ammonia by converting it into urea for excretion into the urine. With liver damage or shunting of blood away from the liver, the urea cycle is compromised, leading to elevation of blood ammonia and decreases in serum/plasma urea nitrogen. Since it readily crosses the blood-brain barrier, ammonia causes **hepatic encephalopathy**. Hyperammonemia can be due to congenital deficiencies of urea cycle enzymes (eg, ornithine transcarbamylase), severe liver failure, renal failure (rising urea diffuses into the gastrointestinal tract, where it is converted to ammonia), **Reye syndrome**, gastrointestinal bleeding (due to bacterial metabolism of blood protein), hepatic immaturity of the newborn (transient hyperammonemia), and **hemolytic disease of the newborn** [ISBN9780683300857, ISBN9781416061649].

Ammonia can also be generated in vitro due to hydrolysis of glutamine in the sample, activation of platelets in the sample, and the lysis of erythrocytes [ISBN9780683300857]. Thus it is essential that blood specimens be placed on ice immediately after collection, rapidly centrifuged, and serum/plasma separated from the red cells. Ammonia analyses should be performed within 30 minutes of specimen collection. Otherwise the samples should be frozen.

12.7.1 Plasma/serum ammonia reference range

Men: 11-51 µMol/L
Women: 16-60 µMol/L

12.8 Aminotransferases

Aspartate aminotransferase (AST) and **alanine aminotransferase (ALT)** catalyze the transfer of an amino group from aspartic acid and alanine, respectively, to α ketoglutarate. These 2 enzymes are among the most sensitive indicators of hepatocyte injury.

The highest activity of AST is found in liver, cardiac tissue, and skeletal muscle with smaller amounts in kidney, pancreas, and erythrocytes. Accordingly, elevations of AST are seen in patients with acute hepatocellular injury, skeletal muscle disorders (eg, muscular dystrophies), and acute myocardial infarction. However, because of its wide distribution, AST has not proven to be a useful biomarker for the diagnosis of myocardial infarction [ISBN9781451118698]. Also, AST is present in both the cytoplasm and mitochondria of the hepatocyte, while ALT is present only in the cytoplasm [ISBN9780683307511].

ALT is considered to be the more liver specific of the aminotransferases, with its highest activity being found in liver, and consequently it is mostly used to evaluate hepatic disorders. Higher ALT activity is found in hepatocellular disorders than in extrahepatic or intrahepatic disorders. In acute inflammatory conditions of the liver (eg, hepatitis), activity is higher than that of AST, and it tends to remain elevated longer than AST due to its longer serum half-life (24 hours) compared to that of AST (16 hours) [ISBN9781451118698].

Elevations of the aminotransferases often precede the development of clinical signs and symptoms of disease. The etiology of the specific disorders may be aided by use of the **De Ritis ratio** (ie, AST:ALT ratio). In health, the ratio is ~1. The ratio is >1 in hepatic cirrhosis, myocardial infarction, and acute skeletal muscle trauma (all due to the greater activity of AST than ALT in these tissues). The ratio is also >1 in alcoholic liver disease (due to low pyridoxal-5-phosphate, a cofactor for ALT, in alcoholics) [ISBN9780683307511]. However, most clinical laboratories now include pyridoxal-5-phosphate in the assay reagents so that the use of the De Ritis ratio in alcoholic liver disease may no longer be helpful. The ratio is <1 in acute viral hepatitis, intrahepatic cholestasis, infectious mononucleosis, and Reye syndrome (all due to the more pronounced elevation of ALT activity relative to that of AST) [ISBN9780683307511].

12.8.1 Plasma/serum aminotransferase reference range
AST: men 0-40 U/L; women 0-32 U/L
ALT: men 0-41 U/L; women 0-33 U/L

12.9 Alkaline phosphatase
Alkaline phosphatase (ALP) is present in liver, bone, intestine, and placenta. In the liver it is located in the canalicular and sinusoidal cell surface membranes. Substantial increases in ALP activity of liver etiology are generally due to hepatobiliary causes such as extrahepatic bile duct obstruction (eg, stone in the common bile duct), intrahepatic biliary cholestasis, and primary biliary cirrhosis. In contrast, patients with hepatocellular damage usually demonstrate only a slight to moderate increase in ALP. Increases in ALP activity of bone etiology include metastatic bone tumors, healing fractures, **Paget disease of the bone**, and physiologic bone growth in children. Placental ALP is the source of ALP activity increases in pregnancy and certain tumors (the so called Regan isoenzyme) [ISBN9780683300857].

While the isoenzymes of ALP can be separated electrophoretically and there is an immunochemical assay for bone ALP, these methods are not widely used. Some laboratories still rely on the heat stability of ALP following heating of the serum/plasma at 56°C for 10 minutes. If the residual activity after heating is <20% of the activity before heating, a bone source of ALP is implicated. If it is >20%, a liver source of ALP is suggested. The most heat stable ALP isoenzyme is placenta, which resists heat denaturation at 65°C for 30 minutes. The heat stability pattern is as follows: bone (least heat stable)<liver<placenta, Regan isoenzyme (most heat stable) [ISBN9781451118698].

12.9.1 Plasma/serum alkaline phosphatase reference range
Adults: 40-120 U/L
Children: 125-530 U/L

12.10 γ glutamyl transferase

γ glutamyl transferase (GGT) is present in liver, kidneys, pancreas, and prostate. Clinical use of GGT activity measurements is confined mostly to evaluation of liver and biliary system disorders. It is elevated in virtually all hepatobiliary disorders (eg, alcohol and drug induced liver damage, acute hepatitis, common bile duct obstruction), making it one of the most sensitive enzyme assays in these conditions [ISBN9780683300857, ISBN9781451118698]. Because of alcohol's effects on GGT activity, increased GGT activity may suggest chronic alcoholism (GGT >2× the upper reference limit). For that reason, the enzyme is often monitored in alcohol treatment programs, returning to normal within 2-3 weeks after abstention from alcohol [ISBN9781451118698].

The measurement of GGT activity is also useful in determining the cause of elevated ALP because, unlike ALP, which is elevated in pregnancy and with bone disorders, GGT is normal in those conditions [ISBN9781451118698].

12.10.1 Plasma/serum γ glutamyl transferase reference range
Men: <61 U/L
Women: <36 U/L

12.11 Tests of specific etiologies

Obviously, myriad tests can be utilized in the workup of specific diseases affecting the liver. These include viral antigens and antibodies (eg, hepatitis A, B, C), elements (eg, copper and iron), autoantibodies (eg, antimitochondrial, antinuclear), fetal antigens (eg, α fetoprotein), and immunoglobulins. However, given their selective use, this discussion is beyond the purview of this chapter.

12.12 References

ISBN9781416061649 Dufour DR [2013] Liver disease. In: Burtis CA, Ashwood ER, Bruns DE, ed. *Tietz Textbook of Clinical Chemistry and Molecular Diagnostics*, 5e. Elsevier Saunders, 1637-94

ISBN9781594251023 Qazi N, Dufour DR [2011] Laboratory diagnosis of liver disease. In: Clarke W, ed. *Contemporary Practice in Clinical Chemistry*, 2e. A Press, 311-22

ISBN9780683300857 Coon DR, Lewandrowski K [2002] Evaluation of hepatic function and disorders of the liver. In: Lewandrowski K, ed. *Clinical Chemistry: Laboratory Management & Clinical Correlations*. Lippincott Williams & Wilkins, 725-749.

ISBN9781451118698 Johnson-Davis KL [2013] Enzymes. In: Bishop ML, Fody EP, Schoeff LE, ed. *Clinical Chemistry: Principles, Techniques, and Correlations*, 7e. Lippincott Williams & Wilkins, 277-81.

ISBN9780683307511 Wu AHB [2002] Diagnostic enzymology and other biochemical markers of organ damage. In: McClatchey KD, ed. *Clinical Laboratory Medicine*, 2e. Lippincott Williams & Wilkins, 288-290

12.13 **Clinical cases**

12.13.1 **Case 1**

A 30-year-old female is seen in her primary care physician's office with fever (102°F) and chills 11 days after returning from central Africa. Since she was not travelling with a tour group, she consumed the local food and water. She developed diarrhea, fever, and mild nausea and vomiting 1 week after arriving in Africa. Laboratory studies obtained on her clinic visit showed serum AST 525 U/L, ALT 615 U/L, total bilirubin 0.4 mg/dL, conjugated bilirubin 0.1 mg/dL, and ALP 111 U/L. A thick smear for malaria was negative, and an infectious mononucleosis screen was negative. The patient has no history of drug abuse. The physical examination was unremarkable.

12.13.1.1 **Questions**

1. What is the most likely diagnosis for this patient?
2. What further tests should be performed to confirm the diagnosis?

12.13.2 **Case 2**

A 45-year-old unemployed male is seen in the emergency department with a chief complaint of severe joint pain for the last 10 months, which has recently made it difficult for him to perform his normal daily activities. He has a history of intravenous drug use. The physical examination was unremarkable except for pain and decreased range of motion of the right arm. The patient was afebrile, and had normal blood pressure and pulse rate. His laboratory studies showed serum AST 201 U/L, ALT 223 U/L, total bilirubin 1.0 mg/dL, conjugated bilirubin 0.1 mg/dL, and ALP 95 U/L.

12.13.2.1 **Questions**

1. What is the most likely diagnosis for this patient?
2. What further tests should be performed to confirm the diagnosis?

12.13.3 **Case 3**

A 65-year-old female with a 20 year history of alcoholism is brought to the emergency department with profound confusion and lethargy. Over the last 18 months, she has developed ataxia and dysarthria. Physical examination reveals a slightly enlarged liver. Laboratory studies showed serum AST 120 U/L, ALT 62 U/L, ammonia 128 μMol/L, total bilirubin 3.5 mg/dL, conjugated bilirubin 0.1 mg/dL, amylase 60 U/L, creatine kinase 251 U/L, prothrombin time 17 sec (control 11 sec), and partial thromboplastin time 48 sec (control 32 sec). Toxicology screening tests and blood cultures were negative.

12.13.3.1 **Question**

What is the most likely explanation for these findings?

12.13.4 Clinical cases answers
12.13.4.1 Case 1 answers

1. AST and ALT are elevated, and the De Ritis ratio is <1 in this patient. Elevated aminotransferases with ratios <1 suggest viral hepatitis, intrahepatic cholestasis, infectious mononucleosis, and Reye syndrome. Intrahepatic cholestasis would cause a very elevated ALP and total bilirubin. This patient has a normal ALP and total bilirubin. The infectious mononucleosis screen was negative, suggesting that this is not the cause. Reye syndrome is usually seen in children and is accompanied by hepatic encephalopathy, not seen in this patient. The clinical history (ingestion of unclean food and water) suggests hepatitis A as the most likely cause of these findings. A less likely cause would be hepatitis E, also spread by ingestion of unclean food and water.

2. Hepatitis A IgM (recent exposure) and (IgM + IgG; immunity) should be ordered; if negative, then IgM and IgG antibodies to hepatitis E could be ordered even though they are not yet FDA approved

12.13.4.2 Case 2 answers

1. Both AST and ALT are elevated, and the De Ritis ratio is <1. Elevated aminotransferases with ratios <1 suggest acute viral hepatitis, intrahepatic cholestasis, infectious mononucleosis, and Reye syndrome. With a normal ALP and total bilirubin, intrahepatic cholestasis is unlikely. Infectious mononucleosis is unlikely with lack of fever and pharyngitis. Reye syndrome is unlikely in an adult, and there is no suggestion of hepatic encephalopathy. Given the history of intravenous drug use and the prolonged time course of his symptoms, chronic hepatitis B and/or hepatitis C are likely. Joint pain is caused by deposition of antigen: antibody complexes in the joints.

2. Tests for hepatitis B surface (S) antigen, e antigen, and IgM to hepatitis core (C) antigen should be obtained. Hepatitis B viral load could also be measured. Additionally, hepatitis C antibody and viral antigen tests should be performed.

12.13.4.3 Case 3 answer

This patient is manifesting the signs and symptoms of hepatic encephalopathy due to chronic alcoholism. Her elevated blood ammonia is suggestive of this, along with elevation of the prothrombin time and partial thromboplastin time (due to inability to make blood coagulation factors) and the low conjugated bilirubin. The De Ritis ratio >1 is also consistent with alcoholic liver disease due to deficiency of pyridoxal-5-phosphate (cofactor for ALT).

The serum creatine kinase may be elevated due to falling since the patient has severe loss of balance.

chapter 13

Tumor markers

13.1 Objectives

At the end of this session, the learner should be able to

➤ describe what constitutes a tumor marker

➤ discuss the uses of tumor markers

➤ name and discuss the use of at least 10 tumor markers

➤ describe the effect of using multiple tumor markers together with respect to sensitivity for detection of cancer

13.2 Key terms

blastula: a hollow sphere of cells surrounding an inner fluid filled cavity in early mammalian embryonic development

choriocarcinoma: a malignant tumor arising from trophoblastic cells within the uterus

endometrium: the inner mucus membrane of the uterus

glycoprotein: a protein containing a carbohydrate moiety

hydatidiform mole: an abnormal cluster of cells that were destined to become placenta and can transform into a malignancy

multiple myeloma: a malignancy of plasma cells, generally involving elaboration of clones of immunoglobulins

neuroblastoma: a childhood tumor arising from immature nerve cells

nonseminomatous germ cell tumor of the testes: a cancer formed from cells that had been destined to become spermatozoa

oncofetal protein: a protein normally found in the fetus but present in some adults with cancer

pheochromocytoma: a neuroendocrine tumor of the adrenal glands that secretes catecholamines

syncytiotrophoblast cell: the outer layer of the trophoblast that invades the uterine wall to form the fetal component of the placenta

trophoblast: the layer of tissue on the outside of the blastula supplying the mammalian embryo with nourishment and destined to become the placenta

13.3 **Background/significance**

Tumor markers are substances produced by cancers or by other cells in response to cancer. Most markers are made by normal cells as well as cancer cells, but are produced at much higher concentrations in cancer. The markers can be proteins, enzymes, hormones, oncofetal antigens, receptors, metabolites, and genetic mutations, and can be detected in blood, urine, other fluids, and solid tissue. Some markers can even be associated with >1 tumor type. Unfortunately, not all people with a particular tumor will have higher levels of the tumor markers associated with that cancer.

The major uses of tumor markers have included screening populations and high risk groups, aiding in diagnosis of cancers (limited utility), staging of cancer, monitoring response to therapy, and checking for recurrence of cancer. The primary use of tumor markers today is in monitoring response to therapy and checking for recurrence of the cancer.

With rapidly evolving analytical technology, more and more substances are being studied and identified as potential tumor markers. This chapter summarizes the use of the more established tumor markers.

13.4 **α fetoprotein (αFP)**

α fetoprotein (αFP), a single chain **glycoprotein** produced by the liver, is a major serum protein in the fetus. As a marker measured in serum, it has been found useful in the evaluation and staging of **nonseminomatous germ cell tumors of the testes** [PMID6158584]. This marker is also associated with hepatocellular carcinoma, with persistently elevated concentrations being indicative of residual disease and rising concentrations being suggestive of disease progression or recurrence. It can also be elevated with pregnancy, acute viral hepatitis, and cirrhosis [PMID21446576].

On the basis of its differential binding to the *Lens culinaris* agglutinin, αFP can be classified into 3 isoforms. The αFP-L3 isoform is associated with hepatocellular carcinoma, and αFP-L3 as a percentage of total αFP (αFP-L3%) is used for patients with chronic liver diseases to evaluate their risk of developing hepatocellular carcinoma. Higher αFP-L3% is associated with increased cancer risk and is also a prognostic indicator for patients who have this cancer. Both αFP and αFP-L3% have been approved by the US Food and Drug Administration (FDA) to be used as tumor markers in diagnosis of liver cancer [ISBN9781594251023].

13.4.1 **Serum αFP reference range (in healthy individuals)**

Total αFP: 0-15 ng/mL
αFP-L3%: 0%-9.9%

13.5 Human chorionic gonadotropin (hCG)

Human chorionic gonadotropin (hCG), produced by the **syncytiotrophoblast cell** after differentiation of the **trophoblast** has been used for >50 years as a serum biomarker in the diagnosis and monitoring of <u>choriocarcinoma</u> and <u>hydatidiform mole</u>. In conjunction with αFP, it can also be useful in the evaluation of therapeutic response and prognosis for <u>nonseminomatous germ cells tumors of the testes</u>. Measurement of the β subunit of hCG is more specific since antibody directed toward the intact hCG cross reacts with many other hormones [ISBN9780683300857]. The use of hCG as a tumor marker is not FDA approved.

13.5.1 Serum hCG reference range (in healthy individuals)

Women (nonpregnant): <6 mIU/mL
Women (pregnant): >10 mIU/mL
Men: <3 mIU/mL

13.6 Cancer antigen 19-9 (CA19-9)

Cancer antigen 19-9 (CA19-9) is a glycoprotein used to monitor response to therapy in patients with <u>pancreatic cancer</u>. This serum biomarker is also elevated with bile duct, gastric, and colon cancers, and even in nonmalignant conditions such as pancreatitis and cystic fibrosis [PMID21446576]. It is FDA approved for use in pancreatic cancer.

13.6.1 Serum CA19-9 reference range (in healthy individuals)

31-42 U/mL

13.7 Cancer antigen 125 (CA125)

Cancer antigen 125 (CA125) is a glycoprotein that is increased in the serum of patients with <u>epithelial ovarian cancers</u> and <u>cancers of the **endometrium**</u>. It can also be increased in patients with other cancers (eg, pancreatic, lung, breast, gastrointestinal), as well as in some benign conditions if the serosal lining is involved (eg, pregnancy, endometriosis, hepatitis) [ISBN9781594251023, Handy 2009]. This biomarker is FDA approved for use with epithelial ovarian cancer.

13.7.1 Serum CA125 reference range (in healthy individuals)

<35 U/mL

13.8 Carcinoembryonic antigen (CEA)

Carcinoembryonic antigen (CEA) is one of the earliest described **oncofetal proteins**. This relatively nonspecific glycoprotein serum marker is elevated with a variety of primary tumor types including colorectal, breast, pancreatic, liver, gastric, lung, ovarian, and uterine cancers. It is also elevated in most cases of metastatic liver cancer [ISBN9781594251023]. This biomarker is FDA approved for use in colorectal cancer.

13.8.1 Serum CEA reference range (in healthy individuals)

Nonsmokers <3.8 ng/mL

13.9 Cancer antigen 15-3 (CA15-3)

Cancer antigen 15-3 (CA15-3) is a serum biomarker utilized in the evaluation of breast cancer, and it is FDA approved for this purpose. This glycoprotein can also be increased in benign liver and breast disease, as well as other cancers (eg, pancreatic, lung, ovarian, colorectal, liver) [ISBN9781594251023].

13.9.1 Serum CA15-3 reference range (in healthy individuals)

0-31 U/mL

13.10 Cancer antigen 27.29 (CA27.29)

Cancer antigen 27.29 (CA27.29), a mucus containing protein, is another serum biomarker used in the evaluation of breast cancer, and it is FDA approved for this purpose. In fact, it is often used in conjunction with CA15-3, and usually the correlation between the 2 markers is good [Handy 2009, ISBN9781594251023].

13.10.1 Serum CA27.29 reference range (in healthy individuals)

0-40 U/mL

13.11 β2 microglobulin (β2M)

β2 microglobulin (β2M) is a low molecular weight protein biomarker found on the surface of all nucleated cells. It is useful in the evaluation of such hematopoietic cancers as **multiple myeloma** and lymphoma [PMID1439309, PMID6189572]. While it can be measured in serum, urine, or cerebrospinal fluid, it is usually monitored in serum to determine the prognosis and follow the response to treatment for these diseases. This biomarker has not been FDA approved for this purpose as of this time.

13.11.1 Serum β2M reference range (in healthy individuals)

0.8-2.4 mg/L

13.12 Human epididymis protein 4 (HE4)

The human epididymis protein 4 (HE4) is overexpressed in ovarian cancer, although it is not specific for ovarian tumors. It has been FDA approved as a serum biomarker for monitoring recurrence and progression of disease in patients with epithelial (but not mucinous or germ cell) ovarian cancer, and in that regard, it is often used in conjunction with CA125 [ISBN9781594251023].

13.12.1 Serum HE4 reference range (in healthy individuals)

0-150 pMol/L

13.13 Chromogranin A (CgA)

Chromogranins are a family of proteins that are major components of the secretory granules of most neuroendocrine cells. Chromogranin A (CgA) is useful as a serum biomarker in the evaluation of neuroendocrine tumors (eg, carcinoid, **pheochromocytoma** and **neuroblastoma**). It is said to be at least as sensitive and specific as plasma catecholamines and urinary metanephrines in the detection of these tumors [ISBN9781416061649]. This marker is not FDA approved for use.

13.13.1 Serum CgA reference range (in healthy individuals)

0-95 ng/mL

13.14 Thyroglobulin (Tg)

Thyroglobulin (Tg), produced in the thyroid gland as a precursor to the thyroid hormones, is an FDA approved serum tumor marker for patients with differentiated thyroid carcinoma [ISBN9781416061649]. Recurrence of tumor is associated with rising concentrations of thyroglobulin.

Unfortunately autoantibodies to Tg are present in the serum of ~25% of patients with differentiated thyroid carcinoma (in contrast to only 10% in the general population) [PMID9543128], and their presence variably compromises the clinical utility of Tg measurements [PMID15985472].

13.14.1 Serum Tg reference range (in healthy individuals)

Adults: 1.3-31.8 ng/mL

13.15 **Calcitonin**

Calcitonin is a 32 amino acid polypeptide hormone produced by the thyroid gland. It is normally secreted in response to elevated serum calcium concentrations, causing calcium to be lowered. In <u>medullary thyroid carcinoma</u>, serum calcitonin is quite elevated. The degree of elevation is associated with tumor size and metastasis [ISBN9781416061649]. This biomarker is not FDA approved for use.

13.15.1 **Serum calcitonin reference range (in healthy individuals)**

Men: 0.0-7.5 pg/mL
Women: 0.0-5.1 pg/mL

13.16 **Prostate specific antigen (PSA)**

Prostate specific antigen (PSA) is a glycoprotein produced by the prostate. Free (unbound, active) PSA and PSA bound to α_1-antichymotrypsin and to α_2-macroglobulin are present in serum. However, PSA bound to α_2-macroglobulin is not measured as a part of the total PSA assay because the binding molecule is so large that it shields the binding site of PSA in the assay. Although PSA is relatively organ specific, it is not cancer specific, and can be elevated with prostatitis and benign prostatic hypertrophy. Total PSA (free plus bound) and free PSA have been approved by the FDA for screening and monitoring <u>prostate cancer</u>. In men with prostate cancer, the free PSA is decreased due to more binding of PSA to α_1-antichymotrypsin [ISBN9781594251023].

In men of age 50 and older, when the total PSA concentration is in the range of 4-10 ng/mL, measurement of free PSA is indicated, and the concentration of free PSA is then linked with the age of the patient to determine the probability of finding prostate cancer on needle biopsy. A free PSA <10% with a total PSA of 4-10 ng/mL generally suggests prostate cancer in all age groups (>50% chance, which increases with the patient's age) [ISBN9781594251023].

The so called PSA density normalizes the PSA for the size of the prostate. The PSA concentration is divided by the prostate volume as estimated by transrectal ultrasonography. Results >0.15 ng/mL/cc suggest a higher risk of prostate cancer, especially when associated with PSA concentrations >4 ng/mL [PMID24926079]. The PSA velocity monitors the change in PSA concentrations with time. It has been suggested that an increase of PSA by ≥0.75 ng/mL per year is shown in more men with prostate cancer than in men without [PMID1372942].

13.16.1 **Serum PSA reference range (in healthy men)**

Total PSA: 0-4 ng/mL

13.17 **Tumor markers in other tissues**

Tumor markers are also monitored in urine and in solid tissues, some of which are listed below:

- ➢ urine (for transitional cell carcinoma of the bladder)
  - ○ bladder tumor antigen (BTA)
  - ○ nuclear mitotic apparatus (NuMA)
- ➢ solid tissues
  - ○ breast tissue
    - ▪ if present, treatment with hormonal therapy is appropriate
      - . estrogen receptors (ERs)
      - . progesterone receptors (PRs)
    - ▪ Her2/neu to determine responsiveness to selected monoclonal antibody therapies
  - ○ epidermal growth factor receptor (EGFR) for various solid tissues to determine responsiveness to EGFR inhibitors

More recent developments include identification of circulating tumor cells in whole blood. Discussion of these specific markers is beyond the purview of this chapter.

13.18 **Use of combinations of tumor markers to improve sensitivity**

The use of several tumor markers together may increase the sensitivity for detection so it is greater than that of the sensitivity of individual markers, particularly for markers that show positivity across a wide variety of cancers. One example is the combined use of CEA and CA19-9 for gastric cancer. The sensitivity for detection of gastric cancer has been reported to be 59% with CEA alone and 76% with CA19-9 alone, while use of both markers together achieves 94% sensitivity [PMID3856076].

13.19 **References**
13.19.1 **Journals**

PMID1372942 Carter HB, Pearson JD, Metter EJ et al [1992] Longitudinal evaluation of prostate specific antigen levels in men with and without prostate disease. *JAMA* 267:2215-20

PMID1439309 Aviles A, Zepeda G, Guzman R et al [1992] [Prognostic importance of β-2-microglobulin in multiple myeloma]. *Rev Invest Clin* 44:215-20

PMID15985472 Spencer CA, Bergoglio M, Kazarosyan M et al [2005] Clinical impact of thyroglobulin (Tg) and Tg autoantibody method differences on the management of patients with differentiated thyroid carcinomas. *J Clin Endocrinol Metab* 90:5566-75

PMID21446576 Rhea JM, Molinaro RJ [2011] Cancer biomarkers: surviving the journey from bench to bedside. *MLO Med Lab Obs* 43 (3):10-2,16,18

PMID24926079 Noguez JH, Fantz CR [2014] Pathology consultation on prostate specific antigen testing. *Am J Clin Pathol* 142:7-15

PMID3856076 Staab HJ, Brummendorf T, Hornung A et al [1985] The clinical validity of circulating tumor associated antigens CEA and CA19-9 in primary diagnosis and follow-up of patients with gastrointestinal malignancies. *Klinische Wochenschrift* 63:106-15

PMID6158584 Lange PH, Nochomovitz LE, Rosai J et al [1980] Serum α-fetoprotein and human chorionic gonadotropin in patients with seminoma. *J Urol* 124:472-8

PMID6189572 Hagberg H, Killander A, Simonsson B [1983] Serum β 2-microglobulin in malignant lymphoma. *Cancer* 51:2220-5

PMID9543128 Spencer CA, Takeuchi M, Kazarosyan M et al [1998] Serum thyroglobulin autoantibodies: prevalence, influence on serum thyroglobulin measurement, and prognostic significance in patients with differentiated thyroid carcinoma. *J Clin Endocrinol Metab* 83:1121-7

Handy B [2009] The clinical utility of tumor markers. *Lab Med* 40:99-103

13.19.2 **Books**

ISBN9780683300857 Schwartz MK [2002] Tumor markers. In: Lewandrowski K, ed. *Clinical Chemistry: Laboratory Management & Clinical Correlations.* Lippincott Williams & Wilkins, 865-76

ISBN9781416061649 Sokoll LJ, Rai AJ, Chan DW [2013] Tumor markers. In: Burtis CA, Ashwood ER, Bruns DE, ed. *Tietz Textbook of Clinical Chemistry and Molecular Diagnostics,* 5e. Elsevier Saunders, 617-68

ISBN9781594251023 Sokoll LJ, Chan DW [2011] Tumor markers. In: Clarke W, ed. *Contemporary Practice in Clinical Chemistry,* 2e. AACC Press, 495-504

chapter 14

The laboratory diagnosis of protein abnormalities

14.1 Objectives

At the end of this session, the learner should be able to

➤ describe the approach to screening for protein abnormalities using serum protein electrophoresis

➤ discuss the identification of specific protein abnormalities using immunofixation electrophoresis

➤ describe the monitoring of specific protein abnormalities using immunoassays

➤ identify acute phase proteins that are elevated in acute inflammation ("positive acute phase reactants")

➤ identify acute phase proteins that are decreased in acute inflammation ("negative acute phase reactants")

➤ discuss C reactive protein and the erythrocyte sedimentation rate as markers of inflammation

➤ describe the frequency of IgG, IgA, and free light chain involvement in multiple myeloma

➤ discuss the causes and findings in Waldenström macroglobulinemia

➤ discuss causes of decreased γ globulins, including congenital and secondary (acquired) causes

➤ discuss causes of increased γ globulins, including polyclonal and monoclonal hypergammaglobulinemias

➤ discuss monoclonal gammopathies of undetermined significance (MGUS)

➤ describe the major serum protein electrophoretic patterns: normal, nephrotic syndrome, acute inflammation, chronic inflammation, α_1-antitrypsin deficiency, agammaglobulinemia, hepatic cirrhosis, and monoclonal gammopathy

➤ describe serum free light chain analysis and how it is used in diagnosis and treatment of multiple myeloma

14.2 Key terms

acute phase reactant: protein whose concentrations increase or decrease with acute inflammation and tissue injury

albumin: the major serum protein; made in the liver

α_1-antitrypsin deficiency: an inherited disorder that causes defective hepatic production of α_1-antitrypsin, leading to defective α_1-antitrypsin activity in blood and lungs with deposition of enzyme in the liver

complement: part of the immune system that assists the antibodies and phagocytic cells in clearing pathogens

cryoglobulin: protein (usually immunoglobulins) that becomes insoluble at reduced temperatures

densitometer: a device that measures the optical density (absorbance) of a semitransparent material

electrophoresis: separation of macromolecules based on size, charge, and adsorptivity to the support medium using an electric field

free light chain: the variable part of the immunoglobulin that is not attached to a heavy chain; used to diagnose and monitor monoclonal immunoglobulin disorders

giardiasis: infection with *Giardia lamblia*

globulins: all serum proteins that are not albumin; determined by subtracting the serum albumin concentration from the total serum protein concentration

immunoglobulins: the γ globulins that are made by plasma cells in the bone marrow and confer humoral immunity

immunofixation electrophoresis: electrophoresis followed by application of specific anti-immunoglobulin antibodies in order to identify the immunoglobulin

monoclonal gammopathy: an abnormal proliferation of B cells leading to overproduction of immunoglobulins of a single clone

multiple myeloma: a cancer of plasma cells, characterized by interference with production of normal blood cells and by production of paraproteins

paraprotein: a monoclonal immunoglobulin or light chain

plasma cells: mature B lymphocytes that produce immunoglobulins; present predominantly in bone marrow

priapism: a sustained erection of the penis

κ and λ light chains: the small polypeptide subunits of an immunoglobulin

14.3 Background/significance

Although **multiple myeloma** accounts for <1% of all new cancer cases and <1% of all cancer related deaths worldwide [PMID21509679], qualitative and quantitative changes to serum proteins are also present in many other conditions, including acute and chronic inflammation, hepatic cirrhosis, nephrotic syndrome, congenital immunodeficiencies, and secondary (acquired) immunodeficiencies. An essential component for the diagnosis of these disorders is the analysis of serum proteins by **electrophoresis**. Thus, a firm understanding of serum proteins in health and disease is important.

14.4 Analytical approach to protein abnormalities

Total serum proteins and serum **albumin** are measured directly in clinical laboratories, usually using dye binding methods on a high volume automated analyzer. Serum **globulins** are inferred by subtraction (globulins = total protein – albumin). Serum proteins can be separated by electrophoresis. The resulting electrophoretic strip can then be scanned with a **densitometer**, the area under the peaks (representing different protein classes) can be integrated, and the percent of each peak's area to the total area can be calculated. By multiplying the percent

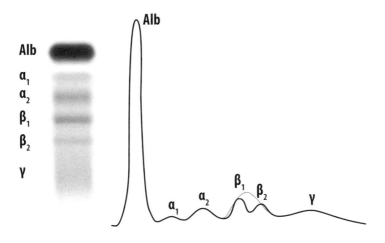

f14.1 Normal serum protein electrophoresis (lighter curve shows lack of split of β-globulin using non-high resolution/ conventional electrophoresis)

of each peak's area by the total protein concentration (determined as described above), the concentration of each protein class can be determined. The peaks present in an electropherogram **f14.1** are defined by the major protein(s) present: albumin, α_1 globulins, α_2 globulins, β globulins, and γ globulins. Note that high resolution electrophoresis splits the β globulins into β_1 (transferrin) and β_2 (C_3 complement) fractions, while conventional protein electrophoresis does not split the β globulin fraction **f14.1**.

Most of the serum proteins are made in the liver, with the exception of **immunoglobulins** (γ globulins), which are made by the **plasma cells** in the bone marrow.

Serum protein electrophoresis is most commonly performed for the diagnosis and monitoring of patients with multiple myeloma. Serum yielding an abnormal serum protein electrophoresis (eg, **monoclonal gammopathy**) can then be reanalyzed along with **immunofixation electrophoresis** to identify the specific immunoglobulin (IgG, IgA, IgM, IgE, IgD) **f14.2**. Quantification of serum **free light chains** is also commonly utilized for diagnosis and to monitor effectiveness of therapy for multiple myeloma patients. Elevation of the concentration of free light chains and abnormal ratios of **κ:λ light chains** indicate increased severity of disease.

14.4.1 Serum free light chain reference range

Free κ: 3.30-19.40 mg/L
Free λ: 5.71-26.30 mg/L
κ:λ: 0.26-1.65

ISBN 978-089189-6548

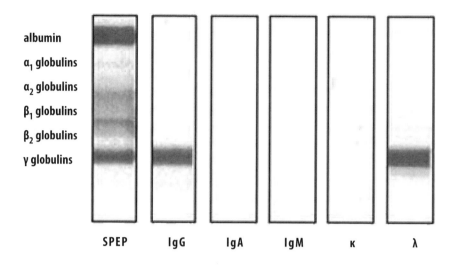

albumin

α₁ globulins

α₂ globulins

β₁ globulins

β₂ globulins

γ globulins

SPEP   IgG   IgA   IgM   κ   λ

f14.2 Abnormal serum protein electrophoresis with simultaneous immunofixation electrophoresis and identifying the monoclonal gammopathy as IgG with λ light chains.

Once the specific monoclonal gammopathy has been identified, it can be monitored by immunoassay for prognostic and therapeutic purposes. Periodic re-evaluation of the serum protein electrophoresis during therapy may also be helpful.

14.4.2 Serum total proteins & albumin reference range

Total proteins = 6.0-8.0 g/dL
Albumin = 3.5-5.2 g/dL

14.5 Other proteins

See **t14.1**

14.6 Acute phase reactants

Inflammation, tissue damage, and infection trigger the so called acute phase response, which results in changes in hepatic synthesis of **acute phase reactants** (proteins). Cytokines, including interleukin-6 (IL6), mediate the reaction [ISBN9781416061649]. The individual acute phase reactants have different time curves, which vary depending on the cause of the reaction. It should be noted that the acute phase response can also occur with chronic diseases such as cancer [PMID20155712].

t14.1 Most important plasma/serum proteins

Protein	Function	Elevated	Decreased
Transthyretin (0.02-0.04 g/dL; prealbumin)	binds T4 and vitamin A: retinol binding protein complex		hepatic damage, widespread tissue necrosis, negative acute phase response; malnutrition
Albumin (3.5-5.2 g/dL)			
Normal	oncotic pressure, transport and buffer, protein reserve; nonspecific carrier of many substances	dehydration; hemoconcentration	hepatic damage, negative acute phase response, protein losing conditions, malnutrition
Variant (bisalbuminemia)	no significant deviation from normal; genetic or acquired		
α_1 globulins (0.1-0.4 g/dL)			
α_1 lipoprotein (HDL; HDL cholesterol >60 mg/dL)	lipid transport	decreased risk of CHD	Tangier disease
α_1 antitrypsin (90-200 mg/dL)	protease inhibitor	acute inflammation; estrogens	hereditary emphysema, hepatic damage, severe nephrotic syndrome
α_1 antichymotrypsin (30-60 mg/dL)	inhibits chymotrypsin	acute inflammation	
Transcortin (1.5-2.0 mg/dL)	binds cortisol	pregnancy, estrogens, oral contraceptives	
α_1 acid glycoprotein (orosomucoid; 47-125 mg/dL)	binds drugs	acute inflammation	
Thyroxine binding globulin (1.3-3.0 mg/dL)	binds T4, T3	pregnancy, administration of estrogens, hereditary	hereditary
α_2 globulins (0.6-1.0 g/dL)			
Ceruloplasmin (15-45 mg/dL)	copper containing protein	pregnancy, administration of estrogen, acute inflammation	Wilson disease (hepatolenticular degeneration), nephrotic syndrome
α_2 macroglobulin (125-410 mg/dL)	protease inhibitor	nephrotic syndrome, estrogens	
Haptoglobin (30-200 mg/dL)	binds free hemoglobin	acute inflammation	in vivo hemolysis
Pre β lipoprotein (VLDL; 2-30 mg/dL)	lipid transport, especially triglycerides	hyperlipidemia	
C4 complement (10-40 mg/dL)	complement	acute inflammation	

t14.1 Most important plasma/serum proteins (continued)

Protein	Function	Elevated	Decreased
β globulins (0.6-1.3 g/dL)			
Transferrin (200-360 mg/dL)	binds iron	iron deficiency anemia, pregnancy, estrogens	chronic liver disease, nephrotic syndrome, malignancies, negative acute phase response, malnutrition
β lipoprotein (LDL; <100 mg/dL)	lipid transport especially cholesterol	hyperlipidemias	
Properdin (20-51 mg/dL)	involved in bactericidal, virus neutralizing reactions		infections, infectious mononucleosis, leukemia, paroxysmal nocturnal hemoglobinuria
C3 component (90-180 mg/dL)	complement	acute inflammation, biliary obstruction	genetic deficiency
Hemopexin (50-115 mg/dL)	binds heme (not hemoglobin)	acute inflammation	hemolytic anemia
β globulin interference Hemoglobin Fibrinogen		specimen hemolyzed specimen not clotted (patient on heparin therapy) or plasma used for electrophoresis, acute inflammation	
γ globulins (0.7-1.5 g/dL)			
Lysozyme (0.9-1.7 mg/dL)	bacterial wall lysis	myelomonocytic leukemias	
C reactive protein (<5mg/L)	synthesized by liver; initiated by antigens	acute inflammation, trauma, bacteria	
Immunoglobulins			
IgA (70-400 mg/dL; between β & γ)	surface immunity	gammopathies (monoclonal, oligoclonal, polyclonal)	selective deficiencies (agammagloblinemia, hypogammaglobu-linemia)
IgM (40-230 mg/dL; mostly in β)	early humoral immunity		
IgG (700-1600 mg/dL; in γ)	late humoral immunity (anamnestic)		
IgD (0-15 mg/dL; between β and γ)	B cell antigen receptor		
IgE (<24 ug/dL; between β & γ)	mast cell binding, histamine release	allergic disorders	

*Reference ranges are for adults; some low concentration proteins are not detectable with electrophoresis (eg, IgD and IgE)

Positive acute phase reactants (proteins that are increased in the acute phase response) include the following [ISBN9781416061649]:

- α_1 globulins
  - α_1-antitrypsin (protease inhibitor protecting tissues from lysosomal enzymes)
  - α_1 acid glycoprotein (binder of small molecules, including drugs)
  - α_1-antichymotrypsin (inhibits proteases; binds prostate specific antigen)
- α_2 globulins
  - haptoglobin (binds free hemoglobin)
  - ceruloplasmin (binds copper)
  - C_4 complement (a major component of the complement system)
- β globulins
  - fibrinogen (coagulation factor I, which is converted to fibrin during clot formation)
  - C_3 complement (a major component of the complement system)
  - hemopexin (binds heme)
- γ globulins
  - C reactive protein (CRP; assists complement binding to foreign and damaged cells and enhances phagocytosis by macrophages)

Negative acute phase reactants (proteins that are decreased in the acute phase response) include the following [ISBN9781416061649]: albumin, transthyretin (formerly called prealbumin; binds thyroxine and retinol binding protein), and transferrin (a β globulin that binds iron).

Because some acute phase reactants increase during the acute phase response while others decrease, the total serum protein concentration may show only little change.

Both CRP and the erythrocyte sedimentation rate (ESR) are elevated with inflammation. However, CRP is very sensitive to short term changes in inflammation, and is considered more accurate than the ESR as an indicator of inflammation since the ESR is influenced by age, sex, and anemia among other factors. In addition, CRP measurements are more easily standardized than are ESR measurements, which depend on reading the millimeter fall in erythrocytes over 1 hour [PMID24187153]. The ESR is elevated in inflammation largely due to the elevation of fibrinogen (an acute phase protein), but the ESR can also be increased with elevated immunoglobulins and **paraproteins**, all of which are positively charged at physiologic pH. These positively charged proteins neutralize the negative surface charge of the erythrocytes, causing them to stack together, thereby increasing the rate of fall **f14.3**. The stacking of erythrocytes can also be observed in a peripheral smear ("rouleax formation") [PMID18782813].

The most important plasma/serum proteins are summarized in **t14.1**.

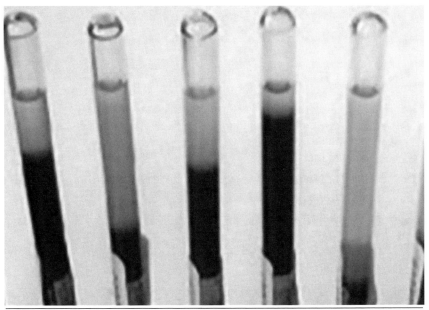

f14.3 Measurement of erythrocyte sedimentation rate (ESR; reference range 0-22 mm/hr for men, 0-29 mm/hr for women)

14.7 Abnormalities of γ globulins

14.7.1 Decreased γ globulins

14.7.1.1 Congenital immunodeficiencies

The congenital immunodeficiencies include the following selective immunoglobulin deficiencies:

➤ selective IgA deficiency is the most common (1:700 incidence); individuals with this disorder have increased incidence of autoimmune diseases and allergies; usually the IgM is increased

➤ combined IgA and IgG deficiency results in recurrent bacterial infection

➤ in combined IgA and IgM deficiency, **giardiasis** is common

➤ IgG deficiency leads to recurrent bacterial infection

➤ IgM deficiency results in increased susceptibility to autoimmune disorders [ISBN9781416061649]

Another congenital immunodeficiency is infantile X linked (Bruton) agammaglobulinemia. Patients with this disorder are usually healthy in the newborn period but have onset of recurrent bacterial infections between 3 and 18 months of age [PMID19302039].

Patients with the so called "hyper IgM syndromes" exhibit low serum IgG, IgA, and IgE concentrations with either normal (paradoxically) or elevated IgM concentrations. They have recurrent bacterial infections [PMID19302039].

Severe combined immunodeficiency (SCID) is a group of disorders resulting in lack of both cellular and humoral immunity. Infants with these disorders have recurrent life threatening infections, often fungal or viral [ISBN9781416061649].

The disorders can be either X linked (seen in males) or autosomal. Afflicted individuals have very low or absent T lymphocytes and may or may not have B lymphocytes.

14.7.1.2 Secondary (acquired) immunodeficiencies

These disorders can result from <u>loss of immunoglobulins</u> (eg, nephrotic syndrome, burns, protein losing intestinal disorders) and from <u>defective synthesis</u> (eg, multiple myeloma, lymphoma, chronic lymphocytic leukemia, neonatal immaturity with delay in immunoglobulin synthesis). With defective synthesis, the IgM declines first, followed by IgA, and then IgG [ISBN9781416061649].

14.7.2 Increased γ globulins

14.7.2.1 Polyclonal hypergammaglobulinemia

Polyclonal hypergammaglobulinemia can be seen with <u>chronic infection</u> (IgA with skin, gut, respiratory, and renal infection; IgM with viral and bloodstream parasites), <u>primary biliary cirrhosis</u> (IgM), <u>chronic active hepatitis</u> (IgG and sometimes IgM), <u>hepatic cirrhosis</u> (IgA, due to its decreased catabolism, and sometimes IgG, causing the so called βγ bridging), and <u>intrauterine infection</u> (IgM) [ISBN9781416061649].

14.7.2.2 Monoclonal immunoglobulinopathies (multiple myeloma)

These disorders result from overproduction of immunoglobulin molecules with a single defined amino acid sequence, often resulting in the appearance of a discrete band (M spike, M protein, monoclonal gammopathy) in the serum protein electrophoresis. These proteins are termed **paraproteins** and can be monomers, polymers, immunoglobulin heavy chains, immunoglobulin light chains, or even fragments of immunoglobulins. Most monoclonal gammopathies are IgG (50%), IgA (25%), or free light chains only (20%) [ISBN9781416061649].

Due to its high molecular weight, the IgM monoclonal gammopathy results in a significant increase in serum viscosity, causing blindness, hypertension, and **priapism** (so called Waldenström macroglobulinemia). IgM can also behave as a **cryoglobulin**, becoming less soluble when exposed to lower temperatures [ISBN9781416061649].

14.7.2.3 Monoclonal gammopathies of undetermined significance (MGUS)

Up to 25% of monoclonal gammopathies may be benign and are termed *monoclonal gammopathies of undetermined significance* (MGUS). They increase in frequency with age of the patient (3% of individuals over 70 years of age have MGUS) and are associated with increased risk for developing multiple myeloma (1% of patients with MGUS convert to multiple myeloma per year; 30% after 25 years) [ISBN9781416061649, PMID20713974]. Thus, patients with MGUS are closely monitored.

Patients with multiple myeloma frequently have what comprises the acronym <u>CRAB</u>: hypercalcemia (C), renal failure (R) due to immunoglobulin and/or light chain nephropathy, anemia (A), and lytic lesions of bone (B) [PMID21156463].

In contrast, patients with MGUS generally are asymptomatic, have <3 g/dL of M protein in the serum, have no or only small amounts of light chains in the urine, have <10% plasma cells in the bone marrow, and do not manifest the features of CRAB [PMID20713974, PMID16110026].

14.8 Serum protein electrophoretic patterns in health & disease

The most common serum protein electrophoretic patterns are shown in **f14.4-f14.11**. It should be noted that, in some institutions, the electropherogram itself is not provided with the laboratory report, and instead, only the concentration of each protein fraction is reported.

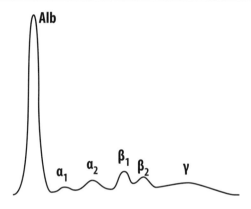

f14.4 Normal pattern

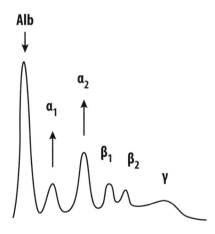

f14.5 Acute inflammation (increase in α_1 globulins due to α_1 antitrypsin; increase in α_2 globulins due to haptoglobin; decrease in albumin)

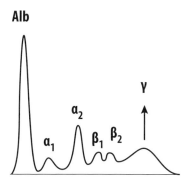

f14.6 Chronic inflammation (diffuse polyclonal increase in γ globulins)

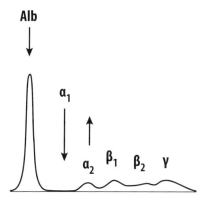

f14.7 α₁ antitrypsin deficiency (decrease in the α₁ globulin fraction; the increase in the α₂ globulin fraction and the decrease in the albumin fraction suggest an acute inflammatory response, perhaps due to pulmonary infection)

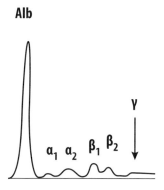

f14.8 Agammaglobulinemia (immunodeficiency state); note the complete absence of γ globulins

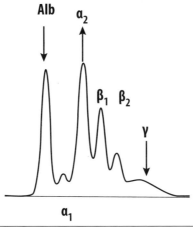

f14.9 Nephrotic syndrome (decrease in albumin, increase in α_2 globulins due to α_2 macroglobulin and lipoproteins, decrease in γ globulins)

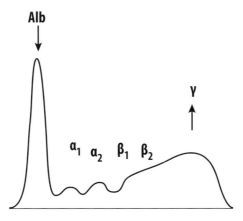

f14.10 Hepatic cirrhosis (decrease in albumin and diffuse increase in immunoglobulins; βγ bridging due to decreased catabolism of IgA)

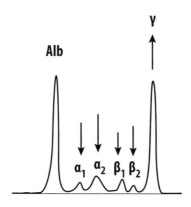

f14.11 Monoclonal protein in γ globulin region with concurrent decrease in the other immunoglobulins

14.9 References

14.9.1 Journals

PMID16110026 Kumar S, Rajkumar SV, Kyle RA et al [2005] Prognostic value of circulating plasma cells in monoclonal gammopathy of undetermined significance. *J Clin Oncol* 33:5668-74

PMID18782813 Raijmakers MTM, Kuijper PHM, Bakkeren DL et al [2008] The effect of paraproteins on the erythrocyte sedimentation rate: a comparison between the StarrSed and TEST 1. *Ann Clin Biochem* 45:593-7

PMID19302039 Conley ME, Dobbs AK, Farmer DM et al [2009] Primary B cell immunodeficiencies: comparisons and contrasts. *Ann Rev Immunol* 27:199-227

PMID20155712 Pang WW, Abdul-Rahman PS, Wan-Ibrahim WI et al [2010] Can the acute-phase reactant proteins be used as cancer biomarkers? *Int J Biological Markers* 25: 1-11

PMID20713974 Wadhera RK, Rajkumar SV [2010] Prevalence of monoclonal gammopathy of undetermined significance: a systematic review. *Mayo Clin Proc* 85:933-42

PMID21156463 Talamo G, Farooq U, Zangari M et al [2010] Beyond the CRAB symptoms: a study of presenting clinical manifestations of multiple myeloma. *Clin Lymphoma Myeloma Leuk* 10: 464-8

PMID21509679 Becker N [2011] Epidemiology of multiple myeloma. *Recent Results in Cancer Research* 183:25-35

Gaujoux-Viala C [2013] C-reactive protein vs erythrocyte sedimentation rate in estimating the 28-join disease activity score. *J Rheumatol* 40:1785-7

14.9.2 Books

ISBN9781416061649 Hortin GL [2013] Amino acids, peptides, and proteins. In: Burtis CA, Ashwood ER, Bruns DE, ed. *Tietz Textbook of Clinical Chemistry and Molecular Diagnostics*, 5e. Elsevier Saunders, 509-64

14.10 Clinical cases

(NOTE: These clinical cases utilize conventional, non-high resolution electrophoresis—no split of the β globulin fraction)

14.10.1 Case 1

An 84-year-old female was seen in the emergency department after experiencing the sudden onset of severe pain in the right clavicular region. She had been in good health and denied falling or having any trauma. The physical examination was unremarkable except for exquisite tenderness over her right clavicle. She denied back pain. Chest X rays revealed a fracture of the right clavicle and a compression fracture of a lower thoracic vertebra. Skeletal X rays showed multiple cortical "punched out" lesions.

The complete blood count showed anemia. A serum chemistry panel showed sodium 139 mMol/L (mEq/L), potassium 5.8 mMol/L (mEq/L), chloride 95 mMol/L (mEq/L), HCO_3^- 20 mMol/L (mEq/L), urea-N 43 mg/dL, and creatinine 4.8 mg/dL

Urinalysis: specific gravity 1.030; protein 3+; 0-1 WBC/HPF; 0-1 RBC/HPF

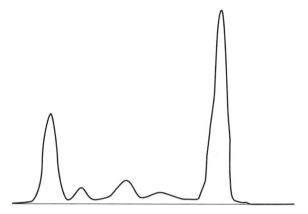

Serum protein electrophoresis results: total protein = 10.4 g/dL; albumin = 2.6 g/dL; globulins (g/dL): α_1 =0.6; α_2 = 1.2; β= 0.7; γ= 5.3

14.10.1.1 Question

What is the most probable explanation for these findings?

14.10.2 Case 2

A 66-year-old male was seen in clinic for a biopsy of his neck mass. On physical examination, in addition to the neck mass, there was a palpable nodule on the right side of the thyroid gland, as well as several palpable right supraclavicular lymph nodes.

The complete blood count showed anemia. The peripheral blood smear showed marked rouleaux formation of the red blood cells. The erythrocyte sedimentation rate (ESR) was 147 mm/hour. The serum viscosity was 5.0 (reference range: 1.4-1.8). Urinalysis was normal, except for 2+ proteinuria.

Biopsy of the thyroid nodule showed follicular adenoma, and biopsy of the neck mass revealed a non-Hodgkin lymphoma.

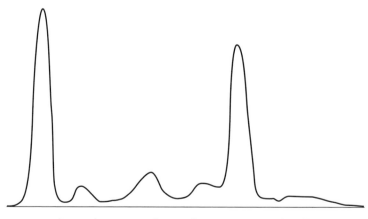

Serum protein electrophoresis results: total protein = 8.3 g/dL; albumin = 2.9 g/dL; globulins (g/dL): α_1 =0.4; α_2 = 1.1; β = 0.7; γ = 3.2

14.10.2.1 Question

What is the most probable explanation for these findings?

14.10.3 Case 3

An 84-year-old male was admitted to the hospital due to complications from advanced chronic obstructive pulmonary disease. Skeletal X rays revealed diffuse areas of patchy demineralization that could represent osteoporosis or early neoplastic disease.

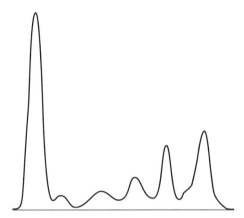

Serum protein electrophoresis results: total protein = 10.4 g/dL; albumin = 3.6 g/dL; globulins (g/dL): α_1 = 0.3; α_2 = 0.8; β = 0.9; γ = 4.8

14.10.3.1 Question

What is the most probable explanation for these findings?

14.10.4 Case 4

A 49-year-old female was admitted to the hospital because of shortness of breath and a massively distended abdomen. She is a chronic alcoholic with previous admissions related to ascites. Her shortness of breath is so severe that she cannot walk more than a half block. She is on a low sodium diet. Physical examination reveals decreased breath sounds at the left base of the chest. She has 3+ edema from her ankles to the abdomen.

Her laboratory studies showed the following: sodium 127 mMol/L (mEq/L), potassium 3.1 mMol/L (mEq/L), chloride 107 mMol/L (mEq/L), bicarbonate 19 mMol/L (mEq/L), and calcium 7.8 mg/dL. The complete blood count showed a white blood cell count of 18,300/mm^3. The platelet count was 110,000/mm^3. Her international normalized ratio (INR) for prothrombin time was 2.9, and her partial thromboplastin time (PTT) was 38.3 seconds (control 31.1 seconds). Her arterial blood gases on room air were pO$_2$ 54 mmHg, pCO$_2$ 29 mmHg, and pH 7.51.

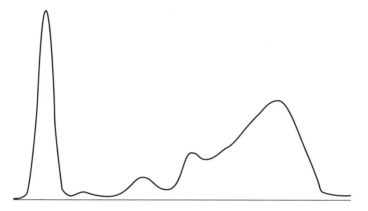

Serum protein electrophoresis results: total protein = 8.0 g/dL; albumin = 2.6 g/dL; globulins (g/dL): $\alpha_1 = 0.3$; $\alpha_2 = 0.5$; $\beta = 0.9$; $\gamma = 3.7$

14.10.4.1 Question

What is the most probable explanation for these findings?

14.10.5 Case 5

A 23-year-old male who abuses intravenous drugs experienced the onset of right lower quadrant pain 1 year ago. He was hospitalized, and a workup for acute appendicitis was negative. However, an elevated serum aspartate aminotransferase (AST 220 U/L) and alanine aminotransferase (ALT 401 U/L) were noted along with a platelet count of 86,000/mm^3. Due to significant splenomegaly and continued low platelet count, his spleen was removed. Now (1 year later) he presents with fever, muscle aches, jaundice, and the following laboratory data: AST 1,460 U/L, ALT 2,351 U/L, total bilirubin 7.9 mg/dL, conjugated bilirubin 4.7 mg/dL, and platelets 220,000/mm^3.

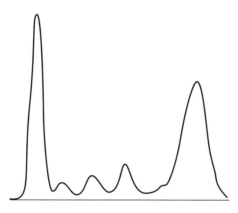

Serum protein electrophoresis results: total protein = 9.2 g/dL; albumin = 3.2 g/dL; globulins (g/dL): $\alpha_1 = 0.3$; $\alpha_2 = 0.6$; $\beta = 0.8$; $\gamma = 4.3$

14.10.5.1 Question

What is the most probable explanation for these findings?

14.10.6 Case 6

A 57-year-old male underwent resection of colorectal adenocarcinoma 1 year ago. Over the ensuing year the man's general condition has deteriorated, and he presents now with the chief complaint of back pain. A bone scan demonstrates numerous skeletal lesions throughout the ribs, long bones, spine, and skull.

A complete blood count shows anemia. The serum aminotransferases were normal, but an alkaline phosphatase was 935 U/L.

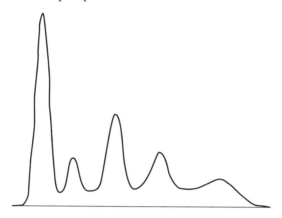

Serum protein electrophoresis results: total protein = 7.9 g/dL; albumin = 2.8 g/dL; globulins (g/dL): α_1=0.8; α_2 = 1.7; β = 1.4; γ = 1.2

14.10.6.1 Question

What is the most probable explanation for these findings?

14.10.7 Case 7

An 18-year-old male in a third world country developed bilateral leg swelling, which was treated with diuretics and steroids without response. Physical examination reveals periorbital edema, pedal edema, and rales in both lung fields.

Laboratory data show serum cholesterol 440 mg/dL, triglycerides 225 mg/dL, serum creatinine 1.2 mg/dL, and urea-N 20 mg/dL.

The urinalysis shows specific gravity 1.042, 4+ protein, and large numbers of hyaline and granular casts.

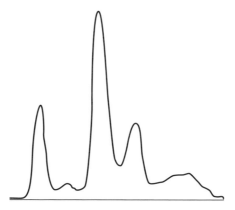

Serum protein electrophoresis results: total protein = 4.6 g/dL; albumin = 0.8 g/dL; globulins (g/dL): α_1 = 0.2; α_2 = 2.0; β = 0.9; γ = 0.7

14.10.7.1 Question

What is the most probable explanation for these findings?

14.10.8 Case 8

A 34-year-old male has had a 5 year history of chronic obstructive pulmonary disease sufficiently severe as to prevent him from working. He has smoked 2 packs of cigarettes per day for 16 years. He has a chronic cough productive of green, blood streaked sputum. Physical examination reveals a hyperresonant chest and scattered wheezes. The chest X ray shows hyperinflation of the lungs consistent with emphysema.

Arterial blood gases showed pO_2 51 mmHg, pCO_2 34 mmHg, and pH 7.43 on room air.

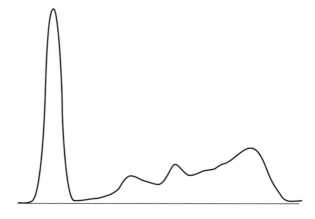

Serum protein electrophoresis results: total protein = 6.0 g/dL; albumin = 2.3 g/dL; globulins (g/dL): α_1 = 0.2; α_2 = 0.7; β = 0.7; γ = 2.1

14.10.8.1 Question

What is the most probable explanation for these findings?

14.10.9 **Case 9**

A 43-year-old male sought treatment for masses in his neck, axilla, and groin 3 years ago. At that time his white blood cell count was 115,000/mm^3 with 89% lymphocytes. He received total body irradiation and chemotherapy for his lymphoma. Because of his weakened condition, he was admitted for hospice care. His white count was 64,000/mm^3 (99% lymphocytes).

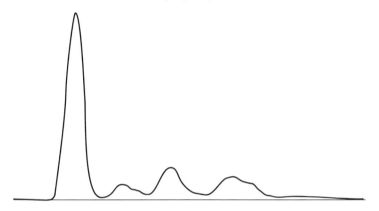

Serum protein electrophoresis results: total protein = 5.1 g/dL; albumin = 3.2 g/dL; globulins (g/dL): α_1=0.3; α_2 = 0.7; β = 0.8; γ = 0.1

14.10.9.1 Question

What is the most probable explanation for these findings?

14.10.10 Clinical case answers

14.10.10.1 Case 1 answer

The serum protein electropherogram suggests a monoclonal gammopathy in the γ globulin region. Upon immunofixation electrophoresis, this was identified as an IgG with κ light chains. Coupled with the radiographic findings of cortical lytic lesions, this confirms multiple myeloma. The clavicular fracture is likely a pathologic fracture due to lytic lesions.

The albumin is decreased due to renal loss from kidney damage from the myeloma. The albumin loss is reflected in the proteinuria and elevated specific gravity noted on urinalysis. The calculated anion gap of 35 and the low bicarbonate suggest metabolic acidosis due to the renal failure. The elevated serum urea-N, creatinine, and potassium are also due to the renal failure. A urea-N:creatinine ratio <10 is consistent with chronic protein loss into the urine since there is less protein to yield amino acids, which, upon deamination, would otherwise be converted into urea.

The slight increase in the α_1 and α_2 globulins may reflect inflammation due to the clavicular fracture. The total protein concentration is elevated due to the large concentration of monoclonal protein in the γ globulin region.

14.10.10.2 Case 2 answer

The serum protein electropherogram suggests a monoclonal gammopathy between the β and the γ globulin regions. Immunofixation electrophoresis identified it as IgM. Together with rouleaux formation of the red cells and the high serum viscosity, this suggests Waldenström macroglobulinemia. The IgM produces the high viscosity and rouleaux formation. The erythrocyte sedimentation rate is increased due to anemia and the presence of IgM, which neutralizes the negative charge on the red cells. The increase in the γ globulin fraction is due to the IgM. The modestly low albumin may be due to renal loss since the urinalysis demonstrated proteinuria.

14.10.10.3 Case 3 answer

The serum protein electropherogram suggests 2 monoclonal gammopathies in the γ globulin region. Immunofixation electrophoresis identified these as IgG and IgA with no light chains. The X rays suggest the possibility of lytic lesions. The chronic obstructive pulmonary disease is unrelated. The patient has multiple myeloma with 2 M proteins.

14.10.10.4 Case 4 answer

The serum protein electropherogram shows βγ bridging, suggestive of hepatic cirrhosis (due to decreased catabolism of IgA). The combination of low serum bicarbonate, low pCO_2, and high pH indicate respiratory alkalosis due to hyperventilation caused by the massive ascites not permitting full movement of the diaphragms. The serum calcium is low due to the low serum albumin, caused by the failure of the diseased liver to synthesize albumin. The calcium would be corrected to the following: $(4.0-2.6)0.8 + 7.8 = 8.9$ mg/dL. The sodium is likely low due to secondary hyperaldosteronism caused by poor renal perfusion (secondary to her ascites and edema), which stimulates the juxtaglomerular cells to secrete renin, which, in turn, stimulates production of aldosterone and leads to retention of sodium and water. Antidiuretic hormone is also secreted in response. The sodium is thus diluted so that the extracellular (serum) sodium is low while the total body sodium is high. In addition, the patient is on a low sodium diet. Secondary hyperaldosteronism causes loss of potassium into the urine. In addition, alcoholics are often malnourished, also contributing to the observed hypokalemia. The platelet count is low due to the toxic effect of alcohol on bone marrow and possibly due to sequestration in the spleen if there is hepatosplenomegaly (often seen in alcoholics). The INR and PTT are elevated due to failed production of blood coagulation factors by the diseased liver. The elevated white blood cell count suggests infection, perhaps in the peritoneum since peritoneal fluid is excellent medium for bacterial growth. The patient's prior admissions for ascites probably involved paracentesis, at which time introduction of bacteria may have occurred. The decreased breath sounds at the left base of the chest suggest pulmonary edema.

14.10.10.5 Case 5 answer

The serum protein electropherogram suggests chronic inflammation (polyclonal hypergammaglobulinemia). The history suggests chronic active hepatitis, given the intravenous drug use of the patient, the elevated total and conjugated bilirubin, and the De Ritis ratio <1. The fact that the liver is conjugating bilirubin suggests that the disease has not progressed to endstage at this time. Hepatitis B and C antigen and antibodies should be ordered.

14.10.10.6 Case 6 answer

The serum protein electropherogram suggests acute inflammation (increased α_1 and α_2 globulins and decreased albumin). The serum alkaline phosphatase is increased due to bone metastasis by the cancer. The acute inflammation is due to metastatic invasion of tissues.

14.10.10.7 Case 7 answer

The serum protein electropherogram suggests nephrotic syndrome (low albumin due to renal loss, high α_2 globulin due to overproduction of α_2 macroglobulin and low density lipoproteins in attempt to restore oncotic pressure). The etiology for the nephrotic syndrome is likely filiriasis (elephantiasis). The cholesterol and triglycerides are elevated due to the overproduction of lipoproteins in attempt to preserve oncotic pressure. The proteinuria reflects the massive loss of albumin into the urine.

14.10.10.8 Case 8 answer

The serum protein electropherogram suggests diminished α_1 globulins although the concentration (0.2 g/dL) is within the reference range. Close examination of the electropherogram suggests that the concentration is due to an artifact of integration (rising baseline). $\beta\gamma$ bridging also present suggests hepatic cirrhosis. This combination of electrophoretic abnormalities along with the clinical history of chronic obstructive pulmonary disease suggests α_1-antitrypsin deficiency. In this congenital condition, α_1-antitrypsin (a protease inhibitor) is not released adequately from the liver, where it is synthesized. The consequent decreased α_1-antitrypsin activity in blood and lung results in the lung not being protected from infection/inflammation, leading to chronic obstructive pulmonary disease. The inadequate release of α_1-antitrypsin from liver may, in many cases, lead to hepatocyte damage and cirrhosis. The low serum albumin is a reflection of this. The altered blood gases reflect difficulty in oxygenation and suggest mild hyperventilation. Measurement of α_1-antitrypsin would be helpful in confirming the diagnosis. Genetic studies can identify whether 1 or 2 copies of the defective allele are present.

14.10.10.9 Case 9 answer

The serum protein electropherogram suggests severe hypogammaglobulinemia likely due to the irradiation and chemotherapy as well as neoplastic infiltration of the bone marrow, thereby reducing production of the immunoglobulins.

chapter 15

Reproductive clinical chemistry

15.1 Objectives

At the end of this session, the learner should be able to

➤ describe the rise and fall of serum human chorionic gonadotropin (hCG) during pregnancy

➤ describe the sensitivity of urine pregnancy tests

➤ describe the sensitivity of serum hCG in diagnosing normal pregnancy

➤ describe the serum hCG concentration changes that occur in normal and ectopic pregnancies

➤ identify the characteristics of normal semen

➤ describe the components of semen analysis

➤ discuss the use of SP10 in the workup of male infertility

➤ describe changes in amniotic fluid volume and chemical composition during pregnancy

➤ discuss the approach to determining fetal lung maturity, including the lecithin:sphingomyelin (L:S) ratio and the lamellar body count in amniotic fluid

➤ describe the use and interpretation of the amniotic fluid ΔOD_{450} in monitoring hemolytic disease of the newborn

➤ discuss the use of fetal fibronectin in monitoring for preterm birth

➤ discuss the use of placental α macroglobulin 1 in monitoring for premature rupture of the membranes

15.2 Key terms

alloimmunization: an immune response to foreign antigens (alloantigens) from members of the same species

alveolar cells: cells lining the air sacs of the lungs

amniocentesis: the process of collecting amniotic fluid

amniotic fluid: substance (mostly fetal urine) that protects the developing fetus

blastocyst: a thin walled hollow structure in early embryonic development containing the inner cell mass from which the embryo develops

decidua: the uterine lining during pregnancy

ectopic pregnancy: a pregnancy in which the embryo develops outside the uterus (eg, fallopian tube)

embryo: a human organism during the period from fertilization of the ovum to the start of the third month of pregnancy

erythroblastosis fetalis: a fetal disease caused by maternal antibody mediated destruction of fetal erythrocytes (also called hemolytic disease of the newborn)

gestation: length of pregnancy measured in weeks from the first day of the last menstrual period

gestational trophoblastic disease: pregnancy related tumors (eg, choriocarcinoma, hydatidiform mole) resulting from uncontrolled proliferation of trophoblasts

human chorionic gonadotropin: a hormone produced by the human placenta and used to maintain pregnancy

immunochromatography: an analytical technique combining chromatography with immunoassay

isoform: a different form/conformation of a protein

kernicterus: brain damage caused by deposition of unconjugated bilirubin in basal ganglia and brain stem nuclei

meconium: the earliest stool of an infant

pulmonary surfactant: a surface active phospholipoprotein elaborated by the type II fetal alveolar cells

respiratory distress syndrome: a disease manifested in premature infants due to lack of sufficient lung surfactant

trophoblast: cells forming the outer layer of the blastocyst

15.3 Background/significance

Laboratory testing for pregnancy has become so commonplace that it is now available to the public in over the counter kits. Going beyond confirmation of pregnancy, the clinical laboratory plays an important role in the diagnosis of male infertility through semen analysis, in the determination and monitoring of fetal lung maturity (FLM) and hemolytic disease of the newborn through analysis of **amniotic fluid**, and in the monitoring of preterm birth and premature rupture of the membranes through analysis of cervicovaginal secretions.

15.4 Pregnancy testing

Pregnancy testing is based on the detection of **human chorionic gonadotropin** (hCG), a peptide glycoprotein hormone synthesized by the placenta during pregnancy. Both the qualitative (urine) and quantitative (serum) tests are "sandwich" immunoassays that detect some or all of the hCG **isoforms**. The analytic variability among assays is considerable, depending on different antibody specificities for the intact hCG molecule, its α and β subunits, and other variants of hCG. Thus, in monitoring patients sequentially, the same assay should be used. Typically a combination of monoclonal antibodies is used in the assays in order to enhance sensitivity and specificity [ISBN9781594251023].

Most over the counter and point of care assays utilize **immunochromatography** to detect hCG in urine. The sensitivity of most of the urine assays is sufficient (50 IU/L) to detect pregnancy by the time of the first missed menses. It should be noted that nonpregnancy related elevations can be noted with **gestational trophoblastic disease** [ISBN9781594251023].

In the clinical laboratory, hCG can be detected in serum (>5 IU/L) 8-11 days after conception and becomes detectable in urine 1-3 days after a positive serum test [ISBN9781416061649a]. The concentration of hCG in serum doubles every 1.5 days for the first 5 weeks of pregnancy, after which it doubles every 40-48 hours, peaking at ~100,000 IU/L between 8 and 11 weeks' **gestation**. The concentrations then decrease in the second and third trimesters of pregnancy, remaining at ~10,000 IU/L until delivery [ISBN9781594251023].

Ectopic pregnancy is an extrauterine pregnancy (~2% of all pregnancies), and is characterized by abdominal cramping, vaginal bleeding, and pain. In this condition, ultrasound results are correlated with serial serum hCG measurements. In normal pregnancy, the serum hCG increases by at least 53% in 2 days, while in ectopic pregnancy, the increase is usually <50% in 2 days. Those pregnancies undergoing spontaneous abortion show a decrease of hCG of at least 20% in 2 days [ISBN9781594251023].

15.4.1 Serum human chorionic gonadotropin reference range
Nonpregnant women: <6 IU/L
Pregnant women: >10 IU/L
Men: <3 IU/L

15.5 Semen analysis
The analysis of semen is an important part of the evaluation of male fertility. The specimen should be submitted to the laboratory within 1 hour of collection. Abstinence from ejaculation for 2-10 days is recommended (shorter periods result in lower sperm counts and reduced volume, while longer periods result in an increase in immotile forms). If semen analysis is normal, it is unlikely that further laboratory testing will be helpful. If it is abnormal, the test should be repeated in ~6 weeks [ISBN9781416061649b].

Semen analysis includes measurement of volume, pH, sperm count, motility, and morphology. A newer approach to evaluation of male infertility uses a monoclonal antibody to sperm protein SP10. This test, available as an over the counter kit, is also used to assess completeness of vasectomy and is considered by some to be equivalent to a sperm count [ISBN9781416061649b].

15.5.1 Semen reference ranges
The World Health Organization has established the following reference ranges for human semen [ISBN9780443045141, ISBN9781416061649b]:

➢ ejaculate volume: >2 mL

➢ pH: 7.2-8.0

➢ sperm count: >20 million/mL (>40 million/ejaculate volume)

➢ motility: >50% forward progression within 60 minutes of ejaculation (viewed on a microscope stage that is heated to body temperature)

➢ morphology: >30% normal forms (Pap stain)

15.6 Laboratory examination of amniotic fluid

In the early stages of gestation, **amniotic fluid** is mostly a dialysate of maternal serum. Later, with development of the kidneys, fetal urine contributes to the composition. The volume of amniotic fluid increases until the 34th week of pregnancy and declines after that. At 16 weeks, it is only 200-300 mL, while at 34 weeks, it ranges broadly from 300 mL to 2,000 mL. At term, it is exchanged at a rate of ~60 mL/hr, resulting in complete exchange of fluid ~2× per day. Toward the end of gestation, the concentration of urea, creatinine, and uric acid increase while the concentration of most other solutes decreases [ISBN9781416061649a].

Analysis of amniotic fluid is primarily directed toward assessment of FLM and the presence and severity of **erythroblastosis fetalis** (hemolytic disease of the newborn). Amniotic fluid is collected by **amniocentesis** using ultrasound guidance.

15.6.1 Tests for fetal lung maturity

During the first 2 trimesters of pregnancy, the amniotic fluid has little **pulmonary surfactant**. However, during the last trimester, the type II **alveolar cells** secrete large quantities of surfactant in order to prepare the fetus for breathing air instead of fluid. With FLM, increases in surfactant based phospholipids such as lecithin occur, so that the ratio of lecithin (L) to nonlung based lipids such as sphingomyelin (S) becomes >2.0. A so called L:S ratio of >2.0 indicates FLM. The ratio can be determined by extraction, thin layer chromatography, and densitometry, but this is very time consuming. Also, contamination with blood and/or **meconium** perturbs the measurement [ISBN9781416061649a].

Beginning at ~28 weeks of gestation, the type II alveolar cells package and store the surfactant into platelet sized (1-5 μm) lamellar bodies, which consist of 90% phospholipids and 10% surfactant. The lamellar body count is a sensitive and specific method used by many laboratories for evaluating FLM. Counts are performed on whole blood counters [ISBN9781594251023]. If the count is low, then the L:S ratio is determined. Delivery of infants without FLM may result in development of **respiratory distress syndrome**.

Other tests such as phosphatidylglycerol (PG; the last surfactant to be produced during fetal lung development) and measurement of microviscosity of amniotic fluid are no longer commonly used in the assessment of FLM.

15.6.1.1 Fetal lung maturity reference ranges

Lamellar body count: >50,000/mm³ indicates FLM
L:S ratio: >2.0 indicates FLM

15.6.2 Diagnosis & monitoring of erythroblastosis fetalis

Alloimmunization during pregnancy results from production of maternal antibodies to fetal antigens. This is most pronounced when the Rh(D) antigen is involved, as might occur with an Rh(D)+ father and an Rh(D)− mother, resulting in a fetus that is Rh(D)+. This leads to **erythroblastosis fetalis**, or hemolytic disease of the newborn. As fetal hemolysis occurs, the hemoglobin is catabolized to bilirubin, which can be detected in the amniotic fluid. Since the fetus is incapable of conjugating bilirubin, the bilirubin in amniotic fluid is unconjugated

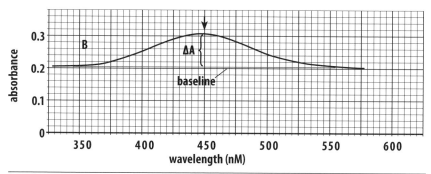

f15.1 Absorption spectrum of amniotic fluid. The arrow depicts bilirubin absorption, and the ΔA (ΔOD450) is the difference between the tangent baseline absorption and the bilirubin absorption; in this example, the ΔA is 0.31 − 0.21 = 0.10

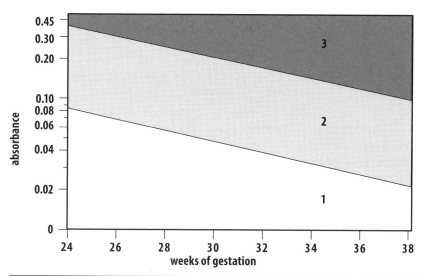

f15.2 The Liley prognostication chart showing the 3 zones of severity: 1 (unaffected/mildly affected); 2 (intermediate); 3 (very severely affected)

but remains in solution due to binding to albumin in the fluid. Unconjugated bilirubin can cross the blood-brain barrier in the fetus, causing **kernicterus**.

The wavelength of maximum absorption for bilirubin is 450 nM so that measurement of the linear difference at 450 nM between a tangent line drawn across the flat portion of the spectrum and the absorption band of bilirubin is proportional to the bilirubin concentration. This is the so called $\underline{\Delta OD}_{450}$ (difference in optical density or absorbance at 450 nM) **f15.1**. The absorbance is interpreted by reference to the Liley Prognostication Chart [PMID14465271]. The chart contains 3 zones that predict severity of the hemolytic disease based on the weeks of gestation and the absorbance at 450 nM: zone 1 (unaffected or mildly affected babies), zone 2 (intermediate zone), and zone 3 (very severely affected babies) **f15.2**. Since bilirubin is photosensitive, it is important that the amniotic fluid be protected from light either by collecting it into an opaque or amber colored tube or into a tube wrapped with foil or masking tape.

Since 1 of the absorption bands of hemoglobin is at 410 nM, hemoglobin, if present, will augment the bilirubin absorbance. Although various correction factors and extraction techniques have been proposed in attempt to mitigate the interference from hemoglobin, they have proved relatively unsuccessful [PMID16707381]. Thus, it is best to repeat the amniocentesis after the blood (either fetal or maternal) has cleared.

15.7 Laboratory monitoring for preterm birth

Fibronectins are adhesive glycoproteins that crosslink to collagen in order to bind cells together. During pregnancy, fetal fibronectin is found in cervicovaginal secretions for the first 22 weeks of pregnancy until the fetal membranes fuse to the maternal **decidua**. By 37 weeks, the fetal fibronectin becomes glycosylated, loses its adhesive properties, and is excreted into the cervicovaginal fluid. Finding fetal fibronectin at >50 ng/mL in women 24-35 weeks pregnant is associated with increased risk of preterm birth [ISBN9781594251023]. A negative test (<50 ng/mL) following a positive test lowers the risk, and a second consecutive negative test returns the risk to baseline [ISBN9781416061649a].

15.7.1 Fetal fibronectin reference range (24-35 weeks' gestation)

No risk pregnancy: negative
Increased risk of preterm birth: >50 ng/mL

15.8 Laboratory monitoring for premature rupture of the membranes

Placental α microglobulin 1 (PAMG1) is a placental glycoprotein that is secreted into the amniotic fluid, where its concentration is much higher than in maternal blood and cervicovaginal fluid. A commercially available immunochromatographic test is used to detect PAMG1 in cervicovaginal fluid. A positive test (>5 ng/mL) before the end of full term pregnancy suggests premature rupture of the membranes. Contamination of cervicovaginal secretions with large amounts of blood will yield a false positive result.

Premature rupture of the membranes is of concern since it often signals a preterm birth and may lead to infection of placental tissues (chorioamnionitis) as well as detachment of the placenta from the uterus.

15.8.1 PAMG1 reference range

Normal: negative
Positive: >5 ng/mL (analytical limit of detection)

15.9 **References**
15.9.1 **Journals**

PMID14465271 Liley AW [1961] Liquor amnii analysis in the management of the pregnancy complicated by rhesus sensitization. *Am J Obstet Gynecol* 82:1359-70

PMID16707381 Bailey DN, Briggs JR [2006] Studies of the extraction of bilirubin from human amniotic fluid. *Am J Clin Pathol* 125:771-3

15.9.2 **Books**

ISBN9780443045141 Glezerman M, Bartoov B [1993] Semen analysis. In: Insler V, Lunenfeld B, ed. *Infertility: Male and Female*, 2e. Churchill Livingstone, 285-315

ISBN9781416061649a Ashwood ER, Grenache DG, Lambert-Messerlian G [2013] Pregnancy and its disorders. In: Burtis CA, Ashwood ER, Bruns DE, ed. *Tietz Textbook of Clinical Chemistry and Molecular Diagnostics*, 5e. Elsevier Saunders, 1991-2044

ISBN9781416061649b Isbell TS, Jungheim E, Gronowski AM [2013] Reproductive endocrinology and related disorders. In: Burtis CA, Ashwood ER, Bruns DE, ed. *Tietz Textbook of Clinical Chemistry and Molecular Diagnostics*, 5e. Elsevier Saunders, 1945-90

ISBN9781594251023 Woodworth A, McCudden CR [2011] Laboratory testing in pregnancy and reproductive disorders. In: Clarke W, ed. *Contemporary Practice in Clinical Chemistry*, 2e. AACC Press, 471-91

chapter 16

Clinical toxicology

16.1 Objectives

At the end of this session, the learner should be able to

➢ differentiate clinical toxicology from forensic toxicology and therapeutic drug monitoring

➢ describe the sample types to submit for clinical toxicology screening

➢ discuss the limitations of a drug "screen"

➢ describe the general treatment of drug overdose

➢ define zero order pharmacokinetics, first order kinetics, serum half-life, and steady state drug concentrations

➢ discuss factors that can alter pharmacokinetics

➢ discuss the features of overdose/poisoning with ethanol, methanol, isopropanol, ethylene glycol, aspirin, acetaminophen, tricyclic antidepressants, benzodiazepines, opiates and opioid agents, cocaine, amphetamines, barbiturates, phencyclidine, other hallucinogens, cannabinoids, designer drugs, other abused agents, carbon monoxide, iron, lead, and organophosphates and carbamates

16.2 Key terms

acetylcholine: a neurotransmitter

acetylcholinesterase: enzyme that hydrolyzes and inactivates acetylcholine

analgesic: relieving pain

antipyretic: relieving fever

anticholinergic effects: the physiological effects when acetylcholine is blocked from binding to its receptor

anxiolytic: diminishing anxiety

apnea: cessation of breathing

arrhythmia: a condition of irregular heartbeat and rhythm

ataxia: lack of voluntary coordination of muscle movements, making it difficult to walk

cathartic: a gastrointestinal purgative agent

diaphoresis: perspiration

dysarthria: unclear articulation of speech

dysphoria: a state of unease or dissatisfaction

emesis: the act of vomiting

gastric lavage: irrigation of the stomach to flush out its contents

hallucinogens: agents that cause altered perception and hallucinations

hematemesis: vomiting of blood

hepatocyte: the chief functional cells of the liver

hyperbaric: referring to high pressure

hyperthermia: increased body temperature

hypothermia: decreased body temperature

hypovolemia: low blood volume

hypoxia: low oxygen content

keratolytic: an agent used to remove warts, corns, and other conditions of epidermal overgrowth

lacrimation: tearing of the eyes

miosis: pupillary constriction

muscarinic receptor: a type of acetylcholine receptor

mydriasis: pupillary dilatation

narcolepsy: uncontrollable sleep

nicotinic receptor: a type of acetylcholine receptor

nystagmus: involuntary and uncontrolled eye movements

pharmacokinetics: the time course for drug absorption, distribution, metabolism, and clearance

pressor agents: medications that raise the blood pressure

rhabdomyolysis: the breakdown of muscle tissues, releasing damaged protein into the blood

serum half-life: the time required for a drug concentration in serum to decline to half of its value

stenosis: narrowing of an orifice

sympathomimetic: mimicking effects of neurotransmitters such as catecholamines and dopamine

tachycardia: rapid heartbeat

tinnitus: ringing in the ears

γ aminobutyric acid: the chief neuroinhibitory transmitter in mammals

16.3 Background/significance

In 2011 there were 5 million drug related emergency department visits in the United States, representing a 100% increase since 2004 [SAMHSA 2011]. Furthermore, poisoning is the leading cause of injury related mortality, with drugs accounting for 90% [PMID22617462, PMID25228059]. Thus, an understanding of laboratory testing in clinical toxicology is important.

16.4 Clinical toxicology in perspective

Clinical toxicology is the measurement and interpretation of drugs and poisons in biological fluids to aid in the treatment of patients suspected of having an adverse reaction or overdose. In contrast, forensic toxicology is the measurement of drugs and toxins in tissues for medicolegal purposes (eg, for determining the cause of death or determining whether or not an individual was impaired while driving). Therapeutic drug monitoring (discussed in Chapter 17) is the measurement of concentrations of drugs in plasma/serum in order to determine whether compliance with medication therapy has been achieved and whether the dosage of the drug needs to be adjusted. For clinical toxicology studies, <u>whole blood or plasma/serum</u> (depending on the analyte) is preferred whenever drug concentrations can be correlated with drug effects and toxicity. <u>Urine specimens</u> are utilized for screening for drugs that have very low concentrations in plasma/serum due to extensive metabolism and renal clearance of the drug (eg, most drugs of abuse). <u>Gastric fluid</u> (eg, from **gastric lavage** or **emesis** is useful for identifying the parent (unmetabolized) drug in overdose cases because it is present in large concentrations following acute ingestion. Finally, <u>artifacts</u> such as pills, powders, tablets, and syringes may be helpful in determining the etiology of the poisoning.

16.5 The drug "screen"

No universal drug screen exists. Every laboratory has its own approach to screening, and thus it is extremely important for the provider to convey the patient history to the laboratory in order to assure that the appropriate drugs/agents are included in the screen. For example, as most laboratories do not include lithium in a drug screen, a laboratory would not include it in a workup if it is not notified that lithium is suspected in an overdose.

A sufficiently broad drug screen that is negative is important because it may prompt the provider to include other studies (eg, imaging studies) to determine the cause of altered mental or physical status.

16.6 General treatment of drug overdose

Patients with drug overdoses respond to supportive care, although a small number require hemodialysis, peritoneal dialysis, hemoperfusion, or other specialized care [PMID9246535]. Such care includes support of the airway (eg, assisted breathing, intubation), heart rate and rhythm (eg, cardioactive agents, cardiac monitoring), and blood pressure (eg, **pressor agents**), as well as removal of the offending agent (eg, activated charcoal for adsorption of the agent, **cathartics** to stimulate fecal excretion of the agent).

16.6.1 Pharmacokinetics

Most drugs follow <u>first order kinetics</u> (a constant <u>percentage</u> of drug is eliminated in a unit of time), and the **serum half-life** can be calculated. Some drugs present in such large concentrations that they saturate the metabolic enzymes and exhibit <u>zero order kinetics</u> (a constant <u>amount</u> of drug is eliminated in a unit of time; eg, ethanol). Drugs that normally follow first order kinetics may convert to zero order kinetics when ingested in massive quantities (overdose).

<u>Steady state drug concentrations</u> are achieved when the overall intake of a drug is in dynamic equilibrium with its elimination. This usually occurs after 4-5× the drug's serum half-life **f16.1**.

Variables that can affect **pharmacokinetics** include <u>renal function</u> (drugs cleared by the kidneys will have elevated serum/plasma concentrations in renal failure), <u>hepatic function</u> (drugs metabolized by the liver will have elevated serum/plasma concentrations in hepatic failure), <u>drug interactions</u> (other coadministered drugs may stimulate, inhibit, or change the protein binding of the

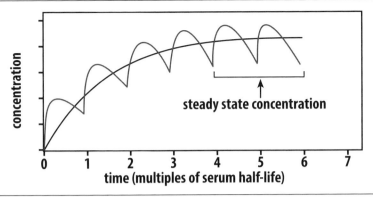

f16.1 Steady state concentration (4-5× the serum half-life)

drug of interest), and <u>saturation effects</u> (drugs present in large amounts may overwhelm the metabolic pathways, leading to conversion to zero order kinetics as noted above).

16.7 Review of specific toxic exposures
This section will briefly review the basic features of the more common toxic exposures. The reader is advised to consult other texts as needed for more comprehensive information.

16.7.1 Ethanol
More than half of adults in the United States report regular use of ethanol [PMID24819891], and it remains the most used and most often abused chemical substance worldwide [ISBN9781416061649]. The effects of ethanol vary with blood concentration and individual tolerance. The blood concentration for legal intoxication in most countries is 80 mg/dL (0.08%). Since it is osmotically active, ethanol contributes substantially to the plasma/serum osmolality, with every 4.6 mg/dL (0.0046%) of ethanol raising the osmolality by 1 mOsm/kg.

Ethanol follows zero order kinetics except at low (<20 mg/dL, <0.02%) and high (>300 mg/dL, >0.300%) concentrations, where it follows first order more closely. In healthy individuals, blood concentrations decline at ~15-20 mg/dL (0.015%-0.020) per hour, while chronic alcoholics may have increased elimination rates due to enzyme induction [ISBN9781416061649]. Ethanol is metabolized by hepatic alcohol dehydrogenase (ADH) to acetaldehyde, which is then metabolized by aldehyde dehydrogenase (ALDH) to acetate **f16.2**. Disulfiram (Antabuse)

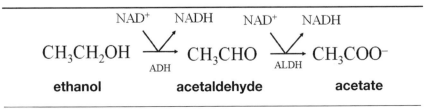

f16.2 Metabolism of ethanol

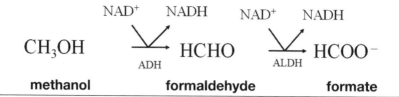

$$CH_3OH \xrightarrow[ADH]{NAD^+ \quad NADH} HCHO \xrightarrow[ALDH]{NAD^+ \quad NADH} HCOO^-$$

methanol **formaldehyde** **formate**

f16.3 Metabolism of methanol

acts by inhibiting ALDH so that acetaldehyde accumulates, producing severe nausea.

Ethanol can be easily measured in plasma/serum and urine by automated spectrophotometric methods.

16.7.2 Methanol

Methanol is available as a solvent (wood alcohol). It is also found in deicers, some antifreeze, and canned fuel (eg, sterno). Its toxicity is due to metabolism to formic acid, which causes a severe metabolic acidosis and an optic neuropathy leading to blindness and death. Methanol is metabolized by hepatic ADH to formaldehyde, which is then further metabolized to formic acid by ALDH f16.3, causing a severe metabolic acidosis. Therapy is aimed at competitively inhibiting the metabolism of methanol by ADH, by administering either fomepizole or ethanol (which is a preferential substrate for ADH). Hemodialysis can then be used to remove unchanged methanol and correct the metabolic acidosis [ISBN9781416061649].

Methanol measurement requires gas-liquid chromatographic analysis and is not generally available routinely.

16.7.3 Isopropanol

Isopropanol is commonly available as "rubbing alcohol" (70% aqueous solution of isopropanol) and has ~2× the central nervous system depressant effect as ethanol. It is rapidly metabolized by ADH to acetone f16.4. Acetone is then eliminated by the lungs and kidneys, but more slowly than isopropanol, so that in isopropanol ingestions, the concentration of acetone often is much greater than that of isopropanol [ISBN9781416061649]. Most cases are treated with supportive care alone.

Isopropanol measurement requires gas-liquid chromatographic analysis and is generally not routinely available.

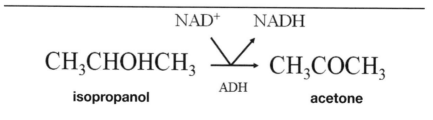

$$CH_3CHOHCH_3 \xrightarrow[ADH]{NAD^+ \quad NADH} CH_3COCH_3$$

isopropanol **acetone**

f16.4 Metabolism of isopropanol

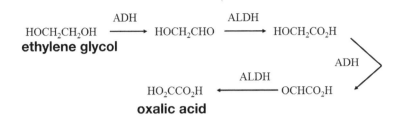

f16.5 Metabolism of ethylene glycol

16.7.4 Ethylene glycol

Ethylene glycol is the active ingredient of most antifreeze. In and of itself, it is relatively nontoxic, and its central nervous system effects are about the same as those of ethanol. However, it is metabolized by ADH to glycoaldehyde, which is further metabolized by ALDH to glycolic acid, which, in turn, is further metabolized by ADH to glyoxylic acid, which is then metabolized by ALDH to oxalic acid, which produces a profound metabolic acidosis **f16.5**. In addition, oxalic acid binds calcium, causing hypocalcemia and oxalate nephropathy as the calcium oxalate crystals are deposited into the tubules [ISBN9781416061649].

Ethylene glycol intoxication has been divided into 3 stages:

1. 6-12 hours: central nervous system involvement (confusion, ataxia, hallucinations, **dysarthria**, coma)

2. 12-24 hours: cardiopulmonary system involvement (**tachycardia**, hypertension, pulmonary edema, hyperventilation)

3. 24-72 hours: renal failure

There is little correlation between the plasma/serum ethylene glycol concentration and the severity of the intoxication because the toxicity is related more to the glycolic acid metabolites. Ethylene glycol measurements are generally used to ascertain clearance of the toxin with therapy. Calcium oxalate crystals in urine are usually of the monohydrate variety (needles) instead of the "envelopes" occasionally seen in normal urinalysis. Treatment involves administration of either ethanol or fomepizole as competitive inhibitors of ADH, followed by hemodialysis [PMID12322772]. Additional treatment includes replenishment of calcium and correction of the metabolic acidosis.

Analysis of ethylene glycol is not routinely available in most clinical laboratories.

16.7.5 Aspirin

Aspirin (acetylsalicylic acid) is a prodrug with **analgesic**, **antipyretic**, and anti-inflammatory activity. It also inhibits platelet aggregation, and for that reason, it is often ingested at small doses (81 mg) to reduce the incidence of thrombus formation and stroke. With therapeutic doses, aspirin is absorbed within 2 hours and is rapidly hydrolyzed to the active form salicylic acid (salicylate), which can be easily measured in serum/plasma. In the case of an overdose, absorption of aspirin can continue for up to 36 hours postingestion due to the formation of pharmacobezoars (a solid mass of pills that can form in the gastrointestinal tract) [PMID15173556]. Given its transient existence in plasma/serum, aspirin itself is not measured. Therapeutic concentrations of salicylate are usually <6 mg/dL for analgesic and antipyretic effects, and 15-30 mg/dL for anti-inflammatory effects [ISBN9781416061649].

In addition to aspirin, salicylic acid can be found in various **keratolytic** compounds, and its methyl ester (methyl salicylate) can be found in oil of wintergreen flavoring for mints and in "witch hazel" after shave lotion.

Early in the time course following an overdose, salicylate stimulates the central respiratory center, causing hyperventilation and subsequent respiratory alkalosis. It also uncouples oxidative phosphorylation, leading to **hyperthermia**, and enhances anaerobic glycolysis, leading to accumulation of organic acids and causing a metabolic acidosis. With high concentrations of salicylate in serum, **tinnitus** occurs [PMID19561730]. This constellation of effects makes salicylate poisoning one of the most complex overdoses. Treatment is directed toward decreasing absorption early on (activated charcoal), increasing renal elimination by alkalinizing urine (to maintain salicylate in its ionized form, thereby reducing its reabsorption), and removing the compound by hemodialysis (which also improves the acid-base balance).

Serum salicylate concentrations are generally not very meaningful if obtained <4 hours after ingestion because significant absorption can still occur. 6 hours after an aspirin overdose, salicylate concentrations of 30-50 mg/dL are suggestive of mild toxicity, 50-70 mg/dL moderate toxicity, and >75 mg/dL severe toxicity [PMID11971828]. Hemodialysis may be indicated when plasma/serum salicylate concentrations exceed 100 mg/dL [ISBN9781416061649].

Salicylate measurements are routinely and quickly available in most clinical laboratories using spectrophotometric procedures.

16.7.6 Acetaminophen

Acetaminophen is both an analgesic and an antipyretic agent, but unlike aspirin, it has very weak anti-inflammatory properties. It is available as an over the counter medication in many formulations (eg, Tylenol). In overdose, acetaminophen causes hepatotoxicity. In the initial phases following ingestion, nausea, vomiting, and abdominal discomfort may be noted. At 24-36 hours, however, hepatic necrosis begins and becomes most severe by 72-96 hours [ISBN9781416061649]. This is manifested by extreme elevation of the aminotransferases (due to hepatocellular necrosis) and prothrombin time (due to diminished liver synthetic capability).

The primary route of acetaminophen metabolism is glucuronidation and sulfation so that the metabolites are excreted into the urine. However, hepatotoxicity is caused by an alternate metabolic mixed function oxidase (MFO) pathway, yielding a toxic electrophilic intermediate (N-acetyl-p-benzoquinone

f16.6 Metabolism of acetaminophen to a toxic imidoquinone (N-acetyl-p-benzoquinone imine [NAPQI])

imine [NAPQI]), which binds to glutathione in the liver **f16.6**. When gluta-thione stores become depleted, NAPQI binds irreversibly to **hepatocytes**, causing necrosis. Hepatic coma and death can occur. Coingestion of agents that induce microsomal enzymes (eg, anticonvulsants) will enhance the formation of NAPQI, and alcoholics, who may already have depleted glutathione stores, may be especially sensitive to the effects of NAPQI [ISBN9781416061649].

Treatment involves administration of intravenous N-acetylcysteine as a source of sulfhydryl groups (-SH) to bind NAPQI before it can destroy the hepa-tocytes. In order to be most effective, this treatment must be initiated before extreme elevation of the aminotransferases. It must be administered over several days and thus requires hospitalization.

Several approaches can be taken in determining the likelihood of hepatic necrosis following a single acute ingestion of acetaminophen (and thus the indi-cation for initiating therapy with N-acetylcysteine). One is based on the so called Rumack nomogram, a semilogarithmic plot of serum/plasma acetaminophen concentration on the Y axis vs time postingestion on the X axis. N-acetylcysteine treatment is indicated if the 4 hour postingestion serum/plasma acetamino-phen concentration is $\geq$200 mg/L or if the 12 hour postingestion serum/plasma acetaminophen concentration is $\geq$50 mg/L [PMID1134886]. The problem with this approach is that the time postingestion is rarely determined accurately.

A better approach has been proposed: obtain 2-3 plasma/serum acetamino-phen concentrations and plot them semilogarithmically on the Y axis against time on the X axis. The first concentration would be "zero time," with subsequent concentrations being the number of hours after the first. The half-life can then be calculated by determining from the plot the amount of time required for a

ISBN 978-089189-6548

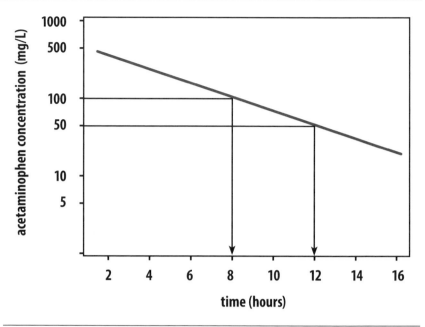

f16.7 Semilogarithmic plot of serum/plasma acetaminophen concentration vs time; in this example, 100 mg/L is at 8 hours while half of that concentration (50 mg/L) is at 12 hours: 12 − 8 hours = 4 hours serum half-life, suggesting hepatotoxicity

serum/plasma concentration to decline to half of its value **f16.7**. Normal individuals exhibit a serum/plasma acetaminophen half-life of 2.0-2.5 hours, while individuals with hepatotoxicity from acetaminophen overdose have half-lives of 4 hours or greater due to hepatic damage [PMID11956504].

Acetaminophen measurements are routinely and quickly available in most clinical laboratories using spectrophotometric methods.

16.7.7 Tricyclic antidepressants

The tricyclic antidepressants (TCAs), eg, amitriptyline, nortriptyline, imipramine, and desipramine, are an older generation of psychoactive medications and have been replaced in many respects with newer classes of drugs such as the selective serotonin reuptake inhibitors. However, TCAs are still used, and given the population for whom they are prescribed, they are involved in overdoses. These drugs block the neuronal uptake of serotonin and norepinephrine, and have both central and peripheral **anticholinergic effects** (eg, urinary retention, **mydriasis**, decreased gastrointestinal motility) [ISBN9781416061649].

In overdose, TCAs manifest serious cardiotoxicity, and death can occur due to **arrhythmias** that lead to cardiac arrest. Even therapeutic concentrations of TCAs can cause electrocardiographic changes, and use of the maximal limb lead QRS interval in the electrocardiogram has been suggested for monitoring TCA overdoses, since plasma/serum concentrations of TCA do not correlate well with the clinical findings [Boehnert 1985]. Serum/plasma TCA measurements are not routinely available in most clinical laboratories.

16.7.8 Benzodiazepines

The benzodiazepines are widely prescribed sedative, hypnotic, **anxiolytic** agents that have fewer side effects and less addictive potential than barbiturates. That said, tolerance does occur, especially with those benzodiazepines that have a shorter half-life, and these drugs have a relatively high addictive potential [ISBN9781416061649]. Some of the drugs (eg, clonazepam) are also used as anticonvulsant agents.

Most benzodiazepines exert their effects by enhancing the affinity of **γ aminobutyric acid** (GABA) for its receptor. Overdose with these drugs is usually treated with supportive care alone, although flumazenil (a competitive inhibitor of benzodiazepines) has been used in selected cases. Caution should be exercised in using flumazenil because it may precipitate withdrawal, which could include symptoms such as seizures in chronic users of benzodiazepines. While quantitative assays for benzodiazepines are available, they are generally not used because serum/plasma concentrations do not predict severity of intoxication. However, qualitative urine immunoassays for this class of drugs can be helpful in diagnosing the cause of sedation [ISBN9781416061649]. Mass spectrometry is also used to confirm the identity of specific benzodiazepines. Examples of benzodiazepines include diazepam, chlordiazepoxide, midazolam, and clonazepam.

16.7.9 Opiates & opioid agents

Opiates are compounds (eg, morphine, codeine) present in opium, which is found in the poppy plant. In contrast, semisynthetic drugs with similar pharmacological actions (eg, hydrocodone, hydromorphone, oxycodone, oxymorphone, fentanyl, meperidine, methadone, tramadol) are termed *opioid agents*. Both opiates and opioid agents have high addictive potential, and in overdose, they cause hypotension, bradycardia, coma, and respiratory arrest. Except for meperidine, all also cause **miosis**. In addition, tramadol and meperidine may cause seizures. Death is usually due to **apnea** and/or pulmonary aspiration of gastric contents [ISBN9780071824866].

Treatment of opiate and opioid agent overdose includes protection of the airway and administration of naloxone, a specific opiate antagonist. Although structurally related to opiates, it has no narcotic effects of its own and can be safely administered to patients suspected of opiate poisoning. Since the duration of naloxone action is only 3-4 hours, it is essential to give repeated dosing and to watch the patient for at least 3 hours after the last dose of naloxone, especially for agents with a long half-life (eg, methadone) [ISBN9780071824866].

While opiates and opioid agents can be quantitated in serum/plasma, they are usually screened qualitatively in urine by immunoassay in the workup of patients suspected of using them. Mass spectrometry is used to confirm the identity of specific opiates.

16.7.10 Cocaine

Cocaine is a naturally occurring alkaloid found in *Erythroxylon coca*, which grows in the South American Andes. It is used medically as a topical anesthetic in ophthalmology and as a vasoconstrictive agent to control bleeding in nasal surgery. Cocaine is one of the most widely abused drugs. It is abused both as a powder (the hydrochloride salt, prepared from coca leaves) and as a solid ("crack," prepared illicitly by dissolving the powder in aqueous alkali, extracting it into a small volume of diethyl ether, and then evaporating the solvent). Since the latter is the free base form of cocaine, it is sufficiently volatile to permit use by smoking, resulting in a particularly rapid absorption of drug. In contrast, the powder is usually administered by nasal insufflation ("snorting") or by injection in solution.

Cocaine is a potent central nervous system stimulant that exerts its effects by blocking the reuptake of dopamine at nerve synapses, thus prolonging the activity of dopamine. It also blocks the reuptake of norepinephrine, thereby producing a **sympathomimetic** effect (**tachycardia**, hypertension, hyperthermia, mydriasis, **diaphoresis**). **Rhabdomyolysis**, renal failure, and disseminated intravascular coagulation can be seen in extreme cases [ISBN9781416061649]. Treatment includes administration of benzodiazepines for agitation and seizures, combined α and β adrenergic blockers for hypertension, and short acting β blockers for hyperthermia [ISBN9780071824866].

Use of ethanol together with cocaine causes transesterification of cocaine from the methyl ester of benzoylecgonine to its ethyl ester (cocaethylene), which has a longer elimination half-life than does cocaine, thus enhancing the toxicity of cocaine [ISBN9781416061649]. Cocaine readily undergoes nonenzymatic hydrolysis to benzoylecgonine, a pharmacologically inactive metabolite. Most testing for cocaine use depends on detection of benzoylecgonine in urine by immunoassay.

16.7.11 Amphetamines

Amphetamine (dextro- or d-amphetamine) and methamphetamine (N-methylamphetamine) are major drugs of abuse that stimulate the central nervous system. They are also used medically to treat **narcolepsy** and various attention deficit disorders. They act centrally by promoting presynaptic release of dopamine, serotonin, and norepinephrine instead of blocking their reuptake. Accordingly, the amphetamines can induce a variety of symptoms, including tachycardia, hypertension, hyperthermia, restlessness, rhabdomyolysis, and a schizophreniform psychosis [ISBN9781416061649]. Like cocaine, amphetamines can also be converted to a solid free base form, which can be smoked. Street terms for methamphetamine include *crystal*, *speed*, and *ice*. Given that the symptoms of cocaine and amphetamine intoxication are similar, the treatment is the same (administration of benzodiazepines for agitation and seizures, combined α and β adrenergic blockers for hypertension, and short acting β blockers for hyperthermia) [ISBN9780071824866]. Methamphetamine is metabolized to amphetamine, and both compounds can be found in urine following use. Amphetamines as a class are easily screened in urine using immunoassay. Immunoassays for amphetamines are subject to cross reactivity to a variety of structurally related analogs. Confirmation by mass spectrometry is recommended in order to identify specific compounds.

16.7.12 Barbiturates

Barbiturates have largely been replaced by benzodiazepines as sedative hypnotic agents because the latter have greater safety. Barbiturates are categorized into 3 classes: long acting (eg, phenobarbital), short acting (eg, pentobarbital, secobarbital), and ultra short acting (eg, thiopental, thiamylal). These terms refer to the duration of the drugs' effect and not their elimination half-life. Barbiturates cause central nervous system depression ranging from mild sedation to anesthesia, and pharmacologic tolerance and addiction are common. Overdose with these agents produces **hypothermia**, coma, hypotension, and cardiorespiratory arrest [ISBN9781416061649]. Barbiturates as a class can be easily detected in urine using immunoassay, and specific compounds can be identified by mass spectrometry.

16.7.13 Hallucinogens

Phencyclidine (aka angel dust, or PCP) is a potent analgesic and anesthetic developed for use in veterinary medicine. Use by humans causes **dysphoria, nystagmus, ataxia**, agitation, paranoia, delusions, hostility, and a schizophreniform psychosis. Because it can cause hallucinations, it has also been classified as a **hallucinogen**. It is abused by inhalation, oral ingestion, and injection. Treatment consists of administration of benzodiazepines for agitation and haloperidol for psychosis. Death can result from the irrational and violent behavior exhibited by users of the drug [ISBN9781416061649]. Phencyclidine can be easily detected in urine by immunoassay, but due to the low prevalence and poor positive predictive value (see Chapter 1), all positive screening tests should be confirmed by a more specific technique such as mass spectrometry.

Other hallucinogens include lysergic acid diethylamide (LSD), peyote/mescaline (cactus), and psilocybin (mushrooms). They produce a wide variety of psychoactive effects. Their toxicity is largely due to the irrational and risky behavior of individuals under the influence of the drugs. They are generally not included in most urine toxicology screens.

16.7.14 Cannabinoids

The cannabinoids are found in the marijuana plant *Cannabis sativa*. Cannabis is among the most abused drugs worldwide [ISBN9781416061649]. The effects of cannabis include euphoria, distorted perceptions, relaxation, and a general feeling of well-being. The primary active ingredient is δ-9-tetrahydrocannabinol (THC). The cannabinoids are generally administered by smoking, although oral ingestion is also used. Other forms are hashish and hemp oil, both isolated from *Cannabis sativa*. After use, THC and its metabolites are released from body fat stores over a prolonged period of time so that they can be detected in casual users up to 7 days and in chronic users for >10 weeks [ISBN9781416061649]. Immunoassays for THC in urine are readily available. Mass spectrometry should be used for confirmation of identity.

16.7.15 Designer drugs

The so called designer drugs are agents that are synthesized ("designed") to mimic effects of conventional drugs. This is usually achieved by making relatively minor alterations in the chemical structure of a drug approved by the US Food and Drug Administration (FDA), thereby creating a drug previously unclassified by the US Drug Enforcement Administration (DEA). The United States Controlled Substance Analogue Enforcement Act of 1986 makes it illegal to manufacture, sell, or possess chemicals that are substantially similar in chemistry and pharmacology to DEA Schedule I and Schedule II drugs [FDA 1986]. Popular examples include the amphetamine structural analogs 3,4-methylenedioxymethamphetamine (MDMA, aka *ecstasy*); 3,4-methylenedioxyamphetamine (MDA); the synthetic cathinones (*bath salts*), which are more potent versions of the FDA approved amphetamines; and the synthetic cannabinoids (*spice*). Earlier drugs included α-methylfentanyl (*China White*) [PMID7109557], marketed as *synthetic heroin*, and the reverse ester of meperidine, marketed as *synthetic Demerol*. For the latter, faulty reaction temperatures and pH created a neurotoxic precursor(1-methyl-4-phenylpyridinium) that produced Parkinson disease in users [PMID6427583].

16.7.16 Other abused agents

A wide variety of other agents has been abused. These include inhalants such as amyl nitrite and its analogs, which can cause rapid vasodilation, producing a sudden drop in blood pressure, experienced as a "high" by the user. Nitrites induce methemoglobinemia and **hypoxia**. These agents are usually not detected as part of the routine drug screen.

16.7.16.1 Carbon monoxide

Carbon monoxide is a colorless, odorless, and tasteless gas that combines tightly with hemoglobin to form carboxyhemoglobin, which can be easily measured by most blood gas instruments. Its affinity for hemoglobin is ~250× that of oxygen. Treatment of carbon monoxide poisoning is fresh air or 100% oxygen. With severe exposure, **hyperbaric** oxygen therapy may be used, although its efficacy has been debated [ISBN9781416061649].

Carboxyhemoglobin (COHb) concentrations are reported as a percentage of total hemoglobin. Concentrations of 15%-25% often cause dizziness and nausea, while those >50% are considered to be life threatening. It is believed that concentrations achieved quickly result in less intense physiological effects than those that are achieved gradually (eg, exposure to a faulty heater). Normal nonsmoking, urban dwelling individuals have background COHb concentrations of 1%-2%, while concentrations in smokers range 5%-6% [ISBN9780962652387].

16.7.16.2 Iron

Iron poisoning is most common in children <5 years old [PMID3784842]. Ingestion of <30 mg/kg body weight usually produces only mild gastrointestinal symptoms, while ingestion of >40-60 mg/kg may cause diarrhea, vomiting, hypotension, fulminant hepatic failure, and metabolic acidosis [ISBN9780071824866].

The clinical course of acute iron poisoning has 4 phases. Phase 1 (up to 6 hours) features acute gastrointestinal irritation with possible **hematemesis** due to the corrosive effects of iron; with severe poisoning there may be impairment of consciousness, convulsions, and metabolic acidosis. Phase 2 (6-12 hours) is characterized by remission of symptoms. Phase 3 (12-48 hours) features shock, metabolic acidosis, renal failure, and hepatocellular necrosis. Phase 4 (2-6 weeks) is only likely to develop in children, and features gastric and duodenal **stenosis** caused by healing of iron induced mucosal ulcers. Usually iron poisoning is not severe enough for patients to progress past phase 2 [PMID3784842].

The metabolic acidosis noted in advanced iron poisoning is due to 1) conversion of iron to ferric hydroxide, leading to generation of hydrogen ions; 2) free radical damage to mitochondrial membranes, leading to development of lactic acidosis; and 3) **hypovolemia** and hypoperfusion related to gastrointestinal fluid losses [PMID3784842].

Treatment of acute iron poisoning involves intravenous administration (15 mg/kg/hour) of deferoxamine when there is 1) any clinical sign of shock; 2) lethargy, coma, or altered mental status; 3) persistent vomiting, diarrhea, hematemesis; 4) metabolic acidosis; 5) a large number of pills on abdominal X ray (iron is radiopaque); 6) a serum iron concentration >500 µg/dL; or 7) an estimated ingested iron dose of >60 mg/kg. Deferoxamine chelates iron to form ferroxamine, which turns the urine to a vin rose color. Most patients require continuous chelation and monitoring of serum iron concentrations for at least 1-2 days [PMID10742921].

16.7.16.3 Lead

Unlike iron poisoning, lead intoxication is usually chronic and may go undiagnosed due to the relative nonspecificity of clinical findings and the lack of documented exposure. Lead intoxication can be characterized by growth failure and impaired intellectual development (children), abdominal pain, behavioral changes, hypochromic microcytic anemia with basophilic stippling, headache, renal dysfunction, hyperuricemia (due to diminished clearance of uric acid), and wrist drop (due to radial nerve damage) [PMID1476518, ISBN9780071668330].

Lead is measured in whole blood because lead resides in the erythrocyte. While no concentration of lead is considered to be nontoxic, the level of concern for blood lead is 5 µg/dL in children. Concentrations of 10-25 µg/dL are associated with impaired neurobehavioral development in children; 25-50 µg/dL with headache, irritability, and subclinical neuropathy; 50-70 µg/dL with moderate toxicity; and >70-100 µg/dL with severe toxicity. Patients with blood lead concentrations >70-100 µg/dL *should* be and those with concentrations 55-70 µg/dL *may* be treated with intravenous edetate calcium disodium (ethylenediaminetetraacetic acid, EDTA; calcium disodium versenate; 50 mg/kg/day) [Boehnert 1985]. The lead chelate is excreted into the urine.

16.7.16.4 Organophosphate & carbamate insecticide poisoning

Organophosphate and carbamate insecticides are widely used and have largely replaced older, environmentally harmful agents such as DDT. They are called anticholinesterases because they inhibit **acetylcholinesterase**, causing an increase in the neurotransmitter acetylcholine at 2 types of acetylcholine receptors: the nicotinic and **muscarinic receptors**. These agents cause abdominal cramping, diarrhea, bronchial hypersecretion, vomiting, diaphoresis, miosis, urination, seizures, skeletal muscle weakness, salivation, and **lacrimation** [ISBN9780071824866]. A helpful pneumonic is "SLUD" (salivation, lacrimation, urination, defecation).

Treatment consists of administration of atropine to reverse muscarinic stimulation and reduce salivation, bronchial hypersecretion, abdominal cramping, and diaphoresis. For organophosphate exposures, administration of pralidoxime reverses organophosphate binding to cholinesterase, thus reactivating the enzyme [ISBN9780071824866].

Acetylcholinesterase (erythrocyte cholinesterase) and butyrylcholinesterase (serum cholinesterase) activities are typically depressed following exposure to these agents with butyrylcholinesterase declining first, followed by acetylcholinesterase [ISBN9781416061649]. Patients become symptomatic when activities are depressed by >50%.

16.8 **References**

16.8.1 **Journals**

PMID10742921 Fine JS [2000] Iron poisoning. *Curr Prob Pediatr* 30:71-90

PMID1134886 Rumack BH, Matthew H [1975] Acetaminophen poisoning and toxicity. *Pediatrics* 55:871-6

PMID11956504 Schiodt FV, Ott P, Christensen E et al [2002] The value of plasma acetaminophen half-life in antidote-treated acetaminophen overdosage. *Clin Pharmacol Ther* 71:221-5

PMID11971828 Dargan PI, Wallace CI, Jones AL [2002] An evidence based flowchart to guide the management of acute salicylate (aspirin) overdose. *Emerg Med J* 19:206-9

PMID12322772 Scalley RD, Ferguson DR, Smart ML et al [2002] Treatment of ethylene glycol poisoning. *Am Fam Physician* 66:807-12

PMID1476518 Needleman H [2004] Lead poisoning. *Ann Rev Med* 55:209-22

PMID15173556 Rivera W, Kleinschmidt KC, Velez LI et al [2004] Delayed salicylate toxicity at 35 hours without early manifestations following a single salicylate investion. *Ann Pharmacother* 38:1186-8

PMID19561730 Samlan SR, Jordan MT, Chan SB et al [2008] Tinnitus as a measure of salicylate toxicity in the overdose setting. *West J Emerg Med* 9:146-9

PMID22617462 Warner M, Chen LH, Makuc DM [2011] Drug poisoning deaths in the United States, 1980-2008. *NCHS Data Brief* 81:1-8

PMID24819891 Blackwell DL, Lucas JW, Clarke TC [2014] Summary health statistics for U.S. adults: national health interview survey 2012. *Vital Health Stat* 10 260:1-161

PMID25228059 Chen LH, Hedegaard H, Warner M [2014] Drug poisoning deaths involving opioid analgesics: United States, 1999-2011. *NCHS Data Brief* 166:1-8

PMID3784842 Proudfoot AT, Simpson D, Dyson EH [1986] Management of acute iron poisoning. *Med Toxicol* 1:83-100

PMID6427583 Centers for Disease Control [1984] Street-drug contaminant causing parkinsonism. *MMWR Morb Mortal Wkly Rep* 33: 351-2

PMID7109557 Gillespie TJ, Gandolfi AJ, Davis TP et al [1982] Identification and quantification of α-methylfentanyl in post mortem specimens. *J Anal Toxicol* 6:139-42

PMID9246535 Vernon DD, Gleich MC [1997] Poisoning and drug overdose. *Crit Care Clin* 13:647-67

Boehnert MT, Lovejoy FH [1985] Value of the QRS duration vs the serum drug level in predicting seizures and ventricular arrhythmias after an acute overdose of tricyclic antidepressants. *N Engl J Med* 313:474-9

Substance Abuse and Mental Health Services Administration (SAMHSA) [2011] Drug Abuse Warning Network: 2011. National estimates of drug related emergency department visits, HHS Publication No. (SMA) 13-4760

16.8.2 Books

ISBN9780071668330 Kosnett MJ [2012] Lead. In: Olson KR, ed. *Poisoning and Drug Overdose*, 6e. McGraw-Hill, 253-58

ISBN9780071824866 Olson KR [2014] Poisoning, In: Papadakis MA, McPhee SJ, Rabow MW, ed. *Current Medical Diagnosis & Treatment*, 53e. McGraw Hill Education, 1509-38

ISBN9780962652387 Baselt RC [2011] Carbon monoxide. In: *Disposition of Toxic Drugs and Chemicals in Man*, 9e. Biomedical Publications, 260

ISBN9781416061649 Langman L, Bechtel L, Holstege CP [2013] Clinical toxicology. In: Burtis CA, Ashwood ER, Bruns DE, ed. *Tietz Textbook of Clinical Chemistry and Molecular Diagnostics*, 5e. Elsevier Saunders, 1109-188.

16.8.3 Other references

US Food and Drug Administration (FDA) [1986] *Controlled Substances Act*, Title 21, United States Code, Chapter 13, Subchapter 1, Part B

16.9 Clinical cases

16.9.1 Case 1

A 23-year-old male is brought to the emergency department by the police. He has the odor of alcohol on his breath, is incoherent, and has ataxia. Laboratory results reveal the following: whole blood: arterial pH 7.15, arterial pCO_2 14 mmHg; plasma: ethanol 217 mg/dL, glucose 63 mg/dL, sodium 129 mMol/L (mEq/L), potassium 4.3 mMol/L (mEq/L), chloride 78 mMol/L (mEq/L), bicarbonate 5 mMol/L (mEq/L), osmolality 376 mOsm/kg, calcium 7.8 mg/dL, and urea-N 30 mg/dL. Molecular weights: ethanol 46; methanol 32; isopropanol 60; ethylene glycol 62.

16.9.1.1 Questions

1. Calculate the osmolal gap.

2. How much of the osmolal gap is due to ethanol?

3. Calculate the anion gap.

4. What potential toxin could explain the results?

5. Using the unexplained osmolal gap, estimate the concentration of the toxin.

6. What additional laboratory tests would be helpful?

7. What therapeutic options should be considered?

 ISBN 978-089189-6548

16.9.2 **Case 2**

A 53-year-old male is brought by friends to the emergency department. He is ataxic and dysarthric, and has the strong odor of alcohol on his breath. The plasma ethanol concentration is 130 mg/dL. The serum osmolality is 320 mOsm/kg. The patient is monitored until he becomes ambulatory and is then discharged.

16.9.2.1 **Questions**

1. What is the significance of the plasma ethanol concentration?

2. Does the plasma ethanol concentration explain the ataxia and dysarthria?

3. Why is the serum osmolality elevated?

4. How long will it take for the ethanol concentration to decrease to lower than the legal level for intoxication (80 mg/dL)?

16.9.3 **Case 3**

A 17-year-old heroin addict lapses into coma shortly after "shooting up." He is found by the police and is brought to the emergency department, where he suffers a respiratory arrest. After resuscitation his pupils are noted to be miotic, and he has very shallow respirations. After administration of 4 ampules of naloxone to the patient, he wakes up and demands to be released.

16.9.3.1 **Questions**

1. Is it safe to discharge the patient at this time?

2. What laboratory tests should be ordered?

3. Can naloxone be administered routinely to the comatose patient?

16.9.4 **Case 4**

A 32-year-old male with a history of depression, alcoholism, hepatitis C, and a past suicide attempt is brought to the emergency department by his friends ~30 minutes after ingesting 100 tablets of acetaminophen, 500 mg. Serum laboratory results showed the following: sodium 141 mMol/L (mEq/L), potassium 3.9 mMol/L (mEq/L), chloride 106 mMol/L (mEq/), bicarbonate 25 mMol/L (mEq/L), urea-N 6 mg/dL, creatinine 0.7 mg/dL, glucose 95 mg/dL, calcium 9.1 mg/dL, and acetaminophen 40 mg/L.

16.9.4.1 **Questions**

1. How should this patient be treated?

2. Does the patient's past medical history have any impact on his condition?

3. After 3 hours in the emergency department, the serum acetaminophen concentration rises to 175 mg/L. What does this suggest?

4. After 2 more hours (5 hours after arrival in the emergency department), the serum acetaminophen concentration rises to 192 mg/L. After 8 more hours (13 hours after arrival), it declines to 105 mg/L. What does this suggest and what should be done?

5. What other laboratory tests should be monitored in this case?

16.9.5 **Case 5**

A 35-year-old female weighing 135 pounds was brought to the emergency department 5 hours after ingesting ~100 ferrous sulfate heptahydrate ($FeSO_4 \cdot 7 H_2O$) pills, 200 mg per pill, in a suicide attempt. In the emergency department, she vomits, and blood and pill fragments are noted in the vomitus. An X ray of the abdomen also shows pill fragments. She complains of epigastric pain. The patient is admitted to the hospital.

Over the next 2 days, her serum laboratory studies reveal the following abnormalities: bicarbonate (decreases from 23-19 mMol/L [mEq/L]); albumin (decreases from 3.9-2.7 g/dL); total bilirubin (increases from 0.3-3.1 mg/dL); direct bilirubin (increases from 0.1-2.1 mg/dL); alanine aminotransferase (increases from 14-4,050 U/L); aspartate aminotransferase (increases from 17-2,417 U/L); prothrombin time (increases from 14.5-51.5 seconds; international normalized ratio increases from 1.0-5.8); iron (increases from 125-557 μg/dL). Her arterial pH dropped from 7.30-7.12. (Conversion factor = 2.2 pounds per kg; atomic weights = Fe 56, S 32, O 16, H 1.)

16.9.5.1 **Questions**

1. How much elemental iron did this patient ingest?

2. Is this a potentially toxic dose of iron?

3. What do the laboratory studies suggest?

4. How should the patient be treated?

5. What other laboratory studies might be helpful?

6. Is this a typical presentation for an iron overdose?

16.9.6 Clinical case answers

16.9.6.1 Case 1 answers

1. Osmolal gap = measured osmolality – calculated osmolality; calculated osmolality = 2(sodium) + glucose/18 + urea-N/2.8 = 2(129) + 63/18 + 30/2.8 = 258 + 3.5 + 10.7 = 272.2; osmolal gap = 376-272 = 104

2. Molecular weight of ethanol = 46; thus, for every 4.6 mg/dL of ethanol, there is a contribution of 1 mOsm/kg to the osmolality. Plasma ethanol = 217 mg/dL; 217/4.6 = 47 mOsm/kg contribution from ethanol

3. Anion gap = (sodium + potassium) – (chloride + bicarbonate) = (129 + 4.3) – (78 + 5) = 133.3-83 = 50

4. Ethylene glycol would be a likely toxin since it produces a metabolic acidosis (increased anion gap; low arterial pH; compensatory hyperventilation, leading to low pCO_2), hypocalcemia due to binding by oxalic acid produced by metabolism of ethylene glycol, and renal failure (increased urea-N), all of which are noted in this case. While methanol ingestion produces acidosis, it does not lead to renal failure and hypocalcemia. Isopropanol ingestion does not lead to any of the abnormal findings noted in this case other than an osmolal gap.

5. Osmolal gap = 104; portion of gap explained by ethanol = 47; unexplained portion of gap = 104-47 = 57. Molecular weight of ethylene glycol = 62. Thus, for every 6.2 mg/dL of ethylene glycol, there is a contribution of 1 mOsm/kg to the osmolality. Thus, the estimated concentration of ethylene glycol is (6.2 × 57) = 353 mg/dL.

6. An ethylene glycol analysis, if available, should be obtained. A serum creatinine measurement should be obtained to confirm renal failure. A urinalysis should be performed to workup renal failure and search for oxalate crystals.

7. The patient should be given fomepizole (he already has ethanol in vivo) to inhibit further metabolism of ethylene glycol to toxic metabolites, and hemodialysis should be considered in order to remove unmetabolized ethylene glycol and to correct the acid-base imbalance

16.9.6.2 Case 2 answers

1. The plasma ethanol concentration of 130 mg/dL is above the legal level for intoxication (80 mg/dL) in most countries; chronic alcoholics can often be coherent with concentrations of that magnitude due to development of tolerance

2. Yes, particularly if the patient is not a chronic alcoholic

3. Ethanol is an osmotically active agent, contributing 1 mOsm/kg for every 4.6 mg/dL concentration

4. Ethanol follows zero order kinetics except at very low (<20 mg/dL) and very high (>300 mg/dL) concentrations, and is eliminated at 15-20 mg/dL/hour; thus the 130 mg/dL ethanol concentration in this patient should decline to 80 mg/dL (a difference of 50 mg/dL) in ~2.5 hours

16.9.6.3 Case 3 answers

1. Since insufficient naloxone may have been administered, the patient should be watched to assure that he does not lapse back into coma and have respiratory depression; further naloxone administration should be considered

2. A toxicology screen of urine should be ordered to confirm the presence of opiates and determine whether other drugs of abuse are present. Since intravenous drug abusers often have hepatitis and acquired immunodeficiency disease, serologic tests for these should be ordered. Blood gases should be ordered to assure that the patient's cardiorespiratory status is resolving

3. Since it has no narcotic activity itself, naloxone can be administered routinely to the comatose patient

16.9.6.4 Case 4 answers

1. Since the patient arrived in <1 hour after ingesting acetaminophen, activated charcoal should be administered in attempt to decrease absorption of acetaminophen; serial acetaminophen concentrations should be obtained

2. The patient's history of alcoholism and hepatitis C suggests that his liver function may already be compromised, putting him particularly at risk for further liver injury

3. The acetaminophen concentration of 175 mg/dL at ~3.5 hours postingestion indicates that, despite aggressive measures to decrease acetaminophen absorption, the patient has absorbed more drug; his acetaminophen concentrations must be followed closely, and intravenous N-acetylcysteine therapy should be contemplated, especially since the 3.5 hour concentration of 175 mg/L is dangerously close to the threshold for toxicity of 200 mg/dL at 4 hours (Rumack).

4. The peak concentration of 192 mg/L at 5 hours after arrival declines to 105 mg/dL at 13 hours after arrival (ie, 8 hours later). This indicates that the observed serum half-life of acetaminophen in this patient is >4 hours (half of 192 mg/L = 92 mg/L, but the patient has a concentration above this 8 hours later). This suggests that hepatotoxicity will occur if the patient is not treated properly (normal serum half-life = 2.0-2.5 hours; hepatotoxicity >4 hours). The patient should be admitted, and intravenous N-acetylcysteine therapy should be initiated

5. Liver function studies should be obtained (alanine aminotransferase, aspartate aminotransferase, prothrombin time, albumin) along with serial serum acetaminophen measurements

16.9.6.5 Case 5 answers

1. Molecular weight of $FeSO_4$ = 56 + 32 + 64 = 152. $FeSO_4$ is complexed with 7 waters. Water has a molecular weight of 18, so the heptahydrate would increase the molecular weight by 126, yielding a molecular weight of 278 for $FeSO_4 \cdot 7\ H_2O$. Then the percentage of elemental iron in $FeSO_4$= 56/278 = 0.20. Amount of $FeSO_4$ ingested = 100 pills × 200 mg/pill = 20,000 mg. Then, 0.20 × 20,000 mg = 4,000 mg. Weight of patient = 135 pounds = 135 pounds/2.2 pounds/kg = 61 kg. Then, 4,000 mg/61 kg = 65 mg/kg ingested

2. Toxic dose >40-60 mg/kg; thus, a toxic dose of elemental iron was ingested

3. The laboratory studies suggest severe iron poisoning as evidenced by the drop in bicarbonate and arterial pH (metabolic acidosis as iron becomes hydrated and poisons the mitochondria), the rise in aminotransferases, fall in albumin, rise in prothrombin time/INR, and rise in total and conjugated bilirubin (liver failure)

4. The patient should be administered intravenous deferoxamine to chelate iron until it is cleared into the urine (vin rose color)

5. Serial serum iron measurements and urine iron measurements would be helpful in evaluating the elimination of iron

6. No; most iron overdoses occur in children <5 years of age

chapter 17

Therapeutic drug monitoring

17.1 Objectives

At the end of this session, the learner should be able to
- define therapeutic drug monitoring
- discuss the rationale for performing therapeutic drug monitoring
- discuss therapeutic monitoring of phenytoin, phenobarbital, primidone, carbamazepine, ethosuximide, valproic acid, theophylline, digoxin, amikacin, gentamicin, tobramycin, vancomycin, cyclosporine A, sirolimus, and tacrolimus

17.2 Key terms

absence seizure: a seizure characterized by brief loss of consciousness

aminoglycoside: a group of antibacterial agents that function by inhibiting protein synthesis in Gram– bacteria and that contain an amino substituted glycoside

ataxia: lack of voluntary coordination of muscle movements, making it difficult to walk

bound drug: the protein bound (inactive) fraction of drug

free drug: the nonprotein bound (active) fraction of drug

gingival hyperplasia: hypertrophy of the gums

glycogenolysis: the conversion of glycogen to glucose in the liver

glycopeptide: a peptide that is glycosylated with carbohydrate residues

glycoside: a sugar bound to another functional group

hypokalemia: low serum/plasma potassium

leukopenia: decreased leukocyte count

nephrotoxicity: renal damage

neuropathic pain: pain caused by damage to the somatosensory nerves

nystagmus: involuntary and uncontrolled eye movements

ototoxicity: loss of hearing

paresthesia: a feeling of numbness and tingling

peak concentration: the highest serum drug concentration following drug dosing (usually within 2-3 hours after a drug is administered orally)

pharmacogenomics: the genetic basis for drug response

pharmacokinetics: the time course for drug absorption, distribution, metabolism, and clearance

serum half-life: the time required for a drug concentration in serum to decline to half of its value

therapeutic drug monitoring: the measurement of drug concentrations in serum/plasma or other body fluids for the purpose of monitoring compliance and for enhancing efficacy through altering drug dosage in response to the measured drug concentration

thrombocytopenia: decreased platelet count

total drug: the sum of free and protein bound drug

trough concentration: the lowest serum drug concentration between multiple doses of a drug (usually measured just before administration of the next dose)

urticaria: hives

γ aminobutyric acid: the chief neuroinhibitory transmitter in mammals

17.3 Background/significance

For many decades **therapeutic drug monitoring** (TDM) has become an accepted practice among providers prescribing medications. Consequently, an understanding of the principles of TDM and how they are applied to specific drugs is important.

17.4 Principles of therapeutic drug monitoring

Tremendous variability in drug disposition exists among individuals, due to differences in demographics (eg, age, body mass, gender, race, genetically based metabolic enzyme polymorphisms); diseases affecting drug absorption, metabolism, and excretion; extracorporeal factors (eg, ongoing dialysis); and concurrent administration of other drugs that can influence the disposition of the drug of interest [ISBN9781416061649].

TDM involves the measurement of drug concentrations in serum/plasma or other body fluids in order to individualize the dosage so that the clinical outcome may be optimized and any side effects minimized.

The characteristics of a drug for which TDM may be useful include the following: the dosage for beneficial effects is near the dosage that produces adverse effects; it has no predictable dose response relationship, so it may produce a beneficial effect in one person and an adverse effect in another; its concentration in serum/plasma cannot be predicted from dose alone; and its efficacy and toxicity correlate with its serum/plasma concentration [Pramod 2014].

More specific reasons that prompt providers to order TDM include the following: concern about potential toxicity, apparent lack of therapeutic response, assessment of compliance/adherence in using the medication, evaluating therapy after a change in dosage regimen, an unexpected change in the clinical state of the patient, potential drug interactions due to change in other administered medications, and differentiation of drug toxicity from toxicity produced by the patient's disease. A relatively limited number of drugs has a better relationship between serum/plasma drug concentrations and response than between drug dose and response [PMID11564048].

This chapter briefly summarizes TDM for some of the most commonly monitored medications. It should be noted that, while measurements of **free** (nonprotein bound, or *active*) **drug** are possible, most TDM involves measurement of **total drug** (sum of free drug plus **bound**, or inactive, **drug**). Measurement of free drug concentrations is reserved for difficult cases, usually involving highly protein bound drugs. Thus, therapeutic serum concentrations provided in this chapter are total drug concentrations.

17.5 Anticonvulsants

17.5.1 Phenytoin (diphenylhydantoin)

Phenytoin, an older anticonvulsant, acts by prolonging the inactivation of the sodium channel and reducing central synaptic transmission, leading to control of abnormal neuronal excitability. The drug has variable absorption and is highly protein bound (>90%), making it a particularly good candidate for TDM. Because hepatic metabolic pathways may become saturated with phenytoin even in therapeutic concentrations, first order kinetics (see Chapter 16) do not apply, and zero order kinetics are observed. Other acidic drugs, such as valproic acid and salicylates, can disrupt protein binding of phenytoin, increasing the free (active) drug fraction, which is then rapidly eliminated, resulting in a decrease in the total (free plus bound) drug concentration, while the free drug concentration (and hence the pharmacological effect) remains stable. Other drugs such as barbiturates and alcohol can induce the metabolism of phenytoin, decreasing its pharmacologic effect, while drugs such as cimetidine and omeprazole can compete with phenytoin metabolism, causing an increase in free (and therefore total) drug concentration and potentiating the pharmacologic effect. The optimal therapeutic concentration for serum/plasma phenytoin is 10-20 mg/L. Concentrations >20 mg/L are associated with **nystagmus** and **ataxia**, while concentrations >35 mg/L are associated with seizure activity. A side effect not associated with serum concentration is **gingival hyperplasia** [ISBN9781416061649].

17.5.2 Phenobarbital

Phenobarbital, introduced in 1912 for use as an anticonvulsant, reduces synaptic transmission, resulting in decreased excitability of the entire nerve cell and causing sedation. It also enhances synaptic inhibition through action on the **γ aminobutyric acid** (GABA) receptor. These actions increase the threshold for seizures, thereby producing an anticonvulsant effect. The drug is 50% bound to proteins, and its **serum half-life** is 70-140 hours. Serum/plasma concentrations increase with coadministration of phenytoin and valproic acid, and decrease with coadministration of other barbiturates, alcohol, and carbamazepine. The optimal therapeutic concentration for serum/plasma phenobarbital is 10-40 mg/L. Concentrations >40 mg/L are associated with sedation, although tolerance to this effect occurs with long term use of the drug [ISBN9781416061649].

17.5.3 Primidone

Primidone is metabolized to phenobarbital, and its anticonvulsant action is similar to that of phenobarbital. It is only 20% protein bound, and its serum half-life is 3-22 hours. The optimal therapeutic concentration for serum/plasma primidone is 5-10 mg/L, and concentrations of its phenobarbital metabolite should be measured concurrently because it has anticonvulsant activity. Concurrent phenobarbital concentrations are usually >40 mg/L. Primidone concentrations >15 mg/L are associated with sedation, nausea, vomiting, dizziness, and ataxia [ISBN9781416061649].

17.5.4 **Carbamazepine**

Like phenytoin, carbamazepine achieves its anticonvulsant effect by modulating the synaptic sodium channel, prolonging its inactivation and controlling abnormal neuronal excitability. It has also been used to treat **neuropathic pain** (eg, postherpetic neuralgia). ~75% of the drug is protein bound, and its serum half-life is 8-12 hours. The active metabolite of carbamazepine is carbamazepine-10,11-epoxide, which in children accumulates in concentrations equal to that of carbamazepine itself. The optimal therapeutic concentration for serum/plasma carbamazepine is 4-12 mg/L. Concentrations >15 mg/L are associated with blurred vision, **paresthesia**, nystagmus, ataxia, drowsiness, and double vision. Side effects not related to serum concentration include depression of the bone marrow (even leading to aplastic anemia) and **urticaria** [ISBN9781416061649].

17.5.5 **Ethosuximide**

Ethosuximide is an anticonvulsant that reduces the flow of calcium through the T type calcium channels. It enjoys almost complete gastrointestinal absorption. It is not protein bound and undergoes extensive metabolism. Its serum half-life is 30-60 hours. The optimal therapeutic concentration for serum/plasma ethosuximide is 40-100 mg/L. Toxicity at high concentrations is rare [ISBN9781416061649].

17.5.6 **Valproic acid**

Valproic acid is a fatty acid primarily used alone to treat **absence seizures**. In combination with other anticonvulsants, it can also be used to manage other types of seizures. It acts by inhibiting GABA transaminase, thereby increasing the concentrations of GABA and inhibiting presynaptic and postsynaptic discharges. It also modulates the synaptic sodium channel by prolonging inactivation and reducing abnormal neuronal excitability. The drug is highly (>90%) protein bound, but the protein binding decreases as the drug concentration increases. The serum half-life is 11-20 hours. Correlation between serum drug concentration and dosage is poor, making TDM very important. Valproic acid modulates the **pharmacokinetics** of many other anticonvulsants, inhibiting the renal clearance of phenobarbital (thus increasing serum phenobarbital concentrations) and competing with phenytoin for protein binding sites (thus increasing the free or active fraction of phenytoin). The effective serum/plasma valproic acid concentration is 50-100 mg/L. Concentrations >100 mg/L have been associated with hepatotoxicity [ISBN9781416061649].

17.6 **Bronchodilators**
17.6.1 **Theophylline**

Theophylline, a methylxanthine that relaxes smooth muscles, is used in the treatment of asthma. It is 50% protein bound, and its serum half-life in nonsmoking adults is 7-9 hours. A minor metabolite of theophylline in adults is caffeine. In neonates, however, this metabolite accumulates and is itself an effective inhibitor of apnea. The optimal serum/plasma theophylline concentration is 10-20 mg/L. Its clearance is dose dependent, with increased doses producing large increases in serum theophylline concentrations when serum concentrations are >20 mg/L.

Toxicity includes nausea, vomiting, headache, diarrhea, insomnia, and irritability. Concentrations >30 mg/L may be associated with cardiac arrhythmias and seizures [ISBN97806833008574, ISBN9781416061649].

In overdose, theophylline stimulates production of catecholamines, leading to hyperglycemia (increased **glycogenolysis**) and **hypokalemia** (potassium is driven into the erythrocyte through stimulation of the sodium-potassium ATPase pump) [PMID3370094, PMID6506685, PMID8308948]. Administration of phenobarbital [PMID6147220] and of phenytoin [PMID3229011] induces the enzymatic metabolism of theophylline, resulting in decreased serum/plasma theophylline concentrations when these drugs are administered together [PMID6147220].

17.7 Cardioactive drugs
17.7.1 Digoxin

Digoxin, a cardiac **glycoside** used in the treatment of arrhythmias and heart failure, inhibits the sodium-potassium ATPase pump and will increase serum potassium (see Chapter 2). It slows the heart rate and increases the strength and velocity of cardiac contractions. Given that its extensive tissue distribution requires several hours, samples for serum/plasma digoxin concentration measurement must be obtained no sooner than 8 hours after the last orally administered dose; otherwise the concentration will be elevated. The drug is eliminated renally, and concentrations are very sensitive to renal function. At equilibrium, ~98% of digoxin is bound to specific cell surface receptors, especially in muscle. When in circulation, the protein binding is ~25%. Optimal serum/plasma digoxin concentrations are 0.9-2.0 mg/L, and the serum half-life is 40 hours. Given the narrow therapeutic range and the severity of digoxin poisoning, therapeutic monitoring of this drug is essential. Concentrations >3.0 mg/L can be associated with nausea, vomiting, tachycardia, ventricular fibrillation, and a green-yellow visual disturbance. When the antiarrhythmic drug quinidine is coadministered with digoxin, it displaces digoxin from its receptors in skeletal muscle and, in addition, diminishes the renal clearance of digoxin, thus increasing digoxin serum concentrations as much as 2-3 fold. Treatment of digoxin poisoning utilizes digoxin antibody fragments (Digibind) [PMID3229011, ISBN9781416061649].

17.8 Antibiotics
17.8.1 Aminoglycosides (amikacin, gentamicin, tobramycin)

The **aminoglycoside** antibiotics act by inhibiting protein synthesis of Gram– bacteria. Due to their poor absorption by the oral route, they are administered parenterally. They are renally cleared as the unmetabolized drug for the most part. Despite their antibiotic efficacy, they exhibit significant toxicity, mostly **nephrotoxicity** and irreversible **ototoxicity**. The major aminoglycoside antibiotics include amikacin, gentamicin, and tobramycin. These drugs demonstrate a "postantibiotic effect," manifesting bactericidal activity even after the drug has cleared [ISBN9781416061649].

The serum half-lives of amikacin, gentamicin, and tobramycin are 2.3, 2.5, and 2.0 hours, respectively, and their protein binding is <10%. Serum/plasma aminoglycoside **peak concentrations** should be measured at 1 hour after infusion, and **trough concentrations** should be measured just before the next infusion or at a minimum of 10-12 hours postinfusion [ISBN9781416061649]. Target peak and trough concentrations are as follows: amikacin (peak 20-25 mg/L, trough 5-10 mg/L); gentamicin (peak 6-10 mg/L, trough 0.5-2.0 mg/L); and tobramycin (peak 6-10 mg/dL, trough 0.5-2.0 mg/L).

17.8.2 Glycopeptides (vancomycin)

The **glycopeptide** vancomycin is effective in treatment of infection by many Gram+ bacteria and some Gram– cocci. It is also used in treatment of methicillin resistant *Staphylococcus aureus* (MRSA). Like the aminoglycosides, it must be administered parenterally. It is usually given by slow intravenous infusion about every 12 hours. It has a serum/plasma half-life of 5.5 hours, and, also like the aminoglycosides, it is excreted renally and can cause ototoxicity and nephrotoxicity, particularly if coadministered with the aminoglycosides. It is 30% bound to serum proteins [ISBN9781416061649, ISBN9781594251023]. Serum/plasma trough concentrations are often targeted to 20 mg/L [PMID21208910]. Peak concentrations are no longer recommended, given the concentration independent pharmacodynamic properties of vancomycin and the lack of data correlating peak concentrations with efficacy and toxicity [PMID19106348].

17.9 Immunosuppressive drugs

17.9.1 Cyclosporine A

Cyclosporine A, a fat soluble cyclic peptide that blocks the activation of T lymphocytes, has been approved for use in kidney, heart, liver, pancreas, and bone marrow transplants. It has also been used to treat psoriasis and rheumatoid arthritis. The drug manifests nephrotoxicity, although liver and central nervous system toxicity can occur. It is highly (90%) protein bound (primarily to lipoproteins in erythrocytes) and extensively metabolized mostly to inactive metabolites. The half-life is 8.4 hours. Because of its binding to the red cell, measurements are performed on whole blood. The drug is manufactured in both oral and intravenous formulations. Therapeutic ranges vary and are dependent on many factors, including the transplanted organ, the assay method, time after transplantation, and coadministration of other immunosuppressive drugs. However, the minimum effective concentration is considered to be 50 µg/dL. Ranges are usually established for each institution and patient [ISBN9781416061649, ISBN9781594251023].

17.9.2 Sirolimus

Sirolimus, a macrocyclic antibiotic with immunosuppressive properties, inhibits T lymphocyte activation and proliferation, and is used in solid organ transplantation. It distributes (>95%) into erythrocytes with only little drug in plasma. Accordingly, TDM of sirolimus is performed on whole blood. Of the amount in plasma, 90% is bound to proteins. Because of its prolonged half-life (62 hours), it is usually administered orally only once daily. The minimum effective immunosuppressant blood concentration is 4 µg/L. The recommended threshold concentration is 13-15 µg/L, above which concentration related toxicity may occur (**thrombocytopenia**, **leukopenia**, and hyperlipidemia). Nephrotoxicity is not seen with sirolimus. Recommended therapeutic ranges vary when other immunosuppressive agents are coadministered [ISBN9781416061649, ISBN9781594251023].

17.9.3 Tacrolimus

Tacrolimus, a macrocyclic lactone that has potent immunosuppressive activity, is administered in both oral and intravenous formulations to patients with liver, kidney, heart, and other solid organ transplants. Its primary toxic effect is nephrotoxicity, although neurotoxicity, hypertension, insomnia, and nausea are occasionally seen. Tacrolimus is found predominately in the erythrocyte, and 85% of the drug in plasma is bound to proteins. Accordingly, TDM is performed on whole blood. The half-life is 21 hours. A therapeutic range of 5-20 µg/L has been suggested [ISBN9781416061649, ISBN9781594251023].

17.10 Future directions in TDM

Future directions in TDM will involve use of a patient's genome to determine which particular drugs will provide optimal response (**pharmacogenomics**). In fact, this is at the core of "individualized," or "personalized," medicine. Already, evaluation of genetic differences in metabolizing such drugs as warfarin is being used in selected cases to optimize dosage regimens [PMID22144632]. Such genetic differences help to explain why the same dosage of a drug yields different serum concentrations in similar individuals so that, traditionally, clinicians have had to adjust dosages empirically and then monitor resulting concentrations.

17.11 References
17.11.1 Journals

PMID11564048 Gross AS [1998] Best practice in therapeutic drug monitoring. *Br J Clin Pharmacol* 46:95-9

PMID19106348 Rybak M, Lomaestro B, Rotschafer JC et al [2009] Therapeutic monitoring of vancomycin in patients: a consensus review of the American Society of Health-System Pharmacists, the Infectious Diseases Society of America, and the Society of Infectious Diseases Pharmacists. *Am J Health Syst Pharm* 66: 82-98

PMID21208910 Liu C, Bayer A, Cosgrove SE et al [2011] Clinical practice guidelines by the infectious diseases society of America for the treatment of methicillin resistant staphylococcus aureus infections in adults and children. *Clin Infect Dis* 52:e18-55

PMID22144632 Carlquist JF, Anderson JL [2011] Using pharmacogenetics in real time to guide warfarin initiation: a clinician update. *Circulation* 124:2554-9

PMID3229011 Adebayo GI [1988] Interaction between phenytoin and theophylline in healthy volunteers. *Clin Exp Pharmacol Physiol* 15: 883-7

PMID3370094 Amitai Y, Lovejoy FH [1988] Hypokalemia in acute theophylline poisoning. *Am J Emerg Med* 6:214-8

PMID6147220 Jonkman JHG, Upton RA [2012] Pharmacokinetic drug interactions with theophylline. *Clin Pharmacokinet* 9:309-34

PMID6506685 Biberstein MP, Ziegler MG, Ward DM [1984] Use of β-blockade and hemoperfusion for acute theophylline poisoning. *West J Med* 141:485-90

PMID8308948 Shannon M [1994] Hypokalemia, hyperglycemia and plasma catecholamine activity after severe theophylline intoxication. *J Toxicol Clin Toxicol* 32:41-7

Pramod K [2014] Review on therapeutic drug monitoring. *Int J Pharmacol Ther* 4:12-18

17.11.2 **Books**

ISBN9780683300857 Yang J [2002] Toxicology testing in the clinical laboratory. In: Lewandrowski K, ed. *Clinical Chemistry: Laboratory Management & Clinical Correlations*. Lippincott Williams & Wilkins, 793-4

ISBN9781416061649 Snozek CLH, McMillin GA, Moyer, TP [2013] Therapeutic drugs and their management. In: Burtis CA, Ashwood ER, Bruns DE, ed. *Tietz Textbook of Clinical Chemistry and Molecular Diagnostics*, 5e. Elsevier Saunders, 1057-1108

ISBN9781594251023 Broussard LA, Hammett-Stabler CA [2011] Therapeutic drug monitoring. In: Clarke W, ed. *Contemporary Practice in Clinical Chemistry*, 2e. AACC Press, 573-85

17.12 **Clinical cases**

17.12.1 **Case 1**

A 67-year-old male treated with digoxin for heart failure is started on quinidine by his cardiologist due to development of an arrhythmia. His serum digoxin concentrations rise to toxic levels. The patient's primary care physician believes that the patient is taking digoxin in excess, but the patient emphatically denies that.

17.12.1.1 **Questions**

1. What has happened?

2. What should be done to correct the situation?

17.12.2 **Case 2**

A 46-year-old male developed shingles ~1 year ago. Since then he has been troubled with postherpetic neuralgia at the site where the lesions had been. His primary care physician prescribes carbamazepine, 200 mg twice per day, for relief of the pain. 4 weeks later the dosage is increased to 600 mg twice per day. ~10 days later, the patient started having nystagmus and difficulty walking. A "stat" serum carbamazepine concentration was 16.3 mg/L.

17.12.2.1 **Questions**

1. Was the patient's carbamazepine dose monitored correctly?

2. Can the nystagmus and difficulty walking be explained by the carbamazepine?

3. How should the patient be treated?

4. What additional laboratory tests should be ordered?

17.12.3 Case 3

A 77-year-old male with a history of a seizure disorder has experienced the onset of falls over the last few weeks as well as generalized unsteadiness and weakness. His medications include phenytoin, phenobarbital, and primidone. In the clinic, his serum phenobarbital concentration was 60 mg/L, and his serum phenytoin concentration was 23 mg/L.

17.12.3.1 Questions

1. Interpret the serum drug concentrations.

2. How would you treat this patient?

17.12.4 Case 4

A 51-year-old male with a seizure disorder treated with phenytoin has experienced confusion and disorientation over the last 4 days accompanied by severe dysarthria, ataxia, and seizures. The man is also a chronic alcoholic and has hypothyroidism. His wife reports that she withheld his phenytoin dose 2 days ago.

Serum laboratory studies obtained in the emergency department show urea-N 14 mg/dL, creatinine 0.8 mg/dL, glucose 101 mg/dL, sodium 139 mMol/L (mEq/L), potassium 4.0 mMol/L (mEq/L), chloride 104 mMol/L (mEq/L), bicarbonate 25mMol/L (mEq/L), calcium 8.9 mg/dL, thyroid stimulating hormone (TSH) 6.23 mIU/mL, and serum phenytoin 47.3 mg/L.

17.12.4.1 Questions

1. What are the most likely causes of the patient's confusion, disorientation, dysarthria, ataxia, and seizures?

2. Explain the elevated serum phenytoin concentration.

3. What additional laboratory tests should be ordered?

4. How should the patient be treated?

17.12.5 **Case 5**

A 75-year-old male with diabetes mellitus type II, asthma, gout, and atrial fibrillation is seen at the urgent care clinic with worsening dyspnea on exertion. His theophylline dose had recently been increased from 600 mg to 800 mg per day. An electrocardiogram shows atrial fibrillation and a heart rate of 135 beats per minute. The patient states that he has taken 6 tablets of 200 mg theophylline in the last 4 hours. In the clinic, the patient suffers a grand mal seizure.

Serum laboratory results show the following: urea-N 31 mg/dL, creatinine 1.8 mg/dL, glucose 242 mg/dL, sodium 134 mMol/L (mEq/L) potassium 2.9 mMol/L (mEq/L), chloride 95 mMol/L (mEq/L), bicarbonate 20 mMol/L (mEq/L), calcium 9.2 mg/dL, and serum theophylline 56 mg/L.

17.12.5.1 **Questions**

1. Explain the seizure activity and atrial fibrillation.

2. Explain the low bicarbonate and the increased anion gap.

3. Explain the elevated urea-N and creatinine.

4. Explain the elevated glucose and the low potassium.

5. How might this situation have been prevented?

17.12.6 Clinical case answers

17.12.6.1 Case 1 answers

1. Quinidine displaces digoxin from its receptors in skeletal muscle and also decreases the renal elimination of digoxin, causing the serum digoxin concentration to rise

2. Either quinidine should be discontinued, or the digoxin dose should be lowered, or both; in cases of severe toxicity, digoxin antibody fragments (Digibind) may be administered. Serum/plasma concentrations of digoxin should be monitored closely.

17.12.6.2 Case 2 answers

1. Prior to increasing the carbamazepine dosage, the physician should have obtained a serum carbamazepine concentration and adjusted the dose based on that measurement

2. Carbamazepine toxicity includes nystagmus and ataxia

3. The carbamazepine dose should be decreased, and after 3-4 days, the drug concentration should be measured again; alternatively, another drug might be substituted for carbamazepine in treatment of the neuropathic pain (eg, amitriptyline)

4. Since carbamazepine can also depress the bone marrow, a complete blood count should be ordered

17.12.6.3 Case 3 answers

1. The serum phenobarbital concentration is significantly higher than the recommended therapeutic range of 10-40 mg/L, and the serum phenytoin concentration is also higher than the recommended therapeutic range, 10-20 mg/L; together these concentrations could certainly explain the patient's unsteadiness and falling

2. The primidone should be discontinued because it will contribute to the phenobarbital concentration due to its metabolism to phenobarbital. The phenobarbital should be discontinued until its serum concentration falls within the recommended reference range (10-40 mg/L). The serum phenytoin dose should be decreased. The serum phenytoin concentrations should then be monitored closely since phenobarbital can induce the metabolism of phenytoin, and decreasing the serum phenobarbital concentration could lead to increased phenytoin concentrations. Also, phenytoin decreases the renal clearance of phenobarbital, causing serum concentrations to increase

17.12.6.4 Case 4 answers

1. The serum phenytoin concentration is significantly higher than the recommended therapeutic range (10-20 mg/L) and could certainly account for the findings. In addition, the patient may be intoxicated with ethanol, leading to ataxia. The seizure activity may be related to phenytoin toxicity and/or alcohol withdrawal if he has not been drinking

2. Although his wife decreased his phenytoin dose 2 days prior, the drug may still saturate the metabolic pathways. In addition, his poorly treated hypothyroidism (evidenced by the elevated TSH) may lead to decreased metabolism of phenytoin, allowing serum phenytoin concentrations to increase. Finally, if he has alcoholic liver disease, he may not be able to metabolize phenytoin appropriately.

3. A serum alcohol measurement and liver function studies should be ordered.

4. Phenytoin should be stopped, and concentrations monitored. The patient should receive thyroid replacement therapy with monitoring of his serum TSH. He should enter alcohol treatment therapy as well.

17.12.6.5 Case 5 answers

1. In overdose, theophylline can produce both cardiac arrhythmias and seizures; since the patient already had a history of atrial fibrillation, the theophylline exacerbated it.

2. The low serum bicarbonate and the increased anion gap suggest metabolic acidosis, which could be secondary to peripheral vasoconstriction from the catecholamine production due to the elevated serum theophylline. Vasoconstriction could induce lactic acidosis. Additionally, the elevated urea-N and creatinine suggest some renal failure, perhaps secondary to the patient's diabetes mellitus or due to decreased renal perfusion due to the vasoconstriction. Renal failure would contribute to the metabolic acidosis as well

3. As noted above, the urea-N and creatinine elevation may be due to diabetic nephropathy or poor renal perfusion secondary to vasoconstriction

4. The hyperglycemia could be due to poorly treated diabetes mellitus, plus the theophylline induced production of catecholamines, which would enhance glycogenolysis. The hypokalemia is due to potassium entering the red cell as a result of the theophylline overdose stimulating the sodium-potassium ATPase pump

5. The patient's serum theophylline concentrations should have been monitored before the dosage was increased

chapter 18

The laboratory diagnosis of thyroid disease

18.1 **Objectives**

At the end of this session, the learner should be able to

- ➢ describe the signs and symptoms of hyperthyroidism
- ➢ describe the signs and symptoms of hypothyroidism
- ➢ discuss the hypothalamic-pituitary-thyroid gland axis
- ➢ describe the causes of hyperthyroidism
- ➢ describe the causes of hypothyroidism
- ➢ describe the binding of thyroxine and triiodothyronine in serum
- ➢ discuss factors that increase the binding of thyroid hormones
- ➢ discuss factors that decrease the binding of thyroid hormones
- ➢ discuss causes of euthyroid hyperthyroxinemia
- ➢ discuss causes of euthyroid hypothyroxinemia
- ➢ discuss the causes of and findings in sick euthyroid syndrome (low T_3 syndrome; nonthyroidal illness)
- ➢ describe concentrations of serum reverse triiodothyronine in acute febrile illness, chronic hepatic cirrhosis, and newborns
- ➢ discuss the use of thyroid stimulating hormone, total thyroxine, free thyroxine, total triiodothyronine, and free triiodothyronine in the workup of thyroid disease
- ➢ discuss the use of antithyroid antibodies in the workup of thyroid disease
- ➢ discuss thyroid stimulating immunoglobulins and their role in Grave disease
- ➢ discuss subclinical hyperthyroidism and its significance
- ➢ discuss subclinical hypothyroidism and its significance
- ➢ describe neonatal thyroid screening
- ➢ discuss changes in serum cholesterol concentration in hyperthyroidism and hypothyroidism
- ➢ discuss changes in serum creatine kinase activity in hyperthyroidism and hypothyroidism

18.2 **Key terms**

atrial fibrillation: a relatively common arrhythmia, characterized by quivering of the atria

bradycardia: slow heartbeat

central hypothyroidism: either secondary (pituitary) or tertiary (hypothalamic) hypothyroidism

dyspnea: shortness of breath

euthyroid: having normal thyroid gland activity

euthyroid hyperthyroxinemia: a condition in which the concentration of total thyroxine in serum/plasma is elevated while the free thyroxine is normal due to elevated binding proteins

euthyroid hypothyroxinemia: a condition in which the concentration of total thyroxine in serum/plasma is low while the free thyroxine is normal due to decreased binding proteins

exophthalmos: abnormal protrusion of the eyeball in Grave disease

Hashimoto thyroiditis: a progressive autoimmune disease of the thyroid gland, usually progressing to hypothyroidism

hyperhidrosis: excessive sweating; diaphoresis

goiter: enlargement of the thyroid gland

Grave disease: thyroid disease usually of autoimmune etiology and characterized by hyperthyroidism, goiter, exophthalmos, and the presence of thyroid stimulating immunoglobulins

primary hyperthyroidism: hyperthyroidism due to overproduction of thyroid hormones by the thyroid gland

primary hypothyroidism: hypothyroidism due to underproduction of the thyroid hormones by the thyroid gland

reverse triiodothyronine: an inactive metabolite of T_4 (rT_3)

secondary hyperthyroidism: hyperthyroidism due to overproduction of thyroid stimulating hormone by the pituitary

secondary hypothyroidism: hypothyroidism due to underproduction of thyroid stimulating hormone by the pituitary

sick euthyroid syndrome (low T_3 syndrome; nonthyroidal illness): a condition in which the triiodothyronine is low due to decreased peripheral conversion of thyroxine to triiodothyronine and characterized by an increase in reverse triiodothyronine

subclinical hyperthyroidism: a persistent decrease in thyroid stimulating hormone when free thyroxine and triiodothyronine concentrations are normal

subclinical hypothyroidism: a persistent increase in thyroid stimulating hormone when free thyroxine and triiodothyronine concentrations are normal

tertiary hypothyroidism: hypothyroidism caused by underproduction of thyrotropin releasing hormone by the hypothalamus

tachycardia: rapid heartbeat

thyroglobulin: a glycoprotein produced by the follicular cells of the thyroid gland and containing the precursors of thyroxine and triiodothyronine

thyroid stimulating hormone (TSH): a hormone secreted by the anterior pituitary gland in response to thyrotropin releasing hormone produced by the hypothalamus; it stimulates the thyroid gland to produce its hormones

thyroperoxidase: an enzyme in thyroid colloid that catalyzes the oxidation of iodide ion to iodine

thyrotropin releasing hormone (TRH): a hormone secreted by the hypothalamus that stimulates the anterior pituitary gland to produce TSH

thyroid stimulating immunoglobulins (TSIs): immunoglobulins with agonist properties at the thyroid stimulating hormone receptor

thyroxine: 3,5,3',5'-tetraiodothyronine (T_4)

thyroxine binding globulin: a serum α_1 globulin that binds thyroxine

triiodothyronine: 3,5,3'-triiodothyronine (T_3)

vitiligo: skin depigmentation

18.3 Background/significance

Thyroid dysfunction is common in adults. The reported prevalence of hypothyroidism is 2%, and of **subclinical hypothyroidism**, up to 17%. The prevalence of hyperthyroidism is 0.2%, and of **subclinical hyperthyroidism** up to 6%. Accordingly, the American Thyroid Association has recommended that adults be screened for thyroid dysfunction beginning at age 35 and every 5 years thereafter [PMID10847249]. An understanding of the laboratory diagnosis of thyroid disease is important to clinical practice.

18.4 Signs & symptoms of hyperthyroidism & hypothyroidism

Hyperthyroidism is characterized by fatigue, weight loss, heat intolerance, **hyperhidrosis**, nervousness, insomnia, tremor, diarrhea, muscle weakness, **dyspnea**, palpitations, **tachycardia**, **atrial fibrillation**, increased deep tendon reflexes, and decreased menses [PMID10847249]. **Vitiligo** is also a feature in some individuals due to autoimmune destruction of the melanocytes.

Hypothyroidism is characterized by fatigue, weight gain, cold intolerance, skin dryness, hair dryness or loss, depression, lethargy, muscle cramps, myalgias, decreased deep tendon reflexes, deepening of the voice, edema, **bradycardia**, constipation, infertility, and menstrual irregularity [PMID10847249].

18.5 Hypothalamic-pituitary-thyroid gland axis & thyroid hormones

The hypothalamus secretes **thyrotropin releasing hormone (TRH)**, which stimulates the anterior pituitary to secrete **thyroid stimulating hormone (TSH)**. In turn, TSH stimulates the thyroid gland to secrete thyroid hormones (**thyroxine**, 3,5,3',5'-tetraiodothyronine [T_4]; **triiodothyronine**, 3,5,3'-triiodothyronine [T_3]). Of the secreted hormones, 80% is T_4, and 20% is T_3. Both T_4 and T_3 exert major negative feedback on TSH and minor negative feedback on TRH. Although the thyroid gland secretes some T_3, most of it is formed from deiodination of T_4 peripherally (mostly in the liver). In fact, substantial evidence suggests that T_3 has the major hormonal activity, so T_4 can effectively be considered to be a prohormone. The T_4 is also deiodinated to yield an inactive metabolite, **reverse triiodothyronine** (rT_3; an isomer of T_3) in about the same amount as T_3

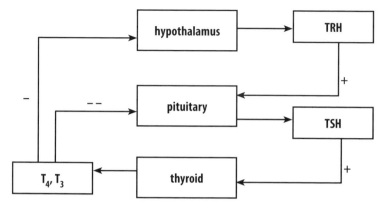

peripherally: $T_4 \to T_3 + rT_3$ (equal amounts); rT_3 is inactive

f18.1 Hypothalamus-pituitary-thyroid gland axis; thyroid hormone production = 80% T_4 (prohormone) and 20% T_3 (active hormone)

T_4

T_3

rT_3

f18.2 Structures of thyroid hormones

[ISBN9781416061649, ISBN9781594251023]. The hypothalamic-pituitary-thyroid gland axis is depicted in **f18.1**, and the structures of the major thyroid hormones are shown in **f18.2**.

18.6 Causes of hyperthyroidism & hypothyroidism

The most common cause of **primary hyperthyroidism** (autonomous excessive secretion of thyroid hormones by the thyroid) is autoantibodies to the thyroid stimulating hormone (TSH) receptor (**Grave disease**). **Exophthalmos** is a prominent finding in this disease, in addition to the other findings of hyperthyroidism previously described. Other causes include thyroid nodules (both nodular and multinodular **goiters**), thyroid follicular adenomas, and congenital hyperthyroidism resulting from a gain of function mutation of the TSH receptor, causing it to stimulate thyroid hormone release. **Secondary hyperthyroidism** (excessive secretion of TSH by the pituitary) can be caused by pituitary adenomas that excessively secrete TSH (rare), and by loss of function mutations in the pituitary T_4 and T_3 receptors so that there is suppression of the feedback inhibition of thyroid hormone release. Finally, transitional gestational thyrotoxicosis occurs in 2%-3% of pregnancies due to TSH receptor sensitivity to human chorionic gonadotropin (hCG). For the same reason, hCG secreting tumors can cause thyrotoxicosis [ISBN9781594251023].

The most common cause of primary endogenous hypothyroidism (hyposecretion of thyroid hormones by the thyroid) is autoimmune destruction of the thyroid gland (**Hashimoto thyroiditis**). Other causes include iodine deficiency, drug or surgery induced dysfunction (eg, in the treatment of hyperthyroidism), and iodine excess (inhibiting thyroid hormone synthesis and release). **Secondary hypothyroidism** (hyposecretion of TSH by the pituitary) can be due to pituitary malignancy or ischemia (infarction), while **tertiary hypothyroidism** (hyposecretion of TRH by the hypothalamus) is caused by hypothalamic dysfunction or infarction. Together, secondary hypothyroidism and tertiary hypothyroidism constitute **central hypothyroidism**. Finally, on rare occasions, there can be peripheral resistance to the effects of thyroid hormones and mutations in the enzymes involved in the deiodination of T_4 to T_3 [ISBN9781594251023].

18.6.1 Thyroid hormone binding

Thyroxine (T_4) binds with high affinity to **thyroxine binding globulin** (TBG; 70%), with low affinity to albumin (ALB; 20%) and transthyretin (TTR; formerly called prealbumin; 10%). The active hormone (free T_4 [FT_4]; 0.03% of total T_4) is unbound. As the concentration of the binding proteins increases, the total hormone concentration (free plus bound) increases, but the free hormone concentration remains within the reference range. Triiodothyronine (T_3) binds with high affinity to TBG (80%), and with low affinity to ALB (10%) and TTR (10%). Free T_3 (FT_3; 0.3% of total T_3) is the active hormone [ISBN9781416061649, ISBN9781594251023].

Euthyroid hyperthyroxinemia is a condition in which the total concentration of thyroxine (T_4) is elevated while the FT_4 is normal, resulting in the patient being **euthyroid**. This condition can result from 1) increased concentration or affinity of thyroid binding proteins: TBG: congenital increases; induction by such drugs as estrogen, tamoxifen, methadone, oral contraceptives; induction by pregnancy; normal elevation in newborns; nonthyroidal illness such as hepatitis, estrogen producing tumors, human immunodeficiency virus infection; TTR: familial increase; ALB: familial dysalbuminemia, in which an abnormal albumin binds excessive amount of T_4; antibodies: autoimmune thyroid disease and hepatocellular carcinoma, in which an excessive amount of T_4 is bound by antibodies; and 2) <u>peripheral resistance to thyroid hormones and/or loss of function mutations in the hormone receptors</u> (resulting in overproduction of thyroid hormones in attempt to overcome the resistance) [ISBN9781416061649].

Euthyroid hypothyroxinemia is a condition in which the total concentration of T_4 is low while the FT_4 is normal, resulting in the patient being euthyroid. Causes of this condition include 1) <u>decreases in TBG concentration</u> (congenital; nonthyroidal illness causing decreased TBG synthesis, as in liver disease, or TBG loss, as in nephrotic syndrome; use of anabolic steroids or large amounts of glucocorticoids); 2) <u>coadministration of drugs that displace T_4 from TBG</u> (eg, salicylates, phenytoin; causing a rise in FT_4, which is then cleared, resulting in a lowered total T_4 concentration, but a normal FT_4); and 3) <u>low transthyretin concentration</u> (eg, with malnutrition or acute inflammation) [ISBN9781416061649].

18.6.2 Sick euthyroid syndrome (low T_3 syndrome; nonthyroidal Illness)

In the so called **sick euthyroid syndrome** (low T_3 syndrome), there is decreased peripheral conversion of T_4 to T_3. This is seen in patients with acute and chronic systemic illness as well as malnutrition, and is thought to be the metabolism responding to the illness by decreasing cellular oxygen demand. The decrease in T_3 is mirrored by an increase in rT_3, because the production of the latter from T_4 is not decreased. The diminished T_3 may result in a slight increase in TSH, but the patient remains essentially euthyroid or only very slightly hypothyroid. With time, the total T_4 may also decrease due to changes in TBG binding affinity [ISBN9781594251023]. Increases of rT_3 are also seen in patients with hepatic cirrhosis [PMID6637968, PMID812882] and acute febrile illnesses [PMID812882], and in newborns [PMID1133163].

18.7 Laboratory testing for thyroid disease
18.7.1 Thyroid stimulating hormone (TSH)

The serum/plasma TSH test is considered to be the most sensitive indicator of thyroid hormone activity, and the current generation of TSH assays is sufficiently sensitive that these assays can be used to assess thyroid status. Thus, the TSH test should be the first performed in evaluation of thyroid function. Low TSH suggests primary hyperthyroidism or central hypothyroidism, while elevated TSH suggests **primary hypothyroidism** or secondary hyperthyroidism.

18.7.1.1 Reference range
TSH: 0.27-4.2 mIU/L

18.7.2 Thyroxine (T_4) & triiodothyronine (T_3)

In patients with primary hyperthyroidism, the serum/plasma total T_4 and T_3 are elevated, while the TSH is decreased. With secondary hyperthyroidism, the TSH, T_4, and T_3 are all elevated. Causes of primary and secondary hyperthyroidism have been described above. Hyperthyroidism can also exist with elevated serum/plasma T_3, but normal T_4 (the so called "T_3 thyrotoxicosis") [PMID4193903].

In patients with primary hypothyroidism, the serum/plasma total T_4 and T_3 are low while the TSH is elevated. With secondary and tertiary hypothyroidism, the TSH, T_4 and T_3 are all low. In earlier years, in order to differentiate secondary from tertiary hypothyroidism, a TRH infusion test was performed. Following intravenous administration of 200 µg of TRH, the serum/plasma TSH was measured. With secondary hypothyroidism, the TSH would not rise, while with tertiary hypothyroidism the TSH rose. However, TRH is no longer available in the United States, and the role of the TRH infusion test in evaluation of central hypothyroidism is limited due to the improved diagnostic sensitivity of serum tests and imaging studies [PMID14646390].

18.7.2.1 Reference ranges (adult)

Total T_4: 4.5-10.9 µg/dL
Total T_3: 80-200 ng/dL
rT_3: 9-27 ng/dL

18.7.3 Free hormones

Measurements of FT_4 and FT_3 are available and provide a better indication of thyroid status than do the respective total hormones. They may be particularly helpful in borderline cases of hyperthyroidism and hypothyroidism. The general approach to the laboratory diagnosis of thyroid disease is to measure a TSH and then perform an FT_4 or FT_3 if the TSH is abnormal.

18.7.3.1 Reference ranges (adult)

FT_4: 0.93-1.7 ng/dL
FT_3: 2.5-430 pg/dL

18.7.4 Antithyroid antibodies

As previously noted, endogenous primary hyperthyroidism is characterized by autoantibodies to various thyroid antigens. In fact, 85% of patients with Grave disease and 95% of patients with Hashimoto thyroiditis have detectable amounts of autoantibodies, mostly directed toward **thyroperoxidase** [ISBN9781594251023].

18.7.5 Thyroid stimulating immunoglobulins (TSIs)

Thyroid stimulating immunoglobulins (TSIs) are antibodies that continuously stimulate the TSH receptor in Grave disease. These antibodies are synthesized in the thyroid gland, bone marrow, and lymph nodes. They can be detected by bioassays or by using an assay for thyrotropin binding inhibiting immunoglobulins [ISBN9780071802154].

18.8 Subclinical hyperthyroidism

Subclinical hyperthyroidism is characterized by decreased serum/plasma TSH concentration (usually <0.1 miU/L) with normal FT_4 and FT_3. Patients with this condition have increased frequency of atrial fibrillation and osteoporosis but, unless they have documented cardiac arrhythmias, decreased bone density, or nodular thyroid disease, there is little indication for treatment [ISBN9781416061649]. There are 2 types of subclinical hyperthyroidism: 1) exogenous (caused by administration of levothyroxine, which should be reduced); and 2) endogenous (not caused by administration of thyroid hormones). These patients should be monitored with thyroid function tests [PMID11519506].

18.9 Subclinical hypothyroidism

Subclinical hypothyroidism is characterized by increased serum/plasma TSH concentration with normal FT_4 and FT_3. This condition affects up to 17% of the population overall and 10% of those over 60 years of age. Individuals with this condition may progress to hypothyroidism, elevated serum/plasma lipids, and cardiovascular disease. If the TSH is persistently >10 miU/L, thyroid hormone replacement therapy is justified. It should be noted that increased TSH with normal FT_4 and FT_3 can also be seen in individuals reinstituting thyroid replacement, as well as in those with poor compliance with replacement therapy and in those with thyroid hormone resistance [ISBN9781416061649].

18.10 Screening for neonatal thyroid disease

Congenital hypothyroidism is found in 1 out of 4,000 newborns. If unrecognized, this condition leads to mental retardation of the newborn (cretinism), and for that reason, most industrialized countries perform neonatal screening for thyroid disease. Most cases of congenital hypothyroidism are due to recessive mutations in thyroperoxidase or **thyroglobulin** [ISBN9780071802154]. Infants are screened at 2-4 days of age or at the time of discharge using eluates of blood collected onto filter paper; and preterm infants are tested within 7 days of birth [PMID16740880]. Most testing in North America involves measurement of T_4. Those infants with the lowest 10% of T_4 concentrations measured that day are subsequently evaluated with a TSH measurement using the same specimen. If the TSH exceeds 60 miU/L after the first 1-2 days of life, the infant is treated with replacement therapy. If the TSH is 20-59 miU/L, the infant is evaluated clinically and repeat testing is performed. If the TSH is <20 miU/L, hypothyroidism is excluded [ISBN9781416061649]. It should be noted that neonatal TSH is usually 20-25 miU/L at 1 day of age, dropping to 9 miU/L at 2-12 weeks of age [PMID16740880]. Some laboratories in Europe use the TSH as the primary test and, if low, measure the T_4 [ISBN9781416061649].

18.11 Nonspecific laboratory findings in thyroid disease

Patients with thyroid disease often manifest nonspecific changes in clinical chemistry tests, including elevation of serum creatine kinase [PMID23105382] and cholesterol [PMID21660244] in hypothyroidism, and depression of serum creatine kinase [PMID23105382] and cholesterol [PMID21660244] in hyperthyroidism. Obviously these endocrine disorders also have profound effect on metabolism of drugs and hormones as well, but a discussion of this is beyond the purview of this chapter.

18.12 References
18.12.1 Journals

PMID10847249 Ladenson PW, Singer PA, Ain KB et al [2000] American thyroid association guidelines for detection of thyroid dysfunction. *Arch Intern Med* 160:1573-5

PMID1133163 Chopra IJ, Sack J, Fisher DA [1975] Circulating 3,3',5'-triiodothyronine (reverse T$_3$) in the human newborn. *J Clin Invest* 55:1137-41

PMID11519506 Toft AD [2001] Clinical practice: subclinical hyperthyroidism. *N Engl J Med* 345:512-6

PMID14646390 Hartoft-Nielsen ML, Lange M, Rasmussen AK et al [2004] Thyrotropin-releasing hormone stimulation test in patients with pituitary pathology. *Horm Res* 61: 53-7

PMID16740880 Rose SR, Brown RS [2006] Update of newborn screening and therapy for congenital hypothyroidism. *Pediatrics* 117:2290-2303

PMID21660244 Rizos CV, Elisaf MS, Liberopoulos EN [2011] Effects of thyroid dysfunction on lipid profile. *Open Cardiovasc Med J* 5:76-84

PMID23105382 Ranka R, Mathur R [2003] Serum creatine phosphokinase in thyroid disorders. *Indian J Clin Biochem* 18:107-10

PMID4193903 Sterling K, Refetoff S, Selenkow HA [1970] T$_3$ thyrotoxicosis: thyrotoxicosis due to elevated serum triiodothyronine levels. *JAMA* 213:571-5

PMID6637968 Kabadi UM, Premachandra BN [1983] Serum T$_3$ and reverse T$_3$ levels in hepatic cirrhosis: relation to hepatocellular damage and normalization on improvement in liver dysfunction. *Am J Gastroenterol* 78:750-5

PMID812882 Chopra IJ, Chopra U, Smith SR et al [1975] Reciprocal changes in serum concentrations of 3,3',5-triiodothyronine (T$_3$) in systemic illnesses. *J Clin Endocrinol Metab* 41:1043-9

18.12.2 Books

ISBN9780071802154 Jameson JL, Mandel SJ, Weetman AP [2015] Disorders of the thyroid gland. In: Kasper DL, Fauci AS, Hauser SL et al, ed. *Harrison's Principles of Internal Medicine*, 19e. McGraw-Hill Education, 2283-2308

ISBN9781416061649 Winter WE, Schatz D, Bertholf RL [2013] The thyroid: pathophysiology and thyroid function testing. In: Burtis CA, Ashwood ER, Bruns DE, ed. *Tietz Textbook of Clinical Chemistry and Molecular Diagnostics*, 5e. Elsevier Saunders, 1905-44

ISBN9781594251023 Bertholf RL [2011] Laboratory evaluation of thyroid function. In: Clarke W, ed. *Contemporary Practice in Clinical Chemistry*, 2e. AACC Press, 431-48

18.13 Clinical cases
18.13.1 Case 1

A 27-year-old female has a serum total thyroxine (T$_4$) of 13.6 µg/dL and total triiodothyronine (T$_3$) of 280 ng/dL. Her serum thyroid stimulating hormone (TSH), cholesterol, and creatine kinase were within the respective reference ranges. The physical examination was within normal limits.

18.13.1.1 Questions

1. What is the most likely explanation for these findings?

2. What other thyroid function test might be obtained in order to confirm the conclusion?

18.13.2 **Case 2**

A 59-year-old female visits her primary care physician and complains of a 30 lb weight gain over the last 8 months, the development of fatigue, "puffiness" around her eyes, dry skin, and a deepening of her voice. Physical examination reveals a diffusely enlarged thyroid gland (1.5× normal size), a heart rate of 56 beats per minute, blood pressure of 130/90 mmHg, and decreased deep tendon reflexes.

Laboratory studies showed serum thyroxine (T_4) 2.6 µg/dL and thyroid stimulating hormone (TSH) 110 mIU/L.

18.13.2.1 **Questions**

1. What is the most likely diagnosis?

2. What additional laboratory studies would be helpful?

18.13.3 **Case 3**

An anxious 49-year-old female with "piercing eyes" but no exophthalmos visited her primary care physician with the chief complaint of tremors. Physical examination revealed tremors of her outstretched hands, a diffusely enlarged thyroid gland, heart rate of 112 beats per minute, blood pressure 140/80 mmHg, and hyperactive deep tendon reflexes.

Laboratory studies showed a serum total thyroxine (T_4) 19.8 µg/dL and a thyroid stimulating hormone (TSH) of 0.04 mIU/L.

18.13.3.1 **Questions**

1. What is the most likely diagnosis for this patient?

2. What additional laboratory studies would be helpful?

18.13.4 **Case 4**

A 55-year-old male visits his primary care physician with complaints of extreme nervousness, fatigue, and weight loss of 20 lb (despite a voracious appetite) over the last 3 months. Physical examination reveals a thin, anxious appearing man with heart rate 115 beats per minute, blood pressure 135/70 mmHg, bilateral exophthalmos so severe that he cannot move his eyes into the superior temporal position, bilateral conjunctival congestion, severe tremor of the outstretched hands, vitiligo, very warm and moist skin, hyperactive deep tendon reflexes, and a firm, symmetrically enlarged thyroid gland with a venous hum heard over the gland.

Laboratory studies show an undetectable serum thyroid stimulating hormone (TSH), total thyroxine (T_4) 18.2 µg/dL, free thyroxine (FT_4) 4.2 ng/dL, positive antithyroid antibodies at 1:1,280 dilution, positive thyroid stimulating immunoglobulins, cholesterol 115 mg/dL, calcium 11.2 mg/dL, phosphorus 5.7 mg/dL, alkaline phosphatase 210 U/L, and fasting glucose 153 mg/dL. A thyroid scan shows enlargement of the gland with a diffuse uptake, and a radioactive iodine uptake is 68% (reference range 5%-28%).

18.13.4.1 Questions

1. What is the most likely diagnosis?

2. What is the most likely cause of this disorder?

3. How might the patient be managed?

4. Why are the calcium, phosphorus, glucose, and alkaline phosphatase elevated?

18.13.5 **Clinical case answers**

18.13.5.1 Case 1 answers

1. The elevated total thyroid hormones with no clinical signs or symptoms of hyperthyroidism suggest euthyroid hyperthyroxinemia caused by increased binding proteins; in a young woman, such increases might be due to use of oral contraceptives

2. A free thyroxine (FT_4) and/or free triiodothyronine (FT_3) would be helpful, and would be expected to be normal

18.13.5.2 **Case 2 answers**

1. The clinical history and laboratory data together indicate that the patient has primary hypothyroidism

2. Additional laboratory studies should include a free thyroxine (FT_4; should be low), a total and free triiodothyronine (T_3 and FT_3; should be low), and antithyroid antibodies (which should be positive if the etiology of the hypothyroidism is Hashimoto thyroiditis, the most common cause of primary endogenous hypothyroidism); if performed, a serum cholesterol and creatine kinase would be elevated

18.13.5.3 **Case 3 answers**

1. The clinical history and laboratory studies together indicate that the patient has primary hyperthyroidism

2. Additional laboratory studies should include a free thyroxine (FT_4, which should be elevated), a total and free triiodothyronine (T_3 and FT_3, which should be elevated), antithyroid antibodies (which should be positive if the patient has Grave disease), and thyroid stimulating immunoglobulins (which should be positive if the patient has Grave disease); if performed, a serum cholesterol and serum creatine kinase should be low

18.13.5.4 **Case 4 answers**

1. The clinical findings, laboratory data, and imaging results indicate Grave disease in "thyroid storm" (thyrotoxicosis); this is confirmed by the massive (68%) uptake of radioactive iodine

2. The cause is the production of thyroid stimulating immunoglobulins (TSIs), which bind to the thyroid stimulating hormone (TSH) receptor, continuously stimulating it; the TSI is not subject to the feedback mechanisms

3. The patient should be started on antithyroid agents such as propylthiouracil or methimazole. Alternate therapy could include radioactive iodine or surgery to ablate the thyroid gland. β blockers such as propranolol can be used to block the effect of thyroid hormones (eg, tachycardia, arrhythmias, tremors, sweating)

4. Thyroid hormones in excess mobilize calcium and phosphorus from bone. The bone stimulation increases bone alkaline phosphatase activity, reflected in the increased serum alkaline phosphatase activity. Thyroid hormones also stimulate glycogenolysis, thus increasing the fasting glucose concentration

19.1 **Objectives**

At the end of this session, the learner should be able to

- ➤ identify the cell types in the islets of Langerhans and the hormones they produce
- ➤ discuss the hormonal regulation of serum/plasma glucose concentrations and provide examples of conditions and diseases that cause hyperglycemia
- ➤ discuss sample collection for measurement of glucose
- ➤ describe the clinical findings in diabetes mellitus type I and type II
- ➤ describe the laboratory findings in diabetes mellitus type I and type II
- ➤ describe the laboratory findings in impaired glucose tolerance
- ➤ discuss the laboratory findings in gestational diabetes
- ➤ discuss maturity onset diabetes of the young
- ➤ discuss ketone bodies in serum and urine
- ➤ discuss the oral glucose tolerance test in diabetes, impaired glucose tolerance, and gestational diabetes
- ➤ describe C peptide and its diagnostic use
- ➤ identify nondiabetic conditions in which glycosuria is not associated with hyperglycemia
- ➤ identify nondiabetic conditions in which glycosuria is associated with hyperglycemia
- ➤ discuss the use of glycated hemoglobin (HbA_{1c}) in management of diabetes mellitus
- ➤ describe the effect of hematologic disorders on the measurement of glycated hemoglobin (HbA_{1c})
- ➤ discuss glycated proteins and their potential use in management of diabetes mellitus
- ➤ describe the use of urinary albumin excretion in management of diabetes mellitus

19.2 **Key terms**

acromegaly: growth hormone excess in adults, characterized by enlargement of features such as the head, hands, and feet

atherosclerosis: the accumulation of fat and cholesterol in artery walls

cortisol: a glucocorticoid secreted by the adrenal cortex that stimulates gluconeogenesis

dyslipidemia: lipoprotein overproduction or deficiency

epinephrine: a catecholamine secreted by the adrenal medulla that increases serum/plasma glucose

Fanconi syndrome: a disease of the proximal renal tubules, resulting in excretion of glucose, phosphate, amino acids, uric acid, and bicarbonate

glucagon: a hormone produced by the α cells of the pancreas and which stimulates gluconeogenesis and glycogenolysis, thereby increasing the serum/plasma glucose

glucagonoma: a tumor producing glucagon

gluconeogenesis: formation of glucose from molecules that are not themselves carbohydrates

glycated hemoglobin: hemoglobin that has a covalent attachment of glucose at 1 or more amino acid residues

glycogenolysis: the conversion of glycogen to glucose

glycosuria: the excretion of glucose into the urine

growth hormone: a hormone secreted by the pituitary and that stimulates gluconeogenesis

hemochromatosis: iron overload, often hereditary, leading to deposition of iron in organs including pancreas, liver, and pituitary

hemoglobin A_{1c}: hemoglobin that has been glycated on the terminal valine of the β chain

hypercortisolism: a condition in which the serum/plasma cortisol is elevated

hyperglycemia: elevated serum/plasma glucose concentration

insulin: a hormone produced by the β cells of the pancreas that lowers serum/plasma glucose

insulinoma: a pancreatic β cell tumor producing insulin autonomously

islets of Langerhans: a group of pancreatic cells secreting hormones

islet cell antibodies: autoimmune antibodies often found in diabetes mellitus type I

ketonemia: excess ketones and ketoacids in the blood

ketonuria: excess ketones and ketoacids in the urine

pheochromocytoma: a neuroendocrine tumor of the adrenal glands producing catecholamines

polycythemia vera: a congenital disorder of the bone marrow, resulting in the production of too many red cells

polydipsia: extreme thirst and fluid intake, which is a symptom of diabetes mellitus

polyphagia: constant hunger, which is a symptom of diabetes mellitus

polyuria: excessive urination, which is a symptom of diabetes mellitus

proinsulin: a precursor to insulin

somatostatin: a hormone produced by the δ cells of the islets of Langerhans that inhibits the release of growth hormone from the pituitary gland and the release of insulin and glucagon from the pancreas, thereby modulating the reciprocal relationship among these hormones

somatostatinoma: a tumor secreting somatostatin

thyroxine: a hormone produced by the thyroid gland that stimulates glycogenolysis

venipuncture: drawing of blood from a vein

19.3 Background/significance

It is estimated that ~250 million people worldwide have diabetes mellitus and that by 2025 this number will reach 280 million, with 80% living in developed countries. Almost 1/3 of individuals with diabetes mellitus are undiagnosed [ISBN9781416061649a]. Accordingly, understanding appropriate laboratory testing for diabetes mellitus is important.

19.4 Glucose regulatory hormones produced in the islets of Langerhans

The **islets of Langerhans** are a cluster of pancreatic cells that occupy ~1%-2% of the volume of the pancreas and collectively weigh ~1-2 g. The islet α cells secrete **glucagon**, the β cells secrete **insulin**, and the δ cells produce **somatostatin** [ISBN9780071622431]. These islet cell hormones regulate serum/plasma glucose concentrations as described below.

19.4.1 Insulin (β cells)

Insulin stimulates the uptake of glucose into muscle and fat, promotes the conversion of glucose to glycogen, and inhibits **gluconeogenesis** in the liver. These effects combine to <u>lower</u> the serum/plasma glucose concentration [ISBN9781416061649a].

19.4.2 Glucagon (α cells)

Glucagon stimulates the production of glucose in the liver by both **glycogenolysis** and gluconeogenesis. These effects combine to <u>increase</u> the serum/plasma glucose concentration [ISBN9781416061649a].

19.4.3 Somatostatin (δ cells)

Somatostatin inhibits the release of growth hormone from the pituitary gland, and the secretion of glucagon and insulin from the pancreas, thereby modulating the reciprocal relationship among these hormones (<u>insulin decreasing glucose, glucagon increasing glucose, and growth hormone increasing glucose</u>) [ISBN9781416061649a].

19.4.4 **Other hormones regulating glucose**

Epinephrine, secreted by the adrenal medulla, stimulates glycogenolysis, decreases glucose utilization, and inhibits insulin secretion, all of which combine to <u>increase</u> serum/plasma glucose [ISBN9781416061649a].

Thyroxine, secreted by the thyroid gland, stimulates glycogenolysis and increases intestinal glucose absorption, both of which <u>increase</u> serum/plasma glucose [ISBN9781416061649a].

Cortisol, secreted by the adrenal cortex, stimulates gluconeogenesis, thereby <u>increasing</u> the serum/plasma glucose [ISBN9781416061649a].

Growth hormone, secreted by the pituitary gland, stimulates gluconeogenesis and antagonizes glucose uptake, resulting in an <u>increase</u> in serum/plasma glucose [ISBN9781416061649a].

19.5 **Diseases producing hyperglycemia**

Diseases and conditions that disrupt the hormonal regulation of glucose may lead to **hyperglycemia**. These include the following:

1. <u>destruction of the pancreas</u> (eg, surgical removal, pancreatic cancer, pancreatic cysts, hemorrhagic pancreatitis, **hemochromatosis**)

2. **acromegaly** (growth hormone excess)

3. **glucagonoma** (glucagon excess)

4. <u>hyperthyroidism</u> (thyroxine excess)

5. **pheochromocytoma** (epinephrine excess)

6. **hypercortisolism** (cortisol excess)

7. **somatostatinoma** (somatostatin excess)

8. <u>exogenous administration of drugs</u> (eg, levothyroxine, glucocorticoids)

19.6 **Monitoring of glucose**

Being a relatively low molecular weight compound, glucose is uniformly distributed in serum/plasma water and the aqueous phase of erythrocytes. However, since serum/plasma contains more water than erythrocytes, glucose concentrations in serum/plasma are 10%-15% higher than they would be in whole blood. Although glucose meters measure glucose in whole blood obtained by finger-stick, they report concentrations calibrated to serum/plasma [ISBN9781416061649a, b].

Samples obtained for analysis of serum/plasma glucose should be centrifuged within 30 minutes of collection because glycolytic enzymes present in erythrocytes and leukocytes will cause a decrease in the glucose concentration (5%-7% per hour at room temperature). If such centrifugation is not possible, blood should be drawn into a gray stoppered vacutainer tube (contains potassium oxalate as the anticoagulant and sodium fluoride as an enzyme inhibitor). However, this blood cannot be used for any other testing due to the enzyme inhibitor and electrolyte content of the anticoagulant and inhibitor [ISBN9781416061649b].

Fasting serum/plasma glucose concentrations are about the same in capillary (fingerstick) blood and simultaneously collected venous (**venipuncture**) blood. However, following a glucose load, capillary blood glucose concentrations are ~20%-25% higher than the corresponding venous blood due to extraction of glucose by tissues in the presence of insulin that is secreted in response to the glucose load [ISBN9781416061649b].

19.7 Classifications of glucose intolerance

19.7.1 Type I diabetes mellitus (formerly called juvenile onset diabetes mellitus)

Type I diabetes mellitus, which accounts for ~10% of all cases of diabetes, is characterized by autoimmune destruction of the insulin secreting pancreatic β cells so that insulin is lacking. The other islets cells are preserved. Such destruction is usually accompanied by the presence of autoantibodies, including **islet cell antibodies** and insulin autoantibodies. The susceptibility to type I diabetes mellitus is inherited, and the disease usually manifests itself in childhood and adolescence. The disease requires insulin in order to prevent hyperglycemia and ketosis [ISBN9781416061649a].

The clinical findings in type I diabetes mellitus are usually of abrupt onset and include **polyuria**, **polydipsia**, **polyphagia**, blurred vision, weight loss, **ketonemia** and/or **ketonuria**, **hyperglycemia** (as defined below), and strong human leukocyte antigen associations with linkage to the DQA and DQB genes [PMID18165339, ISBN9780071824866, ISBN9781416061649a].

19.7.2 Type II diabetes mellitus (formerly called adult or maturity onset diabetes mellitus)

Type II diabetes mellitus, which accounts for ~90% of all cases of diabetes, is caused by insulin resistance and relative insulin deficiency. At the time of diagnosis, patients have minimal symptoms and are not prone to ketosis because they make insulin. The patients are usually >40 years old, are often obese, and as the disease progresses may develop polyuria, polydipsia, hypertension, blurred vision, **dyslipidemia**, and **atherosclerosis** [PMID18165339, ISBN9780071824866, ISBN9781416061649a]. Insulin treatment is not usually required to prevent ketonuria, and insulin concentrations can be quite variable, given the resistance to insulin [ISBN9781416061649a].

19.8 Laboratory diagnosis of diabetes mellitus

Laboratory diagnosis of diabetes mellitus requires one or more of the following: a fasting serum/plasma glucose of ≥126 mg/dL (on >1 occasion), a random glucose of ≥200 mg/dL, a 2 hour postprandial glucose of ≥200 mg/dL during an oral glucose tolerance test using a glucose load of 75 g of glucose [PMID18165339, ISBN9780071824866], or a **hemoglobin A$_{1c}$** ≥6.5% (see below). Fasting is defined as no food intake for at least 10-16 hours. Prior to the oral glucose tolerance test, the patient should be ambulatory (bedrest causes glucose intolerance) and on a 150-200 g carbohydrate diet for at least 3 days (carbohydrate deprivation causes glucose intolerance). The hyperglycemia in diabetes usually results in a glycated hemoglobin $A_{1c} \geq 6.5\%$ (see discussion of glycated hemoglobin below) [PMID18165339, ISBN9780071824866, ISBN9781416061649a]. It should be noted that early in the evolution of type II diabetes mellitus, the fasting serum/plasma glucose concentration may actually be normal as the developing resistance to insulin causes the pancreas to secrete more insulin in attempt to control the hyperglycemia. However, the postprandial glucoses are elevated. By comparison, the reference ranges for nondiabetic individuals are as follows [ISBN9780071824866]:

➢ fasting: <100 mg/dL
➢ 2 hour postprandial: <140 mg/dL
➢ nondiabetic hemoglobin A_{1c}: <5.7%

19.8.1 Impaired glucose tolerance (formerly called prediabetes)

Impaired glucose tolerance is diagnosed in people with fasting serum/plasma glucoses less than that required for diagnosis of diabetes but greater than that in normal individuals. The fasting serum/plasma glucose is 100-125 mg/dL, and the 2 hour postprandial glucose is 140-199 mg/dL [ISBN9781416061649a]. The hemoglobin A_{1c} is 5.7%-6.4% [ISBN9780071824866].

19.8.2 Gestational diabetes

Gestational diabetes is defined as any sign of glucose intolerance that develops during pregnancy. Its frequency ranges from 1% to 14% of pregnancies. Oral glucose tolerance tests on pregnant women are performed with a 100 g glucose dose, following which at least 2 serum/plasma glucose concentrations should exceed the following: fasting, 95 mg/dL; 1 hour, 180 mg/dL; 2 hours, 155 mg/dL; and 3 hours, 140 mg/dL. A variation involves a preliminary test using a 50 g dose of glucose and a 1 hour glucose measurement. If the serum/plasma glucose exceeds 140 mg/dL, then the 100 g test is performed [ISBN9781416061649a].

19.8.3 Maturity onset diabetes of the young (MODY)

Maturity onset diabetes of the young (MODY) is a rare group of autosomal dominant disorders. The clinical presentation can be quite varied, ranging from asymptomatic hyperglycemia to more acute presentation [ISBN9780071824866, ISBN9781416061649a]. The disorder's name reflects the fact that it is noninsulin dependent (similar to type II diabetes, formerly called maturity onset diabetes), but it is usually diagnosed in patients <25 years of age (young). The patients are nonobese, and the hyperglycemia is due to genetic defects of pancreatic β cell function. 6 types of MODY have been described (MODY1 through MODY6). MODY3 is the most common type (2/3 of all cases) and ultimately leads to progressive β cell failure with insulin dependence. In contrast, MODY2, another common form, is relatively mild and manifests only slight fasting hyperglycemia. It responds well to oral antidiabetic agents and dietary control [ISBN9780071824866].

f19.1 Ketone body formation

19.8.4 **Ketone bodies**

Ketone bodies are formed from free fatty acids from the adipose stores. Under normal conditions, the fatty acids are taken up by the liver, where they are esterified to form triglycerides. They are then either stored in the liver or incorporated into very low density lipoproteins and returned to the serum/plasma. Low concentrations of insulin cause an increase in free fatty acids in the serum/plasma. The increased glucagon:insulin ratio in type I diabetes enhances fatty acid oxidation in the liver to yield β-hydroxy-β-methylglutaryl-CoA, which is further metabolized to yield the ketone body acetoacetate, which, in turn, is further converted to β-hydroxybutyrate. Acetocetate also spontaneously loses carbon dioxide to form acetone **f19.1** [ISBN9781416061649a].

With prolonged insulin deficiency, the predominant compound is β-hydroxybutyric acid, which is not detected by conventional urinalysis dipstick or tablet tests (see Chapter 6). Acetone is only weakly reactive and also highly volatile. Thus, practically speaking, a positive *ketone body* test in serum or urine suggests acetoacetate. Paradoxically, this can result in an increasingly positive test for ketone bodies in patients who are being treated for ketoacidosis as β-hydroxybutyric acid (which is not reactive in most tests for ketone bodies) is converted to acetoacetate, which is detected [ISBN9781416061649a].

19.8.5 **C peptide**

Insulin is first synthesized as the precursor **proinsulin**, which consists of an A&B chain connected by C peptide. The proinsulin is converted in the pancreatic β cells to insulin, which is secreted together with C peptide in equimolar amounts. Although neither insulin nor C peptide concentrations has a role in the routine workup of diabetes mellitus, the measurement of C peptide has been performed in evaluating fasting hypoglycemia (as may be caused by an **insulinoma**), assessment of β cell activity, and the diagnosis of factitious hypoglycemia caused by use of insulin. Exogenous insulin does not contain C peptide because it does not arise from proinsulin [ISBN9781416061649a].

19.8.6 Glycosuria

Glycosuria is found when the serum/plasma glucose concentration exceeds the renal threshold for reabsorption of glucose. In nondiabetic individuals, this threshold is 160-180 mg/dL [ISBN9781416061649a]. Nondiabetic causes of glycosuria with normal serum/plasma glucose concentration include the following: familial renal glycosuria in which the renal tubular reabsorption of glucose is impaired so that serum/plasma glucose concentrations as low as 100 mg/dL may be associated with glycosuria, **Fanconi syndrome**, and pregnancy [ISBN9780071824866, ISBN9781416061649a]. Of course, nondiabetic diseases causing hyperglycemia described previously will also cause glycosuria when the serum/plasma glucose exceeds 160-180 mg/dL. Testing for glucose is an integral part of the routine urinalysis (see Chapter 6).

19.8.7 Glycated hemoglobin

Hemoglobin becomes glycosylated by glucose through the nonenzymatic, largely irreversible, posttranslational attachment of glucose to the terminal valine of the β globin chain of hemoglobin, yielding hemoglobin A_{1c} (HbA_{1c}) or **glycated hemoglobin**, which is reported as percent of total hemoglobin that is glycated. The concentration of HbA_{1c} reflects a time weighted average of the concentration of glucose in blood over the lifetime of the erythrocyte (120 days). However, because the rate of glycosylation depends on the concentration of blood glucose, the HbA_{1c} reflects the glucose concentration over the preceding 8-12 weeks. Obviously interpretation of HbA_{1c} depends on individuals having a normal erythrocyte lifespan. People with shortened red cell lifetimes (eg, those with hemolytic anemia, those with unstable hemoglobins such as SS) will have decreased HbA_{1c}, while those with conditions that prolong the erythrocyte lifespan (eg, **polycythemia vera**, splenectomy) will have increased HbA_{1c}. In addition, acute significant blood loss will result in decreased HbA_{1c} due to the presence of a higher fraction of young red blood cells. Patients with iron deficiency anemia have higher HbA_{1c} due to a higher proportion of older erythrocytes [ISBN9781416061649a].

The presence of hemoglobin variants (eg, hemoglobins F, S, and C) may affect the measurement of HbA_{1c} depending on the method used. Among the various methods, boronate affinity chromatography is relatively unaffected by hemoglobin variants [ISBN9781416061649a] because it measures total glycated hemoglobin instead of HbA_{1c} alone.

As previously noted, the HbA_{1c} reflects the mean serum/plasma glucose concentration over the prior 8-12 weeks. Averaged over a population, they have a linear relationship, so that 5% HbA_{1c} reflects an average glucose concentration of 97 mg/dL; 6%, 126 mg/dL; 7%, 154 mg/dL; 8%, 183 mg/dL; 9%, 212 mg/dL; 10%, 240 mg/dL; 11%, 269 mg/dL; and 12%, 298 mg/dL [ISBN9780071824866]. Despite this linear relationship, a large degree of variability is possible. For example, in a population of subjects with an HbA_{1c} of 7%, the average glucose ranged from 125 to 200 mg/dL [PMID19114619]. As previously noted, nondiabetic individuals have HbA_{1c} <5.7%. Significantly, in 2009, the American Diabetes Association endorsed the recommendation that an HbA_{1c} ≥6.5% could be used as a decision point for diagnosis of diabetes, with HbA_{1c} of 5.7%-6.4% indicating individuals at high risk for developing diabetes [ISBN9781416061649a].

19.8.8 Glycated proteins (fructosamine)

In some individuals for whom HbA_{1c} measurement may not be accurate (eg, due to hemolytic anemia) or assessment of shorter term glucose control is required, the measurement of glycated proteins may be a suitable alternative. The generic name for glycated proteins is *fructosamine*, but because serum albumin is the predominant protein, fructosamine largely represents glycated albumin. Because serum proteins have shorter lifespans than erythrocytes (half-life of serum albumin 20 days), the concentration of fructosamine reflects serum/plasma glucose concentrations over the preceding 2-3 weeks. Currently there is lack of consensus about the clinical utility of fructosamine for routine use in managing diabetes mellitus [ISBN9781416061649a].

19.8.9 Urinary albumin excretion

One of the most serious effects of diabetes mellitus is kidney damage. In fact, diabetes is the most common cause of endstage renal disease in the United States and Europe [ISBN9781416061649a]. Consequently, close monitoring of the renal function of diabetics is critically important. Part of such surveillance is the determination of urinary albumin excretion because the first sign of impending nephropathy is the excretion of small concentrations of albumin (formerly termed *microalbuminuria*). Due to these small concentrations, which are not detectable by routine urinalysis, special, more sensitive analytical methods are used. The decision to start angiotensin converting enzyme inhibitors often depends on the results of this test. 2 out of 3 tests should be positive over a 3-6 month period to confirm the presence of urinary albumin [ISBN9781416061649a].

19.8.9.1 Urinary albumin reference range [ISBN9781416061649a]

Normal: <30 mg albumin/g creatinine; <2 mg/dL (random urine) or <30 mg/dL (24 hour)

Increased: 30-300 mg albumin/g creatinine; >2 mg/dL (random urine) or >30 mg/dL (24 hour)

Clinical albuminuria: >300 mg albumin/g creatinine

19.9 **References**
19.9.1 **Journals**

PMID18165339 American Diabetes Association, Bantle JP, Wylie-Rosett J, et al [2008] Nutrition recommendations and interventions for diabetes: a position statement of the American Diabetes Association. *Diabetes Care* 31Suppl1:S61-78

PMID19114619 Nathan DM, Kuenen J, Borg R et al [2008] Translating the A1c assay into estimated average glucose values. *Diabetes Care* 31:1473-78

19.9.2 **Books**

ISBN9780071622431 Masharani U, German MS [2011] Pancreatic hormones and diabetes mellitus. In: Gardner DG, Shoback D, ed. *Greenspan's Basic & Clinical Endocrinology*, 9e. McGraw-Hill, 573-656

ISBN9780071824866 Masharani U [2014] Diabetes mellitus and hypoglycemia. In: Papadakis MA, McPhee SJ, Rabow MW, ed. *Current Medical Diagnosis & Treatment*, 53e. McGraw Hill Education, 1165-1216

ISBN9781416061649a Sacks DB [2013] Diabetes mellitus. In: Burtis CA, Ashwood ER, Bruns DE, ed. *Tietz Textbook of Clinical Chemistry and Molecular Diagnostics*, 5e. Elsevier Saunders, 1415-56

ISBN9781416061649b Sacks DB [2013] Carbohydrates. In: Burtis CA, Ashwood ER, Bruns DE, ed. *Tietz Textbook of Clinical Chemistry and Molecular Diagnostics*, 5e. Elsevier Saunders, 1483-1530

19.10 **Clinical cases**
19.10.1 **Case 1**

A 10-year-old male, in excellent health until 1 month ago, is noted to have become irritable and have bouts of lethargy after meals. Because his 15-year-old brother has type I diabetes mellitus, the parents ask the pediatrician to evaluate the boy for diabetes.

Fasting plasma glucose on 2 occasions is 130 mg/dL and 140 mg/dL. A random plasma glucose in the afternoon is 190 mg/dL, and the HbA_{1c} is 8.5%. Islet cell antibodies are present at a titer of 1:4.

19.10.1.1 **Questions**

1. Should the patient be considered to have diabetes, and, if so, what type?

2. How should the patient be treated?

19.10.2 **Case 2**

A 68-year-old obese female is brought comatose to the emergency department. She has a history of seizures and hypertension for which she has been treated with anticonvulsants and diuretics. Her clinical history does not include diabetes.

Blood pressure is 100/50 mmHg, and the heart rate is 118 beats per minute. Serum laboratory results show the following: glucose 1080 mg/dL, sodium 144 mMol/L (mEq/L), potassium 4.4 mMol/L (mEq/L), chloride 113 mMol/L (mEq/L), bicarbonate 23 mMol/L (mEq/L), and urea-nitrogen 60 mg/dL.

19.10.2.1 **Questions**

1. Calculate the serum osmolality.

2. Calculate the anion gap.

3. What is the effect of the hyperglycemia on the serum sodium?

4. Is there evidence of ketoacidosis?

5. Why are the serum urea-N and chloride increased?

6. Why is the patient comatose?

7. Why is the blood pressure low and the heart rate elevated?

19.10.3 Clinical case answers

19.10.3.1 Case 1 answers

1. The boy has diabetes based on the fact that the fasting and random plasma glucose concentrations and the HbA_{1c} exceed normal values; it is type I based on his age, family history, and the finding of autoantibodies

2. The boy should probably be started on insulin therapy if a trial of oral antidiabetic agents is ineffective. Fasting plasma glucose and HbA_{1c} concentrations should be monitored along with urine albumin excretion. Home glucose monitoring should be performed daily. Regular diabetic monitoring (including eye exams, foot exams) should be performed

19.10.3.2 Case 2 answers

1. Serum osmolality = 2 (sodium) + glucose/18 + urea-N/2.8
   = 2 (144) + 1080/18 + 60/2.8 = 288 + 60 + 21 = 369 (reference range, 275-300 mOsm/kg)

2. Anion gap = (sodium + potassium) − (chloride + bicarbonate)
   = (144 + 4.4) − (113 + 23) = 148-136 = 12 (reference, 12-20).

3. Serum glucose concentrations decrease the serum sodium by 1.6-2.4 mMol/L for every 100 mg/dL of glucose above normal of 100 mg/dL. In this case, the glucose concentration is 980 mg/dL above normal (or 9.8 increments of 100 mg/dL) causing a depression of sodium by 16-24 mMol/L. The corrected sodium would be (144 + 16) to (144 + 24) = 160-168 mMol/L. The elevated glucose concentration causes hemodilution of the sodium due to an extracellular shift of water and an intracellular shift of sodium

4. There is no evidence of ketoacidosis since the anion gap is normal

5. The serum urea-N and chloride are elevated due to dehydration, which is evidenced by the elevated corrected serum sodium. The tremendous osmotic effect of the elevated serum glucose has caused an osmotic diuresis, which has dehydrated the patient. Note that, being comatose, the patient was not drinking water but was still urinating, which ultimately led to dehydration

6. The high serum osmolality has caused dehydration, altering consciousness, which condition is known as hyperglycemic hyperosmolar nonketotic coma

7. The blood pressure is low and the heart rate is elevated due to dehydration

20.1 **Objectives**

At the end of this session, the learner should be able to

➢ describe the signs and symptoms of hypercortisolism

➢ describe the changes in serum/plasma potassium, glucose, and acid-base balance in hypercortisolism

➢ describe the signs and symptoms of hypocortisolism

➢ describe the changes in serum/plasma sodium, potassium, glucose, urea-nitrogen, and acid-base balance in hypocortisolism

➢ discuss the hypothalamic-pituitary-adrenal cortex axis

➢ describe the causes of hypercortisolism

➢ describe the causes of hypocortisolism

➢ discuss the use of serum/plasma cortisol in the workup of hypercortisolism and hypocortisolism

➢ discuss the use of urinary free cortisol in the workup of hypercortisolism

➢ describe the use of serum adrenocorticotrophic hormone (ACTH) in determining the cause of hypercortisolism, in differentiating primary from central (secondary and tertiary hypocortisolism), and in demonstrating ectopic ACTH production before clinical symptoms of hypercortisolism appear

➢ discuss the short (overnight), low dose, and high dose dexamethasone suppression tests and interpretation of results

➢ describe the short and long ACTH stimulation tests and their use in distinguishing primary from central (secondary and tertiary) hypocortisolism

➢ discuss the corticotropin releasing hormone (CRH) stimulation test and its use in distinguishing secondary from tertiary hypocortisolism; also discuss the patterns observed with Cushing disease, and with ectopic ACTH production

➢ describe the metapyrone test and its use in monitoring the integrity of the pituitary-adrenal cortex axis

➢ discuss congenital adrenal hyperplasia and the findings in 21-hydroxylase deficiency and in 11-β-hydroxylase deficiency; discuss the diagnostic workup of congenital adrenal hyperplasia

➢ discuss primary hyperaldosteronism (Conn syndrome) and its causes; describe serum aldosterone and renin concentrations in primary hyperaldosteronism

➢ discuss secondary hyperaldosteronism and its causes; describe serum aldosterone and renin concentrations in secondary hyperaldosteronism

20.2 **Key terms**

Addisonian crisis: acute adrenal gland failure (a life threatening emergency)

Addison disease (primary hypocortisolism): primary adrenal insufficiency due to destruction or dysfunction of the adrenal glands

adenoma: a noncancerous (benign) tumor

adrenocorticotropic hormone (ACTH): hormone secreted by the anterior pituitary gland; acts on the adrenal cortex to induce secretion of cortisol

aldosterone: the major mineralocorticoid hormone secreted by the adrenal cortex; controls salt and water balance in the kidney

amenorrhea: lack of menses

congenital adrenal hyperplasia (adrenogenital syndrome): a group of hereditary diseases resulting from enzyme deficiencies in the steroid hormone production pathways

corticotropin releasing hormone (CRH): hormone secreted by the hypothalamus causing release of ACTH from the anterior pituitary gland

cortisol: the major adrenal cortex glucocorticoid; affects metabolism of glucose, proteins, and lipids, and in excess, has mineralocorticoid activity

Cushing syndrome: hypercortisolism

glucocorticoid: one of a group of steroid hormones (the major one being cortisol), secreted by the adrenal cortex and regulating carbohydrate metabolism

hirsutism: excessive growth of hair, especially on women

hyperaldosteronism: increased secretion of the mineralocorticoid aldosterone by the adrenal cortex because of increased renin secretion (secondary hyperaldosteronism) or because of autonomous adrenocortical secretion (primary hyperaldosteronism, Conn syndrome)

melanocytes: pigment producing cells in human skin

mineralocorticoids: steroid hormones (the major one being aldosterone) secreted by the adrenal cortex that stimulate the reabsorption of sodium and water and the excretion of potassium and hydrogen ion in the distal tubules of the kidney

plethora: a red or ruddy colored complexion

polycystic ovary syndrome: a major androgen excess disorder in women

renin-angiotensin-aldosterone system: a regulatory system for aldosterone secretion by the adrenal cortex

striae: irregular areas of banding or stripes on skin

20.3 **Background/significance**

Cushing syndrome (hypercortisolism) affects 10-15 of every 1,000,000 people each year, while **congenital adrenal hyperplasia (adrenogenital syndrome)**, affects 1 in 15,000 births. **Addison disease (primary hypocortisolism)** afflicts 1-4 of every 100,000 people, and Conn syndrome (**primary hyperaldosteronism**) affects >10% of all people with hypertension [NICHD 2013]. Given the incidence and severity of most adrenocortical diseases, a firm understanding of laboratory testing for these disorders is important.

20.4 **Hypercortisolism (Cushing syndrome) & hypocortisolism**

20.4.1 **Signs & symptoms**

Hypercortisolism is characterized by central obesity, thin skin, moon shaped facies, hypertension (due to sodium and water retention), purple skin **striae**, **hirsutism**, menstrual disorders (usually **amenorrhea**), **plethora**, impotence, mental disturbances, and a "buffalo hump" (dorsal fat pad) [ISBN9780071802154, ISBN9780071824866]. Hyperglycemia (cortisol excess stimulating gluconeogenesis), hypokalemia (**mineralocorticoid** effect of excess cortisol causing potassium and hydrogen ion loss), and metabolic alkalosis are noted on routine laboratory testing [ISBN9780071824866].

Hypocortisolism is characterized by fatigue, weakness, anorexia, weight loss (loss of water with sodium), nausea and vomiting, abdominal pain, amenorrhea, skin hyperpigmentation (primary adrenal insufficiency only, Addison disease; due to excess stimulation of **melanocytes** by the precursor protein of **adrenocorticotropic hormone**, especially in areas of skin creases, pressure areas, and nipples), and hypotension (due to volume loss). Hypoglycemia (cortisol lack), hyponatremia (due to lack of cortisol and **aldosterone**), hyperkalemia (due to lack of cortisol and aldosterone), metabolic acidosis (due to retention of hydrogen ion), and elevated serum/plasma urea-nitrogen (due to volume loss/dehydration) are noted on routine laboratory testing [ISBN9780071802154, ISBN9780071824866].

20.4.2 Hypothalamic-pituitary-adrenal cortex axis

The hypothalamus secretes **corticotropin releasing hormone (CRH)** in response to stress (both physical and psychological), exercise, and hypoglycemia. The CRH stimulates the anterior pituitary gland to secrete **adrenocorticotropic hormone (ACTH)**, which, in turn, induces the adrenal cortex to synthesize and secrete **cortisol**, the major **glucocorticoid**. Cortisol exerts major negative feedback on the hypothalamus (CRH) and to a lesser extent on the pituitary (ACTH) [ISBN9781416061649]. The hypothalamic-pituitary-adrenal cortex axis is depicted in **f20.1**.

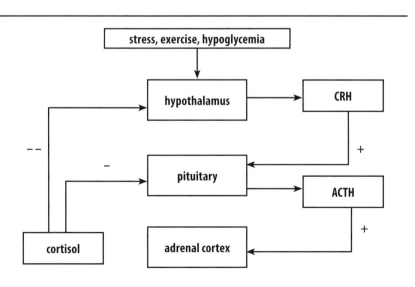

f20.1 Hypothalamus-pituitary-adrenal cortex axis

20.4.3 Causes

Hypercortisolism (Cushing syndrome) is caused endogenously by an ACTH producing pituitary **adenoma** (benign tumor; 75% of cases; the classical Cushing disease), ectopic production of ACTH by tumors (15%; eg, pancreatic carcinoid tumors, bronchial tumors, small cell lung cancer), a cortisol producing adrenal adenoma (9%), and a cortisol producing adrenal carcinoma (<1%) [ISBN9780071802154]. Exogenously the condition can be caused by excess administration of glucocorticoids.

Hypocortisolism can be primary (Addison disease; defect in the adrenal gland), secondary (defect in the pituitary gland), or tertiary (defect in the hypothalamus). Causes of primary hypocortisolism are autoimmune processes (eg, "autoimmune adrenalitis"; 70% of cases in the Western world), systemic disorders (eg, neoplastic destruction of the adrenal glands, hemochromatosis), inborn metabolic errors (eg, enzyme deficiencies including **congenital adrenal hyperplasia**), vascular disorders/hemorrhage, and infection (a large cause of primary hypocortisolism worldwide; eg, tuberculosis, fungal infections, cytomegalovirus infections).

Secondary hypocortisolism is caused by pituitary failure due to trauma, tumor, infiltrative diseases (eg, amyloidosis), inflammation, hemorrhage, hemochromatosis, infarction, and congenital malformations [ISBN9781416061649]. Tertiary hypocortisolism is caused by hypothalamic malfunction due to congenital malformations, trauma, hemorrhage, inflammation, and infection [ISBN9781416061649].

20.5 Laboratory tests of adrenocortical function
20.5.1 Serum/plasma cortisol

The major glucocorticoid cortisol, produced in the zona fasciculata of the adrenal cortex, is bound 90% to corticosteroid binding globulin (CBG; transcortin), an α_1 globulin, and ~8% to albumin. Although as a glucocorticoid, cortisol promotes gluconeogenesis, in excess it has mineralocorticoid activity, stimulating the excretion of potassium and hydrogen ion and the retention of sodium and water. As with other hormones, the free (unbound) fraction (~2% of total cortisol) is the "active" hormone. Agents that increase the transcortin (eg, pregnancy, oral contraceptives) will increase the total cortisol concentration while the free cortisol remains normal [ISBN9781416061649]. Serum/plasma cortisol is also increased in patients who have chronic alcoholism, stress, infection, depression, starvation, and **polycystic ovary syndrome** [ISBN9781451118698].

Serum/plasma cortisol shows wide diurnal variation in normal individuals, reflecting secretion of ACTH in bursts. Cortisol is highest between 6 AM and 8 AM and 50%-80% lower between 10 PM and 12 AM. In hypercortisolism, this diurnal variation is often lost; however, this is not a consistent finding. Random serum/plasma cortisol measurements are of little value in diagnosis of hypercortisolism because concentrations in normal individuals vary widely during the day and may overlap with those seen in hypercortisolism. Generally speaking, the morning concentrations are also of little diagnostic value unless they are clearly above the reference range. In contrast, a single midnight cortisol concentration >7.5 µg/dL suggests loss of diurnal variation and is 90%-96% sensitive and 100% specific for hypercortisolism, provided that the patient has remained in the same time zone for at least 3 days and has an indwelling intravenous line inserted in advance of the blood drawing [ISBN9780071824866, ISBN9781416061649, ISBN9781451118698].

In hypocortisolism (primary, secondary, tertiary) serum/plasma cortisol concentrations are low (AM <3 µg/dL). Random measurements are only useful in excluding the diagnosis of hypocortisolism when the serum/plasma cortisol is >20 µg/dL [ISBN9780071824866, ISBN9781451118698].

Saliva has also been used in the measurement of cortisol concentrations in many institutions, especially for assessment of midnight cortisol because it is easier to collect. Concentrations are much lower in this matrix.

20.5.1.1 Reference ranges
20.5.1.1.1 Serum/plasma cortisol
AM: 6.2-19.4 µg/dL; PM: 2.3-11.9 µg/dL

20.5.1.1.2 Saliva cortisol
PM: <0.11 µg/dL

20.5.2 Urinary free cortisol
Measurement of 24 hour urine cortisol concentration reflects free cortisol concentration. In normal individuals, <2% of secreted cortisol appears in the urine. In most people, concentrations <50 µg/24 hour are sufficient to exclude the diagnosis of hypercortisolism [ISBN9781416061649]. Urine free cortisol measurement is normal when total serum/plasma cortisol is elevated due to elevated transcortin. The measurement of urinary free cortisol is not helpful in the workup of hypocortisolism.

20.5.2.1.1 Reference range
Adult women: ≤45 µg/24 hour
Adult men: ≤60 µg/24 hour

20.5.3 Serum/plasma adrenocorticotropic hormone (ACTH)
The measurement of ACTH in serum or plasma is most helpful in determining the cause of hypercortisolism (<10 pg/mL suggesting a cortisol secreting adrenal adenoma or carcinoma due to suppression of ACTH by the excess cortisol production and >50 pg/mL suggesting Cushing disease, pituitary adenoma due to stimulation of cortisol production by the adrenal), in differentiating primary from central (secondary and tertiary) hypocortisolism (>150 pg/mL suggesting primary hypocortisolism due to the negative feedback loop trying to drive cortisol production; low concentrations suggesting either secondary hypocortisolism due to the inability of the pituitary gland to produce ACTH or tertiary hypocortisolism due to lack of hypothalamic CRH stimulation of the pituitary gland), and in the diagnosis of ectopic ACTH producing tumors before the Cushing syndrome develops clinically (ACTH elevated) [ISBN9781416061649].

20.5.3.1.1 Reference range
Adult women: 6-58 pg/mL
Adult men: 7-69 pg/mL

20.6 Provocative tests of adrenocortical function

20.6.1 Dexamethasone suppression test for the workup of hypercortisolism

Dexamethasone is a synthetic fluoride containing corticosteroid that is 25× more potent than cortisol, including its negative feedback action on the pituitary to inhibit ACTH secretion. Because it is given in small doses and is structurally different than cortisol, it does not interfere with the measurement of serum/plasma cortisol. This provides the basis for a useful test in the diagnostic workup of hypercortisolism.

The short (overnight) dexamethasone suppression test is performed by administering 1 mg of dexamethasone orally between 10 PM and 12 PM. A serum/plasma sample for cortisol measurement is obtained at 8 AM. Normal individuals will show suppression of serum/plasma cortisol to <5 µg/dL as the dexamethasone inhibits ACTH release from the pituitary.

If the concentrations are >10 µg/dL (most cases of hypercortisolism), the test is continued as the low dose dexamethasone suppression test, in which 0.5 mg of dexamethasone is administered orally every 6 hours for 48 hours. Normal individuals will show suppression of serum/plasma cortisol to <2.2 µg/dL on the morning following the last dose and urine free cortisol to <25 µg/day.

If suppression is not noted (most cases of hypercortisolism), the test is continued as the high dose dexamethasone suppression test, which can be performed either overnight or over several days. In the overnight test, 4 mg of dexamethasone is administered orally at midnight. In patients with Cushing disease, the serum/plasma cortisol concentration at 8 AM should be suppressed by at least 50% below the baseline (predexamethasone) concentration due to the small size of most pituitary adenomas. If such suppression is not noted, then the high dose overnight test is repeated using 8-24 mg of dexamethasone. If no suppression is noted, then either an adrenal adenoma or carcinoma producing cortisol, or a tumor producing ACTH is suspected. These can be differentiated by measuring serum/plasma ACTH (low with adrenal adenoma or carcinoma, high with tumors producing ACTH). The multiday high dose dexamethasone suppression test is performed by administering 2 mg of dexamethasone orally every 6 hours for 48 hours. Serum/plasma cortisol and 24 hour urine free cortisol concentrations are suppressed in most patients with pituitary adenoma (Cushing disease), but not in patients with adrenal adenoma or carcinoma or in patients with tumors secreting ACTH. Some clinicians combine the low dose and high dose tests over the course of 6 days, obtaining baseline cortisol measurements in both serum/plasma and 24 hour urines on days 1 and 2, then performing the low dose test over days 3 and 4, and the high dose test over days 5 and 6 [ISBN9781416061649].

20.6.2 ACTH stimulation test for the workup of hypocortisolism

The ACTH stimulation test evaluates the ability of the adrenal cortex to respond to ACTH stimulation by producing cortisol. Thus it differentiates primary from central (secondary and tertiary) hypocortisolism. There are 2 versions of this test: the short ACTH stimulation test and the long ACTH stimulation test.

In the short ACTH stimulation test, a baseline serum/plasma cortisol measurement is obtained. Then 250 µg of cosyntropin, a synthetic polypeptide analog of ACTH, is administered either intramuscularly or intravenously. Additional serum/plasma cortisol measurements are obtained at 30 minutes and at 60 minutes after the cosyntropin administration. In normal individuals the serum/plasma cortisol should peak at ≥18-20 µg/dL with an increase of 7-10 µg/dL over the baseline cortisol concentration [ISBN9781416061649]. With primary hypocortisolism, minimal or no response is noted. If the patient with suspected hypocortisolism has been treated with glucocorticoids or if there is longstanding central (pituitary or hypothalamic) hypocortisolism, the resulting hypoplastic adrenal cortex may need stimulation over a longer period of time in order to respond. In those instances, the long ACTH stimulation test is performed.

In the long ACTH stimulation test, 250 µg of cosyntropin is administered parenterally on each of 3 days, followed by an 8 hour infusion of cosyntropin. Serum/plasma cortisol and 24 hour urine free cortisol concentrations are then measured. A serum/plasma cortisol concentration >18-20 µg/dL excludes primary hypocortisolism. In patients whose adrenal cortex has become hypoplastic due to lack of stimulation over time, a staircase rise in concentration may be noted as the adrenal cortex begins to produce cortisol due to the stimulation by cosyntropin. A CRH stimulation test is then performed to differentiate secondary from tertiary hypocortisolism (see below). There are 2 and 5 day variations of the long ACTH stimulation test [ISBN9781416061649].

20.6.3 CRH stimulation test

In this test, synthetic CRH, 1 µg/kg of body weight, is administered as an intravenous bolus injection at either 9 AM or 8 PM. Blood samples for measurement of cortisol and ACTH are obtained 15 minutes before the injection, and then at 5, 15, 30, 60, 120, and 180 minutes postinjection. In normal individuals, serum/plasma ACTH should peak at 30 minutes postinjection (80 ± 7 pg/mL at 9:30 AM or 29 ± 2.6 pg/mL at 8:30 PM), and serum/plasma cortisol should peak at 60 minutes (13 ± 1 µg/dL at 10 AM or 17 ± 0.7 µg/dL at 9 PM). Patients with secondary hypocortisolism will have decreased ACTH and cortisol responses. Patients with tertiary hypocortisolism will have prolonged ACTH responses with a smaller rise in cortisol.

The CRH stimulation test can also be used to differentiate between hypercortisolism caused by ectopic production of ACTH by tumors and hypercortisolism caused by pituitary adenoma (Cushing disease). Tumors producing ACTH will not respond to CRH infusion because cortisol production is already maximally stimulated, while pituitary adenomas (Cushing disease) will show either a normal or an excessive increase in ACTH and cortisol [ISBN9781416061649].

20.6.4 Metapyrone test for evaluation of pituitary-adrenal cortex axis

Although not widely utilized, the metapyrone test can be used to test the ability of the pituitary gland to produce ACTH and to check the integrity of the pituitary-adrenal cortex axis. Metapyrone inhibits 11-β-hydroxylase, an enzyme in

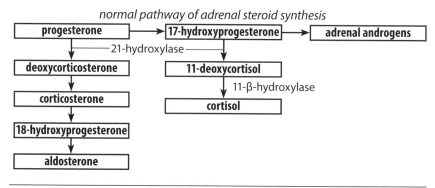

f20.2 Biochemical pathway for congenital adrenal hyperplasia disorders

the adrenal cortex that catalyzes the conversion of 11-desoxycortisol to cortisol (the last step in the formation of cortisol) f20.2. Since cortisol is not formed, the secretion of ACTH by the pituitary gland is stimulated (in attempt to drive cortisol production). Due to the enzyme inhibition, the cortisol precursor 11-desoxycortisol accumulates in serum/plasma, in which it is measured. The test is performed by administering metapyrone orally, 30 mg/kg body weight, at midnight. At 8 AM, blood is drawn for measurement of 11-desoxycortisol, cortisol, and ACTH. In normal individuals, following metapyrone administration, the serum/plasma 11-desoxycortisol increases from a baseline of <1 µg/dL to a value >7 µg/dL. Cortisol concentrations should decline while ACTH concentrations should exceed 150 pg/mL due to the negative feedback from lack of cortisol. Failure to respond to metapyrone suggests central hypocortisolism (lack of ACTH production) and/or that the adrenal gland cannot respond to ACTH by generating the 11-desoxycortisol precursor of cortisol (primary hypocortisolism). In patients with tumors secreting ACTH, 11-desoxycortisol does not increase further, because it is at its maximum already due to continuous stimulation by the ectopic production of ACTH. The test should be performed with extreme caution in patients with suspected primary hypocortisolism, since metapyrone diminishes cortisol concentration and may precipitate an **Addisonian crisis** [ISBN9781416061649] due to decreasing the synthesis of cortisol. 2 and 3 day versions of the metapyrone test are also available for inpatient use.

20.7 Congenital adrenal hyperplasia (adrenogenital syndrome)

Congenital adrenal hyperplasia, the most common cause of hypocortisolism in newborn infants, results from autosomal recessive loss of function mutations in 1 of more of the 6 adrenocortical enzymes responsible for cortisol production. The most common cause of this disorder is 21-hydroxylase deficiency (95% of cases). This enzyme is essential for the synthesis of both cortisol (converts 17-hydroxyprogesterone to 11-desoxycortisol, which is then converted by 11-β-hydroxylase to cortisol) and **aldosterone** (converts progesterone to deoxycorticosterone in the aldosterone synthetic pathway). Thus infants with the severe form of this disorder suffer from both life threatening hypocortisolism and hypoaldosteronism, manifested by hyponatremia (due to salt loss) and hyperkalemia. Because of the negative feedback control by cortisol, the pituitary secretes excessive ACTH, and due to the enzymatic deficiency, 17-hydroxyprogesterone (17OHP) accumulates. Measurement of this compound is used in the diagnosis of 21-hydroxylase deficiency. The 17OHP is a precursor to androgen formation, which causes anomalous genital development in girls (ambiguous genitalia) and precocious pseudopuberty in boys—hence the name *adrenogenital syndrome*. In addition to the severe (salt losing) form of 21-hydroxylase deficiency (depletion of both cortisol and aldosterone), a milder form is characterized by mild hypocortisolism with sufficient aldosterone synthesis to prevent salt loss [ISBN9781416061649].

The second most common cause of congenital adrenal hyperplasia is 11-β-hydroxylase deficiency, which results in virilization, depressed cortisol, elevated 11-desoxycortisol and 17OHP, but no abnormalities in aldosterone [ISBN9781416061649].

The biochemical pathways are depicted in **f20.2**.

20.8 Hyperaldosteronism

In primary hyperaldosteronism (Conn syndrome) the adrenal gland secretes excessive amounts of aldosterone, resulting in suppression of renin due to the **renin-angiotensin-aldosterone system** feedback loop (see Chapter 8). This causes retention of sodium and water and loss of potassium and hydrogen ion, resulting in hypertension and a hypokalemic metabolic alkalosis in many patients. In fact, 5%-12% of cases of hypertension are believed to be due to this disorder. In most cases, this condition is caused by bilateral hypertrophy of the zona glomerulosa. Less common causes are an aldosterone secreting adrenal adenoma or carcinoma. The laboratory diagnosis involves demonstration of suppressed serum/plasma renin and elevated serum/plasma aldosterone that cannot be suppressed with volume expansion, particularly in the setting of metabolic alkalosis and hypokalemia. In the early phase of the disease, the serum/plasma potassium may be normal. Ingestion of older versions of black licorice candy causes primary aldosteronism because it contains glycyrrhetinic acid, which has a mineralocorticoid effect [ISBN9780071802154, ISBN9781416061649].

In contrast, secondary hyperaldosteronism can be seen in patients with volume depletion, edema, and hypokalemic alkalosis (eg, patients with hepatic cirrhosis/ascites, congestive heart failure, nephrotic syndrome). This causes release of renin from the juxtaglomerular cells of the kidney stimulating secretion of aldosterone, which elevates both serum/plasma renin and aldosterone [ISBN9781416061649].

20.9 The role of imaging

Imaging studies are also important in the diagnosis of many of the conditions described above, particularly those involving adenomas and carcinomas. In some instances, interventional studies, such as cannulation of vessels, to monitor hormone concentrations emanating from tumors may be helpful. However, a discussion of these techniques is beyond the purview of this chapter.

20.10 **References**

20.10.4.1 **Books**

ISBN9780071802154 Arlt W [2015] Disorders of the adrenal cortex. In: Kasper DL, Fauci AS, Hause SL et al, ed. *Harrison's Principles of Internal Medicine*, 19e. McGraw Hill Education, 2309-29

ISBN9780071824866 Fitzgerald PA [2014] Endocrine disorders. In: Papadakis MA, McPhee SJ, Rabow MW, ed. *Current Medical Diagnosis & Treatment*, 53e. McGraw Hill Education, 1112-124.

ISBN9781416061649 Bertholf RF, Jialal I, Winter WE [2013] The adrenal cortex. In: Burtis CA, Ashwood ER, Bruns DE, ed. *Tietz Textbook of Clinical Chemistry and Molecular Diagnostics*, 5e. Elsevier Saunders, 1847-1904.

ISBN9781451118698 Mitchell TC, Meikle AW [2013] Adrenal function. In: Bishop ML, Fody EP, Schoeff LE, ed. *Clinical Chemistry: Principles, Techniques, and Correlations*, 7e. Lippincott Williams & Wilkins, 453-71

20.10.4.2 **Other resources**

Eunice Kennedy Shriver National Institute of Child Health and Human Development (NICHD) [2013] How many people are affected by or at risk of adrenal gland disorders? https://www.nichd.nih.gov/health/topics/adrenalgland/conditioninfo/pages/risk.aspx

20.11 Clinical cases

20.11.1 Case 1

A 43-year-old female has experienced fatigue, muscle weakness, facial puffiness, and easy bruising for 18 months. Physical examination reveals hypertension, round facies, muscle wasting, and numerous purpuric lesions. Laboratory studies show a midnight plasma cortisol of 21 µg/dL. Urine free cortisol is 85 µg/24 hours. After administration of 4 mg of dexamethasone at midnight, the 8 AM cortisol is 6 µg/dL.

20.11.1.1 Questions

1. What is the most likely cause for these findings?
2. What additional studies should be performed?

20.11.2 Case 2

A 26-year-old female vaginally delivered a normal term infant. However, the delivery was complicated by uterine atony (lack of contraction of the uterine muscles), bleeding, and shock. 5 days after delivery, the patient developed anorexia, nausea, vomiting, and confusion. Her blood pressure was 80/40 mmHg, and her heart rate was 112 beats per minute.

Laboratory studies showed anemia, plasma sodium 121 mMol/L (mEq/L), potassium 5.2 mMol/L (mEq/L), and glucose 56 mg/dL.

20.11.2.1 Questions

1. What is the most likely diagnosis?
2. What additional studies should be performed?

20.11.3 Case 3

A 52-year-old male has had general malaise and muscle weakness for 6 months. Over the last 3 months he has complained of "fullness" and dull pain in the right side of his abdomen. He has also noted weight loss. His midnight plasma cortisol was 31 µg/dL, and his 24 hour urine free cortisol was 110 µg/24 hours. An overnight high dose (4 mg) dexamethasone suppression test did not suppress the plasma cortisol.

20.11.3.1 Questions

1. What is the most likely diagnosis?
2. What additional studies should be performed?

ISBN 978-089189-6548

20.11.4 **Clinical case answers**

20.11.4.1 **Case 1 answers**

1. The results are consistent with a pituitary adenoma (Cushing disease); other causes of hypercortisolism, such as an ectopic ACTH secreting tumor and cortisol secreting adrenal adenomas and carcinomas, would not be suppressed by the overnight high dose dexamethasone suppression test

2. A plasma ACTH should be elevated; imaging studies should be performed in attempt to visualize the pituitary adenoma

20.11.4.2 **Case 2 answers**

1. The clinical history suggests pituitary infarction (Sheehan syndrome) due to the complicated delivery, which has resulted in diminished ACTH production, resulting in deficient cortisol production; the lack of glucocorticoid effect causes the decreased plasma glucose, while the lack of mineralocorticoid effect causes hyperkalemia and hyponatremia

2. Additional studies should include plasma bicarbonate (should be low due to retention of hydrogen ion with potassium, yielding a hyperkalemic acidosis), a plasma cortisol (should be low), a thyroid stimulating hormone (should be low), a plasma ACTH (should be low), and imaging studies of the pituitary. The patient is also likely dehydrated due to the resulting adrenal insufficiency (lack of ACTH), accompanied by sodium and water loss. This is evidenced by the low blood pressure and rapid pulse rate. The anemia is due to bleeding and would be even worse if the patient were hydrated

20.11.4.3 **Case 3 answers**

1. The lack of suppression of cortisol by the overnight high dose dexamethasone suppression test suggests either a cortisol secreting adrenal adenoma or carcinoma or an ectopic ACTH producing tumor

2. A plasma ACTH measurement should be obtained. If elevated, this would suggest an ectopic ACTH producing tumor. If decreased, this would suggest an adrenal adenoma or carcinoma. Appropriate imaging studies should then be obtained

chapter 21

The laboratory diagnosis of lipid disorders

21.1 Objectives

At the end of this session, the learner should be able to

➢ describe the structure of lipoprotein particles

➢ discuss the composition and function of chylomicrons

➢ discuss very low density lipoproteins (VLDLs) and their role

➢ discuss intermediate density lipoproteins (IDLs) and their role

➢ discuss low density lipoproteins (LDLs) and their role

➢ discuss high density lipoproteins (HDLs) and their role

➢ discuss the National Cholesterol Education Program (NCEP) and the United States Preventive Services Task Force (USPSTF) guidelines for cholesterol screening

➢ describe the NCEP risk factor stratification scheme for establishing LDL cholesterol targets and therapy

➢ describe the requirements for fasting for lipid testing

➢ calculate LDL cholesterol using the Friedewald formula

➢ calculate the non-HDL cholesterol and discuss its advantages over LDL cholesterol

➢ discuss reference ranges for total cholesterol, LDL cholesterol, HDL cholesterol, non-HDL cholesterol, and triglycerides

➢ discuss the primary ("familial") dyslipidemias (Fredrickson classification) and the findings for each type

➢ describe the major causes of secondary ("acquired") hyperlipidemias

21.2 Key terms

apolipoprotein: a protein that binds lipids to form lipoproteins

arcus senilis: a white, blue, or gray ring in the corneal margins, caused by fat deposition

atheroma: accumulation of degenerative material (eg, macrophages, calcium, lipids, connective tissue) in the inner walls of arteries

atherosclerosis: atheroma formation

cholesterol: a lipid that is an essential part of animal cell membranes and is a precursor for synthesis of steroid hormones, vitamin D, and bile acids; the principle sterol synthesized by animals

chylomicron: the largest lipoprotein, containing 99% lipid and 1% protein; transports dietary triglycerides from the gastrointestinal tract into the circulation

dyslipidemia: a disorder of lipoprotein metabolism

Fredrickson classification: a classification of the hyperlipidemias based on the pattern of lipoproteins on electrophoresis or ultracentrifugation

high density lipoprotein (HDL): a lipoprotein that removes fat and cholesterol from cells; when bound to cholesterol, it is known as *HDL cholesterol*

intermediate density lipoprotein (IDL): a lipoprotein that carries cholesterol esters and triglycerides and is present in low concentrations in the circulation

intrahepatic cholestasis: interruption in the excretion of bile

low density lipoprotein (LDL): a lipoprotein that transports fat molecules into artery walls and attracts macrophages, thereby driving atheroma formation; when bound to cholesterol, it is known as *LDL cholesterol*

lipemia retinalis: a creamy appearance of the retinal blood vessels

lipid: a class of hydrophobic compounds that are soluble in many organic solvents but insoluble in water

lipoprotein: a protein containing lipid; transports lipids in the circulation

lipoprotein lipase: an enzyme that hydrolyzes triglycerides in lipoprotein

lipoprotein X: an abnormal lipoprotein found in cholestasis

phospholipid: a class of lipid present in cell membranes that forms lipid bilayer

triglyceride: an ester derived from glycerol and 3 fatty acids

very low density lipoprotein (VLDL): a lipoprotein that contains nondietary (endogenous) triglycerides

xanthelasma: a marked yellowish deposit of fat under the skin, often around the eyelids

xanthoma: a deposit of cholesterol rich yellow fat in body tissues, especially tendons

21.3 Background/significance

Most adults in the United States are affected by some type of **lipid** abnormality, many having elevations of the low density lipoprotein (LDL) cholesterol, which increases the risk of cardiovascular disease [PMID22836069]. Knowledge of laboratory testing for **dyslipidemias** is important in their diagnosis and treatment.

21.4 Circulating lipoproteins

Cholesterol and **triglycerides** are the major lipids in serum/plasma, with ~70% of the cholesterol being esterified.

Lipoproteins are comprised of a polar, water soluble outer shell consisting of cholesterol, **phospholipids**, and **apolipoproteins** (proteins that bind lipid to form **lipoproteins**). The polar hydroxyl group of cholesterol, the phosphate group of phospholipids, and the polar surface of the apolipoproteins are oriented toward the outside of the lipoprotein particle so that it is water soluble and can be transported in serum/plasma. The lipophilic (nonwater soluble or hydrophobic) groups of these 3 entities are oriented toward the interior of the particle.

The apolipoproteins are important in activating enzymes in the lipoprotein metabolic pathways, maintaining the structural integrity of the lipoprotein, and facilitating uptake of the lipoprotein into cells.

Chylomicrons are among the largest lipoproteins, are 99% lipid and 1% protein, and mostly contain dietary (exogenous) triglycerides, which they transport from the gastrointestinal tract into the circulation. In the periphery, small amounts of free fatty acids are released from the triglyceride component of the chylomicron and taken up by muscle and adipose cells. This cleavage of triglyceride is mediated through interactions with **high density lipoprotein (HDL)** cholesterol (see below), which supplies apolipoprotein CII to the chylomicron. Apolipoprotein CII activates **lipoprotein lipase**, which cleaves free fatty acids from triglyceride molecules. The chylomicron remnants are then catabolized by the liver.

The **very low density lipoprotein (VLDL)** is synthesized by the liver and contains endogenous (nondietary) triglycerides. In a manner similar to release of free fatty acids from chylomicrons, apolipoprotein CII activates lipoprotein lipase, which hydrolyzes the triglycerides and releases free fatty acids into the endothelial cells.

The remainder of the VLDL can either be taken back up by the liver or can be converted into **intermediate density lipoprotein (IDL)**, which contains both triglycerides and cholesterol esters, and into **low density lipoproteins (LDLs)**, which contain cholesterol esters and transport fat into artery walls, driving the formation of **atheroma**. The cholesterol in LDL is known as *LDL cholesterol*.

The HDL is synthesized by the liver and predominantly contains phospholipids. It serves to remove fat and cholesterol from cells, returning the cholesterol to the liver. The cholesterol carried by HDL is known as *HDL cholesterol*.

A summary of the circulating lipoproteins is shown in **t21.1** [ISBN9781594251023].

t21.1 Circulating lipoproteins

Lipoprotein	Lipid:protein content ratio	Contents	Role
Chylomicrons	99:1	triglycerides (exogenous, dietary)	transferring fatty acids from digestive tract to liver
High density lipoprotein (HDL)	50:50	phospholipids, cholesterol	removing fat and cholesterol from cells
Low density lipoprotein (LDL)	80:20	cholesterol	transporting fat into artery walls and attracting macrophages (promoting atherosclerosis)
Very low density lipoprotein (VLDL)	90:10	triglycerides (endogenous)	precursor to IDL and LDL; internal transport mechanism for lipids
Intermediate density lipoprotein (IDL)	85:15	triglycerides (endogenous) and cholesterol	transporting triglycerides and cholesterol into artery walls (promoting atherosclerosis); due to low concentration, is less important than LDL in this regard

21.5 **Cholesterol screening guidelines**

The National Cholesterol Education Program (NCEP) recommends screening of all individuals age 20 or older for high serum/plasma cholesterol, with follow-up screening every 5 years, while the United States Preventive Services Task Force (USPSTF) suggests beginning at 20 years of age only if there is increased risk of coronary heart disease. For men without increased risk, the USPSTF recommends screening starting at age 35, but makes no recommendation for screening for women and for men aged 20-35 [ISBN9780071824866].

The NCEP stratifies individuals without cardiovascular disease according to the following risk factors: 1) men age 45 or older; 2) women age 55 or older; 3) those with family history of myocardial infarction or sudden cardiac death before age 55 in a first degree male relative or before age 65 in a first degree female relative; 4) hypertension (whether treated or not); 5) current cigarette smoking (10 or more cigarettes per day); and 6) serum HDL cholesterol <40 mg/dL. 1 risk factor is subtracted if the HDL cholesterol is >60 mg/dL because HDL cholesterol is protective. Patients with 2 or more of the above risk factors are then further stratified by evaluating their risk of developing coronary heart disease using the Framingham projections of 10 year risk. Treatment decisions are then based on the serum LDL cholesterol, the patient's risk profile factor, and the estimated 10 year risk. Patients with 2 or more risk factors ("intermediate risk") are usually treated with diet therapy/therapeutic lifestyle changes (eg, increased physical activity, weight control) if the LDL cholesterol is >130 mg/dL. However, if those patients' LDL cholesterol is either >160 mg/dL (even with a 10 year risk for coronary heart disease <10%), or if the LDL cholesterol is >130 mg/dL and their 10 year risk is 10%-20%, drug treatment is recommended. Individuals with 0-1 risk factor and an estimated 10 year risk of <10% are treated with diet/therapeutic lifestyle changes if the LDL cholesterol >160 mg/dL, and with drug therapy if the LDL cholesterol >190 mg/dL [PMID11368702, ISBN9780071824866].

21.6 **Laboratory testing for hyperlipidemias**

Serum/plasma triglyceride and LDL cholesterol concentrations should be measured in specimens obtained from patients who have been fasting for 12 hours, while cholesterol and HDL cholesterol measurements may be performed in either the fasting or nonfasting state.

Total serum/plasma cholesterol is the sum of HDL cholesterol, LDL cholesterol, and VLDL cholesterol. (Chylomicrons and IDL carry only minimal cholesterol.) Thus, serum/plasma LDL cholesterol = total cholesterol − HDL cholesterol − VLDL cholesterol. Since the mass of triglycerides in VLDL is 5× that of cholesterol, the VLDL cholesterol can be estimated by dividing the measured triglyceride concentration by 5, so that serum/plasma LDL cholesterol can be calculated as follows:

LDL cholesterol = total cholesterol − HDL cholesterol − triglycerides/5

This is the so called Friedewald formula, for which the concentration units of all analytes are mg/dL. When serum/plasma triglyceride concentrations exceed 400 mg/dL, however, the triglyceride:VLDL ratio is altered so that direct measurement of LDL cholesterol is performed [ISBN9781416061649]. In order to use the

Friedewald formula, serum/plasma must be collected from patients who are in a fasting state.

More recently the non-HDL cholesterol calculation has gained favor, since this fraction contains all of the apolipoprotein B containing lipoproteins, which are the major contributors to **atherosclerosis.** It is thought to represent all atherosclerotic particles better than LDL cholesterol, especially in the setting of elevated triglycerides. Also, it is believed to be less affected by nonfasting because it does not include triglycerides in the calculation. The non-HDL cholesterol is calculated as follows [ISBN9781416061649]:

Non-HDL cholesterol = total cholesterol − HDL cholesterol

The target concentration of non-HDL cholesterol for introduction of lipid lowering strategies is ~30 mg/dL higher than that for LDL cholesterol.

21.6.1 Serum/plasma reference ranges for adults (not stratified for risk factors) [PMID11368702, ISBN9781594251023]

Total cholesterol: desirable (<200 mg/dL), borderline (200-239 mg/dL), undesirable (≥240 mg/dL)

Triglyceride: desirable (<130 mg/dL), borderline (130-159 mg/dL), undesirable (>160 mg/dL)

LDL cholesterol: optimal (<100 mg/dL), near or above optimal (100-129 mg/dL), borderline high (130-159 mg/dL), high (160-189 mg/dL), very high (≥190 mg/dL)

HDL cholesterol: optimal (≥60 mg/dL), desirable (40-59 mg/dL), undesirable (<40 mg/dL)

21.6.2 Hyperlipidemias

The hyperlipidemias are categorized as either primary (familial or genetic) or secondary (acquired). The primary hyperlipidemias are caused by genetic defects, while the secondary are due to other diseases (eg, diabetes mellitus). Occasionally hyperlipidemia may be idiopathic. The hyperlipidemias are also classified by the type of lipid that is elevated (eg, hypertriglyceridemia).

21.6.2.1 Primary (familial, genetic) hyperlipidemia

These disorders are categorized according to the **Fredrickson classification**, which is based on the pattern of lipoproteins on electrophoresis or ultracentrifugation [ISBN9781594251023].

Type I hyperlipidemia (1 in 1,000,000 incidence), which usually presents in childhood, is often associated with acute pancreatitis, abdominal colic, **lipemia retinalis**, eruptive skin **xanthomas**, and hepatosplenomegaly. The elevated lipoprotein is the chylomicron fraction, while the predominant serum lipid elevation is the triglyceride fraction. The serum triglyceride concentration usually exceeds 1,000 mg/dL and can be as high as 25,000 mg/dL. The serum forms a creamy layer on top with clear serum below, after sitting under refrigeration. The condition is treated by dietary control.

Type II hyperlipidemia is the most common form. Subtype IIa (familial hypercholesterolemia), caused by a mutation in the LDL receptor, is characterized by an elevated LDL, and the predominant lipid elevation is the LDL cholesterol, due to lack of uptake of LDL by its receptor. The serum appears clear after sitting under refrigeration. Patients frequently have **xanthelasma**, **arcus senilis**, xanthomas, and premature cardiovascular disease. The incidence is 1 in 500 for heterozygotes and 1 in 1,000,000 for homozygotes. Subtype IIb ("familial combined hyperlipidemia"), caused by overproduction of triglycerides, an increase in apolipoprotein B100 synthesis, and/or decreased clearance of LDL, is characterized by an elevation of both LDL and VLDL. The predominant lipid elevation is the LDL cholesterol and triglycerides. The serum may appear slightly turbid after sitting under refrigeration. The incidence is 1 in 100. Both subtypes are treated with statins (to inhibit cholesterol synthesis and decrease LDL cholesterol), fibrates (to decrease triglycerides and increase HDL cholesterol), and niacin (to decrease VLDL and LDL cholesterol and to increase HDL cholesterol).

Type III hyperlipidemia, aka familial dysbetalipoproteinemia, is due to the apolipoprotein E E2/E2 genotype and abnormal functioning of the apolipoprotein E receptor, and results in cholesterol rich VLDL. The IDL is increased. The condition is associated with an increase in triglycerides and LDL cholesterol. The main symptoms are xanthomas on the palms, elbows, and knees, and often, early onset of cardiovascular disease. The incidence is 1 in 10,000. The serum may appear slightly turbid after sitting under refrigeration. Patients are treated with statins and fibrates.

Type IV hyperlipidemia (familial hypertriglyceridemia) is due to an autosomal dominant increased VLDL production and decreased elimination of VLDL. Onset is usually in adulthood. Accordingly, the VLDL concentration is elevated. The serum triglyceride concentration is in the range of 200-1,000 mg/dL. Affected individuals frequently develop acute pancreatitis. The serum after sitting under refrigeration may appear turbid. The incidence of this disorder is 1 in 500. Treatment is with statins and fibrates.

Type V hyperlipidemia (mixed hyperlipoproteinemia) is similar to type I but has high VLDL along with increased chylomicrons. Onset is usually in adulthood. The defect is increased VLDL production and decreased lipoprotein lipase. Affected individuals may have xanthomas, lipemia retinalis, pancreatitis, and an abnormal glucose tolerance with hyperinsulinemia. The serum triglyceride concentration usually exceeds 1,000 mg/dL. The serum after sitting under refrigeration appears creamy on top and turbid below. The incidence is 1 in 500. Treatment is with niacin and fibrates.

The primary hyperlipidemias are summarized in **t21.2** [ISBN9781416061649, ISBN9781594251023].

t21.2 Fredrickson classification of primary hyperlipidemias

Type (treatment*)	Incidence	Clinical findings	Increased lipoprotein	Elevated lipid
I (diet)	1/1,000,000 (childhood onset)	acute pancreatitis, abdominal colic, lipemia retinalis, xanthomas, hepatosplenomegaly	chylomicrons (serum: creamy layer on top when refrigerated)	triglycerides (>1,000 mg/dL)
IIa; familial hypercholesterolemia (statins, fibrates, niacin)	1/500 (heterozygotes); 1/1,000,000 (homozygotes)	xanthelasmas, arcus senilis, xanthomas, premature cardiovascular disease	LDL (serum clear when refrigerated)	LDL cholesterol
IIb; familial combined hyperlipidemia (statins, fibrates, niacin)	1/100	no unique findings	LDL; VLDL (serum slightly turbid when refrigerated)	LDL cholesterol; triglycerides
III; familial dysbetalipoproteinemia (statins, fibrates)	1/10,000	xanthomas; early onset of cardiovascular disease	IDL (serum slightly turbid when refrigerated)	LDL cholesterol; triglycerides
IV; familial hypertriglyceridemia (statins, fibrates)	1/500	acute pancreatitis	VLDL (serum turbid when refrigerated)	triglycerides (200-1,000 mg/dL)
V; mixed hyperlipoproteinemia (niacin, fibrates)	1/500	xanthomas, lipemia retinalis, pancreatitis, abnormal glucose tolerance with hyperinsulinemia	VLDL; chylomicrons (serum: creamy layer on top and turbid below when refrigerated)	triglycerides (>1,000 mg/dL)

*Statins inhibit cholesterol synthesis and decrease LDL cholesterol; fibrates decrease triglycerides and increase HDL cholesterol; niacin decreases VLDL and LDL cholesterol and increases HDL cholesterol. Other agents are indicated for selected use (bile acid binding resins such as cholestyramine bind bile acids in the intestine and decrease LDL cholesterol; and cholesterol absorption inhibitors such as ezetimibe inhibit the cholesterol transporter)

21.6.2.2 Secondary (acquired) hyperlipidemias

The secondary (acquired) hyperlipidemias result in the same risks as the primary hyperlipidemias described above.

Some of the more common causes of secondary hyperlipidemia include the following [ISBN9780071802154, ISBN9781416061649]:

Hypothyroidism decreases the hepatic LDL receptor function and the clearance of LDL, thereby causing increased LDL cholesterol. Nephrotic syndrome causes an increase in VLDL and other lipoproteins in attempt to compensate for the loss of albumin, resulting in increased cholesterol and triglycerides. Hypercortisolism increases VLDL, causing an increase in triglycerides. Smoking produces a decrease in HDL cholesterol. Alcohol use inhibits the hepatic oxidation of free fatty acids, and promotes the synthesis of triglycerides and the secretion of VLDL, resulting in increased triglycerides; however, it also raises HDL cholesterol. Chronic kidney disease causes an increase in VLDL, resulting in increased triglycerides. Diabetes mellitus and obesity cause insulin resistance, increased triglycerides, and decreased HDL cholesterol.

Intrahepatic cholestasis is usually accompanied by the appearance of **lipoprotein X**, which increases the LDL cholesterol. Drugs (eg, cyclosporine, β blockers, anabolic steroids, thiazide diuretics) can exert variable effects on lipids, causing increased LDL, increased VLDL, and decreased HDL, depending on the specific drug or drug combinations involved.

21.7 **References**

21.7.1 **Journals**

PMID11368702 Expert Panel on Detection, Evaluation, and Treatment of High Blood Cholesterol in Adults [2001] Executive Summary of the Third Report of the National Cholesterol Education Program Expert Panel (NCEP) on Detection, Evaluation, and Treatment of High Blood Cholesterol in Adults (Adult Treatment Panel III). *JAMA* 285(19):2486-97

PMID22836069 Toth PP, Potter D, Ming EE [2012] Prevalence of lipid abnormalities in the United States: the national health and nutrition examination survey (2003-2006). *J Clin Lipidol* 6:325-30

21.7.2 **Books**

ISBN9780071802154 Rader DJ, Hobbs HH [2015] Disorders of lipoprotein metabolism. In: Kasper DL, Fauci AS, Hauser SL et al, ed. *Harrison's Principles of Internal Medicine*, 19e. McGraw Hill Education, 2435-2449

ISBN9780071824866 Baron RB [2014] Lipid disorders. In: Papadakis MA, McPhee SJ, Rabow MW, ed. *Current Medical Diagnosis & Treatment*, 53e. McGraw Hill Education, 1202-211.

ISBN9781416061649 Remaley AT, Rifai N, Warnick GR [2013] Lipids, lipoproteins, apolipoproteins, and other cardiovascular risk factors. In: Burtis CA, Ashwood ER, Bruns DE, ed. *Tietz Textbook of Clinical Chemistry and Molecular Diagnostics*, 5e. Elsevier Saunders, 731-806.

ISBN9781594251023 Winter WE, Carter C, Harris NS [2011] Lipoprotein disorders. In: Clarke W, ed. *Contemporary Practice in Clinical Chemistry*, 2e. AACC Press, 285-98

21.8 **Clinical case**

A 72-year-old male with congestive heart failure, hyperlipidemia, and hypothyroidism has been treated with simvastatin, digoxin, and levothyroxine for 5 years. He visits the urgent care center complaining of generalized muscle weakness.

Physical examination reveals decreased deep tendon reflexes and decreased muscle strength in the extremities. Serum laboratory studies show total creatine kinase 74,350 U/L (CKMB 81.5 ng/mL), troponin I <0.07 ng/mL, potassium 5.3 mMol/L (mEq/L), thyroid stimulating hormone (TSH) 42.1 mIU/L, free thyroxine 0.42 ng/dL, aspartate aminotransferase 1,471 U/L, and digoxin 3.0 ng/mL. Urinalysis revealed amber colored urine positive for heme protein.

21.8.1 **Questions**

1. Explain the elevated creatine kinase and CKMB.

2. Explain the elevated aspartate aminotransferase.

3. Explain the elevated serum potassium.

4. Explain the amber colored urine.

5. Explain the general muscle weakness in this patient.

21.8.2 **Clinical case answers**

1. The elevated CK and CKMB are from muscle due to apparent rhabdomyolysis caused by the chronic statin therapy. In addition, the patient's serum TSH reflects that he is hypothyroid, further contributing to elevation of CK. The troponin I is normal, so a myocardial source of CKMB can be ruled out. Large muscle contains CKMB, and the apparent rhabdomyolysis has liberated it from large muscle.

2. Muscle contains aspartate aminotransferase, and the rhabdomyolysis has liberated it

3. Digoxin inhibits the sodium-potassium ATPase pump and increases the serum potassium; in fact, the patient's serum digoxin concentration is elevated

4. Rhabdomyolysis releases myoglobin from muscle, which colors the urine amber; since it is a heme protein, it reacts with the urinalysis dipstick

5. The general muscle weakness and decreased deep tendon reflexes are likely due to both the hypothyroidism and the adverse effect of the statin therapy (rhabdomyolysis)

A.1 Preparation of laboratory sessions

A.1.1 Blood drawing laboratory

The blood drawing laboratory should be offered within the first 2 weeks of the course with discussion of the results of the laboratory testing to be held as a class session ~4-6 weeks after the laboratory. The intervening period will allow time to perform the laboratory testing, to review the results, to perform any confirmatory testing needed, and for a physician to review and provide written comments on each of the panels. It will also allow time for students to learn some baseline clinical chemistry before interpreting panels.

A.1.1.1 Purpose

The blood drawing session has several purposes: 1) to familiarize students with phlebotomy using both the Vacutainer system and the "butterfly" system; 2) to obtain samples for discussion of blood panels; 3) to stimulate interest in learning clinical chemistry; and 4) to provide an opportunity for students to obtain a "wellness" panel.

A.1.1.2 Laboratory session (2 hours) followed by discussion of results 4-6 weeks later (2 hours)

Students should draw blood using the conventional Vacutainer system and the "butterfly" system. Blood should be drawn for the following tests: glucose, ureanitrogen, creatinine, potassium, sodium, chloride, bicarbonate, hemoglobin A_{1c}, aspartate aminotransferase, alanine aminotransferase, total bilirubin, albumin, alkaline phosphatase, cholesterol, triglycerides, LDL cholesterol (calculated), HDL cholesterol, vitamin D, calcium, phosphate, and thyroid stimulating hormone. Although fasting is desirable, if the blood drawing session cannot be held in the morning, students should be permitted to be nonfasting. (*Note: In our course we also draw blood for a complete blood count because this is of interest to most students; however, hematology is beyond the purview of this book.*)

Prior to the phlebotomy, the instructor/phlebotomist should discuss the art of phlebotomy and demonstrate it on volunteers. The instructor also should discuss the different types of Vacutainer tubes, their contents, and their use [see figure]).

This is an opportunity to also discuss the difference between plasma (which contains clotting factors) and serum (which does not). It should be emphasized that, due to the advent of gel separator tubes, plasma can be easily separated and removed from blood cells; therefore it has become in many laboratories the preferred matrix for clinical chemistry analyses because it does not require time for clotting.

Students should have opportunity to pair up and to draw one another's blood. A trained phlebotomist should be available to assist the students and perform venipunctures in the event that a student fails to obtain blood or does not wish to be drawn by his or her colleagues. To perform all of the above tests and allow for confirmatory testing, 2 4.5 mL yellow serum separator tubes and one 4 mL lavender tube (ethylenediaminetetraacetate) should be obtained from each student.

A.1.1.2.1 Supplies
- Vacutainer holders (with 21 gauge needles)
- butterfly blood collection devices (with 21 gauge needles)
- tourniquet tubing
- sterile gauze
- alcohol wipes
- name labels for blood collection tubes
- examination gloves
- bandages
- Vacutainer tubes
  - 2 yellow serum separator tubes, 4.5 mL (all chemistry tests except for hemoglobin A_{1c}) for each student
  - 1 lavender tube (ethylenediaminetetraacetate), 4 mL (hemoglobin A_{1c}) for each student
- for demonstration use only: multiple types of Vacutainer tubes (see fA.1).

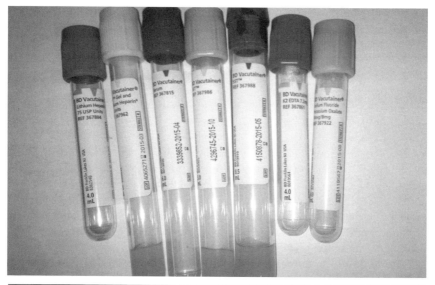

fA.1 Some commonly used Vacutainer tubes in clinical chemistry. From left to right: green (lithium heparin); green (lithium heparin with plasma separator gel); red (no anticoagulant); yellow (no anticoagulant and with serum separator gel); red ("tiger eye") (no anticoagulant and with serum separator gel); lavender (ethylenediaminetetraacetate); and gray (potassium oxalate plus sodium fluoride as inhibitor of glycolysis). Note that red and green tubes are used for general clinical chemistry tests; lavender tubes are used for whole blood studies (eg, hemoglobin A1c, erythrocyte folate) as well as complete blood counts; gray tubes are used for glucose when the sample cannot be separated from plasma within 30 minutes and for other analytes that may undergo enzymatic degradation

In the subsequent 2 hour discussion of the blood drawing session (which should take place ~4-6 weeks after the laboratory), the specific tests performed should be discussed during the first hour, with emphasis on those tests that have not yet been covered in the course. (*Note: Students with abnormal laboratory results should be contacted immediately once results are available after testing.*)

The results of student panels should be distributed in a confidential manner after this discussion. In our experience, when test results are distributed prior to the discussion, students focus on those rather than the instructor's overview of the tests. The instructor should then display the deidentified panels and discuss each one. Following the session, the instructor should be available to discuss individual panels confidentially with students who may wish to do so.

Students should calculate their own estimated glomerular filtration rates using the Cockcroft-Gault formula (Chapter 5) because their demographic information will not be known by the analytical laboratory performing the analyses. They should also calculate their own non-HDL cholesterol concentrations (Chapter 21).

A.2 Urinalysis laboratory

The urinalysis laboratory session should be offered immediately after the urinalysis lecture (Chapter 6). Students will be afforded the opportunity to perform urinalysis on pooled patient urines and on their own individual urines.

A.2.1 Purpose

The laboratory will serve 1) to familiarize students with the urinalysis procedure; 2) to stimulate interest in clinical chemistry; and 3) to provide them with opportunity to obtain their own urinalysis results.

A.2.2 Laboratory session (2 hours)

2 pooled patient urine samples (Pool A and Pool B, 1 liter volume of each) should be provided in order to maximize the opportunity of finding abnormal results.

Students should perform the macroscopic, chemical, and microscopic examinations of the pooled urines, and have the opportunity to analyze their own urines. In addition to dipstick measurement, specific gravity should be determined by at least 1 additional method (eg, hydrometer and/or refractometer).

A.2.2.2.1 Supplies
- Microscopes (at least 1 should have 2 heads, which facilitates teaching)
- conical plastic centrifuge tubes (15 mL)
- urine collection containers
- hydrometer
- refractometer
- urine dipsticks
- examination gloves
- sulfosalicylic acid, 3% (W/V) in water

➢ pooled urine; samples should be augmented as follows within 4 hours of the laboratory session:

  ○ Pool A (1 L)

  ▪ protein

    • dissolve 1.8 g reagent grade albumin in 50 mL water; mix well
    • then add the solution to the 1 L of urine; mix well

  ▪ heme protein: to the 1 L urine, add 10 μL of a blood sample drawn into a lavender Vacutainer tube and for which a normal complete blood count has been obtained; mix well

  ▪ glucose: Add 4 g D-glucose to the 1 L of urine; mix well

  ▪ ketone bodies: add 250 mg acetoacetate, lithium salt, to the 1 L of urine (note: lithium acetoacetate is unstable and must be kept frozen prior to use; once opened and used, it should be discarded)

  ○ Pool B (1 L)

  ▪ protein

    • dissolve 360 mg reagent grade albumin in 50 mL water; mix well
    • then add the solution to the 1 L of urine; mix well

  ▪ heme protein: to the 1 L of urine, add 2 μL of a blood sample drawn into a lavender vacutainer tube and for which a normal complete blood count has been obtained; mix well

  ▪ glucose: add 0.8 g D-glucose to the 1 L of urine; mix well

  ▪ calcium oxalate crystals:

    • add 160 μL of 0.1 N calcium chloride to 200 μL of saturated ammonium oxalate; a cloudy suspension should result
    • allow the suspension to sit overnight to permit formation of calcium oxalate crystals
    • then add the contents to the 1 liter of urine

Prior to use of Pool A and Pool B, they should each be submitted to automated urinalysis to establish target values.

Outline of the differential diagnosis for selected abnormal clinical chemistry tests

I. Alkaline phosphatase elevation
   A. extrahepatic bile duct obstruction
   B. intrahepatic biliary cholestasis
   C. primary biliary cirrhosis
   D. metastatic bone tumors
   E. bone fractures
   F. Paget disease of the bone
   G. pregnancy
   H. primary hyperparathyroidism
   I. secondary hyperparathyroidism
   J. acromegaly

II. Aminotransferase elevation
   A. acute hepatocellular injury (following liver injury, ALT is elevated longer than AST due to longer half-life of ALT than AST)
   B. drugs (eg, acetaminophen overdose, valproic acid overdose; toxins, eg, carbon tetrachloride)
   C. viral infections (eg, hepatitis, infectious mononucleosis; DeRitis ratio <1)
   D. intrahepatic cholestasis (DeRitis ratio <1)
   E. Reye syndrome (DeRitis ratio <1)
   F. Hepatic cirrhosis (DeRitis ratio >1)

III. Amylase elevation
   A. acute pancreatitis
   B. spasm of sphincter of Oddi
   C. renal failure
   D. sialitis
   E. perforated peptic ulcer
   F. intestinal obstruction
   G. cholestatis
   H. ruptured ectopic pregnancy
   I. mesenteric infarction
   J. acute appendicitis
   K. ectopic production by tumors
   L. diabetic ketoacidosis
   M. macroamylasemia

IV. Anion gap depression
   A. hypoalbuminemia (eg, nephrotic syndrome, liver failure, burns)
   B. paraproteins
   C. hypercalcemia (see causes below)
   D. hypermagnesemia (see causes below)
   E. hemodilution
V. Anion gap elevation
   A. ketoacidosis
   B. renal failure
   C. lactic acidosis
   D. exogenous substances ingested or transfused
VI. Aspartate aminotransferase elevation
   A. drugs (eg, acetaminophen, valproic acid; toxins, eg, carbon tetrachloride)
   B. skeletal muscle injury (DeRitis ratio >1)
   C. myocardial infarction (DeRitis ratio >1)
   D. acute hepatocellular injury
   E. hepatic cirrhosis (DeRitis ratio >1)
VII. Bicarbonate depression
   A. respiratory alkalosis (eg, hyperventilation due to anxiety, ascites, obesity, living at high altitudes)
   B. metabolic acidosis (eg, ketoacidosis, lactic acidosis, retention of acid in renal failure, loss of base via diarrhea)
XIII. Bicarbonate elevation
   A. respiratory acidosis (eg, central nervous system depression, chronic obstructive pulmonary disease, paralysis of respiratory musculature, airway disease, sleep apnea, cardiac disease with hypoperfusion)
   B. metabolic alkalosis (eg, uncontrollable vomiting, excessive nasogastric suction, hypercortisolism, hyperaldosteronism, massive blood transfusion, administration of excess base, chronic diuretic use)
IX. Bilirubin elevation, conjugated plus unconjugated
   A. nonend stage cirrhosis
   B. acute hepatitis
   C. cholestasis
   D. posthepatic obstruction
   E. Dubin-Johnson syndrome
   F. rotor syndrome
X. Bilirubin elevation, unconjugated
   A. hemolytic anemia
   B. end stage cirrhosis
   C. Crigler-Najjar syndrome types I and II
   D. Gilbert syndrome
XI. Cerebrospinal fluid: cells
   A. neutrophils: bacterial meningitis
   B. lymphocytes: viral, fungal, tuberculous meningitis; neurosyphillis
XII. Cerebrospinal fluid: differentiation from other fluids
   A. rhinorrhea, otorrhea, and tears: assay β2 transferrin (present only in CSF and not in these other fluids; serum has β1 transferrin; also assay glucose: present in CSF but not in these other fluids)
XII. Creatine kinase elevation
   A. acute myocardial infarction

    B. skeletal muscle injury; higher than acute myocardial infarction (most substantial is electrocution)

    C. myocarditis

    D. polymyositis

    E. dermatomyositis

    F. cardiac surgery

    G. rhabdomyolysis

    H. muscular dystrophies

    I. malignant hyperthermia

    J. shock

    K. severe angina

    L. hypothyroidism

    M. vigorous exercise

    N. drugs (eg, statins, antiretroviral drug therapy for human immunodeficiency virus infection)

XIV. Creatinine elevation

    A. acute glomerulonephritis (SUN: CR >20, decreased GFR, mild proteinuria)

    B. chronic glomerulonephritis (SUN: CR <10, decreased GFR, proteinuria, hyperkalemia, hyponatremia, oliguria, hypermagnesemia, hypocalcemia, hyperphosphatemia, hyperuricemia, metabolic acidosis due to retention of hydrogen ion with potassium)

    C. postrenal obstruction

XV. Digoxin elevation

    A. renal failure

    B. digoxin dose high

    C. coadministration of quinidine

    D. coadministration of amiodarone

    E. drawing before 8 hours after the last dose

XVI. Glycosuria with normal plasma glucose

    A. familial renal glycosuria

    B. Fanconi syndrome

    C. pregnancy

XVII. Hypercalcemia

    A. primary hyperparathyroidism

    B. tertiary hyperparathyroidism

    C. malignancy (bone lesions, PTHrP, lymphomas stimulating calcitriol production)

    D. hypothyroidism

    E. hyperthyroidism

    F. hyperalbuminemia

    G. granulomatous diseases

    H. vitamin D excess

    I. excess calcium ingestion

    J. vitamin A excess

    K. thiazide excess

    L. milk alkali syndrome

    M. chronic lithium therapy

    N. prolonged immobilization

    O. familial hypocalciuric hypercalcemia

    P. multiple endocrine neoplasia

XVIII. Hypercortisolism
    A. exogenous steroids
    B. pituitary adenoma (Cushing disease)
    C. adrenal adenoma or carcinoma
    D. ACTH secreting tumor (ectopic)
XIX. Hyperglycemia
    A. diabetes mellitus
    B. hypercortisolism
    C. hyperthyroidism
    D. glucagonoma
    E. pheochromocytoma
    F. somatostatinoma
    G. acromegaly
    H. pancreatic destruction (eg, surgery, hemochromatosis, cancer, cysts, hemorrhagic pancreatitis)
    I. theophylline overdose
    J. drugs (eg, levothyroxine, glucocorticoids)
XX. Hyperkalemia
    A. spurious
        1. refrigeration of intact blood samples
        2. contamination with EDTA (but calcium negligible)
        3. fist pumping during phlebotomy
        4. prolonged application of the tourniquet during phlebotomy
        5. thrombocythemia
        6. polycythemia vera
        7. iatrogenic or surreptitious
    B. hypoadrenalism
    C. dehydration
    D. metabolic acidosis (eg, diabetic ketoacidosis)
    E. tumor lysis
    F. tissue trauma
    G. rhabdomyolysis
    H. renal failure
    I. decreased renal perfusion (eg, dehydration, shock, congestive heart failure)
    J. digoxin overdose
    K. angiotensin converting enzyme inhibitors
    L. aldosterone inhibitors
    M. massive transfusion of old blood
XXI. Hyperlipidemia
    A. primary
        1. type I
        2. types IIa and IIb
        3. type III
        4. type IV
        5. type V

B. secondary
1. hypothyroidism
2. nephrotic syndrome
3. hypercortisolism
4. smoking
5. alcohol use
6. chronic kidney disease
7. diabetes mellitus
8. obesity
9. intrahepatic cholestasis
10. drugs (eg, cyclosporine, β blockers, anabolic steroids, thiazide diuretics)

XXII. Hypermagnesemia
A. iatrogenic (treatment of pre-eclampsia and eclampsia)
B. excessive ingestion (especially with renal failure)
C. milk alkali syndrome
D. rhabdomyolysis
E. tumor lysis

XXIII. Hypernatremia
A. dehydration
B. hypercortisolism
C. hyperaldosteronism
D. renin producing tumors
E. diarrhea with water loss

XXIV. Hyperphosphatemia
A. increased phosphate intake
B. excessive vitamin D
C. milk alkali syndrome
D. renal failure
E. hypoparathyroidism
F. pseudohypoparathyroidism
G. acromegaly
H. prolonged immobilization
I. thyrotoxicosis
J. tumor lysis
K. metabolic acidosis (cellular release of phosphate)
L. rhabdomyolysis

XXV. Hyperthyroxinemia
A. primary hyperthyroxinemia (autoantibodies to TSH receptor; thyroid nodules, thyroid follicular adenoma, gain of function mutation of TSH receptor which is usually congenital)
B. secondary hyperthyroxinemia (pituitary adenoma; loss of function mutation in pituitary thyroxine and T3 receptors)
C. gestational hyperthyroxinemia (TSH receptor sensitivity to hCG)
D. hCG secreting tumors
E. increased thyroid binding proteins (eg, thyroxine binding globulin due to oral contraceptives, tamoxifen, methadone, pregnancy, hepatitis, estrogen producing tumors; transthyretin due to familial increase; albumin due to familial dysalbuminemia; antibodies that bind thyroxine)
F. peripheral resistance to effects of thyroid hormones and/or loss of function mutations in the hormone receptors

 ISBN 978-089189-6548

XXVI. Hypocalcemia
    A. chronic renal failure
    B. primary hypoparathyroidism
    C. pseudohypoparathyroidism
    D. pseudohypohyperparathyroidism
    E. deficient vitamin D action
    F. secondary hyperparathyroidism
    G. healing bone ("hungry bone")
    H. drugs (eg, bisphosphonates)
    I. intestinal malabsorption
    J. hemorrhagic pancreatitis
    K. dietary deficiency
    L. thyroidectomy/parathyroidectomy with inadequate replacement therapy
    M. hypoalbuminemia
    N. fluoride poisoning
    O. ethylene glycol poisoning
    P. metabolic alkalosis (ionized calcium goes down and total calcium goes down)
    Q. spurious (EDTA contamination but high potassium)

XXVII. Hypocortisolism
    A. primary hypocortisolism (eg, autoimmune, neoplastic, hemochromatosis, congenital deficiencies, vascular disorders and hemorrhage, infection)
    B. secondary hypocortisolism (eg, infarction, trauma, tumor, amyloidosis, inflammation, hemorrhage, hemochromatosis, congenital malformations)
    C. tertiary hypocortisolism (eg, congenital malformations, trauma, hemorrhage, inflammation, infection)

XXVIII. Hypoglycemia
    A. malnutrition
    B. hypocortisolism
    C. hypothyroidism
    D. endstage liver failure
    E. reactive hypoglycemia
    F. surreptitious use of oral antidiabetic drugs and/or insulin
    G. spurious; intact blood sample sitting; leukocytosis
    H. insulinoma

XXIX. Hypokalemia
    A. malnutrition
    B. diarrhea
    C. vomiting
    D. hypercortisolism (including use of exogenous glucocorticoids)
    E. hyperaldosteronism
    F. renin producing tumors
    G. theophylline overdose
    H. ingestion of original black licorice
    I. diuretic use
    J. familial hypokalemic periodic paralysis

XXX. Hypomagnesemia
    A. malabsorption
    B. alcohol use
    C. poor renal tubular reabsorption

  D. "hungry bone" syndrome
  E. nephrotoxic drugs (eg, amphotericin, aminoglycoside antibiotics)
  F. malnutrition
  G. vomiting
  H. nasogastric suction
  I. diarrhea
  J. drugs (thiazide diuretics, proton pump inhibitors)
  K. hyperthyroidism
  L. primary hyperaldosteronism
  M. osmotic diuresis
XXXI. Hyponatremia
  A. spurious (hyperlipidemia with indirect ion selective electrode measurements; dilutional hyponatremia due to hyperglycemia)
  B. overhydration
  C. hypoadrenalism
  D. renal disease
  E. diabetic ketoacidosis
  F. syndrome of inappropriate antidiuretic hormone
  G. potassium sparing diuretics
  H. compulsive water drinking
  I. hypothyroidism
  J. secondary hyperaldosteronism
  K. aldosterone inhibitors and angiotensin converting enzyme inhibitors
XXXII. Hypophosphatemia
  A. malnutrition
  B. vitamin D deficiency
  C. redistribution of phosphate into cells (eg, acute respiratory alkalosis, insulin administration, healing bone)
  D. renal loss (eg, hyperparathyroidism, Fanconi syndrome)
  E. gastrointestinal loss (eg, vomiting, diarrhea, phosphate binding antacids, malabsorption)
XXXIII. Hypothyroxinemia
  A. primary hypothyroidism (eg, Hashimoto thyroiditis; autoimmune destruction of thyroid, iodine deficiency, surgery, iodine excess)
  B. secondary hypothyroidism (pituitary tumor, pituitary infarction)
  C. tertiary hypothyroidism (hypothalamic infarction or dysfunction)
  D. decreased thyroid binding proteins (congenital, decreased thyroxine binding globulin synthesis as with liver disease or TBG loss as in nephrotic syndrome; anabolic steroid use or large amounts of glucocorticoids)
  E. drugs that displace thyroxine from thyroxine binding globulin (eg, salicylates, phenytoin)
  F. low transthyretin (eg, acute inflammation, malnutrition)
XXXIV. Iron elevation
  A. oral contraceptives
  B. iron overload (eg, hereditary hemochromatosis, excessive iron ingestion)
  C. hepatitis

XXXV. Lipase elevation
   A. acute pancreatitis
   B. cholecystitis
   C. perforated peptic ulcer
   D. intestinal obstruction
   E. peritonitis
   F. pancreatic trauma
   G. renal failure
   H. spasm of the sphincter of Oddi
XXXVI. Nonglucose reducing substance in urine
   A. lactose
   B. galactose
   C. glucose
   D. fructose
   E. pentose
   F. ascorbic acid
   G. homogentisic acid
   H. aspirin
XXXVII. Urea-nitrogen elevation
   A. high protein diet
   B. tissue trauma
   C. gastrointestinal bleeding
   D. muscle wasting diseases
   E. intraperitoneal extravasation of urine
   F. urinary enteric fistulas
   G. decreased glomerular filtration rate (eg, glomerulonephritis, decreased blood flow to the kidney as with shock or congestive heart failure, dehydration, postrenal obstruction, malignant nephrosclerosis)
XXXVIII. Urine specific gravity/osmolality depression
   A. chronic glomerulonephritis (isosthenuria)
   B. overhydration
   C. diabetes insipidus
XXXIX. Urine specific gravity/osmolality elevation
   A. dehydration
   B. syndrome of inappropriate antidiuretic hormone

The differential diagnosis of some of the most common clinical chemistry abnormalities encountered by pathology residents taking night call

For >30 years, DNB has conducted clinical chemistry callbook conferences for the pathology residents of the University of California, San Diego. These didactic sessions highlight illustrative cases for which the residents received night call. The calls have ranged from a simple report of critical values by the laboratory staff, to clinicians seeking advice about next steps in diagnostic workup of an abnormality, to clinicians asking for interpretation of the results. In the conferences, these cases were used as springboards for discussion of the differential diagnosis for the abnormal results. We believe that the conditions discussed below represent some of the most common clinical chemistry abnormalities encountered by pathology residents taking night call. The pathophysiology of and findings in the conditions have been previously discussed in various chapters of this book. Further testing should be performed as indicated.

In addition to the categorical conditions below, we have included several specific interesting cases taken by the pathology residents on night call.

C.1 Categorical conditions

C.1.1 Elevated creatine kinase

C.1.1.1 Case

A 67-year-old woman with Alzheimer disease was noted to have a serum/plasma total creatine kinase activity of 446 U/L.

C.1.1.2 Signs, symptoms & findings

The signs, symptoms, and findings of elevated serum/plasma creatine kinase are related to the specific pathophysiology causing the elevation (eg, myocardial infarction, vigorous exercise, rhabdomyolysis).

C.1.1.3 Differential diagnosis

Elevation of serum/plasma creatinine kinase can be seen with myocardial infarction (usually <450 U/L), myocarditis, polymyositis, dermatomyositis, cardiac surgery, electrocution (massive elevation), rhabdomyolysis, malignant hyperthermia, shock, severe angina, vigorous exercise, hypothyroidism, coronary insufficiency, and certain drugs (statins and highly active antiretroviral drug therapy for human immunodeficiency virus infection).

C.1.1.4 Present case

In the present case, the cause of the elevated serum/plasma creatine kinase was not apparent from the clinical history.

C.1.2 Elevated digoxin

C.1.2.1 Case

An 87-year-old male with ischemic cardiomyopathy, atrial fibrillation, complete heart block, obstructive uropathy, and urinary retention is found to have a serum/plasma digoxin concentration of 3.9 ng/mL.

C.1.2.2 Signs, symptoms & findings

Patients with digoxin overdose may exhibit nausea, vomiting, bradycardia, ventricular fibrillation, hyperkalemia, and a green-yellow visual disturbance.

C.1.2.3 Differential diagnosis

Digoxin is eliminated renally so that any reduction in renal function will lead to elevation of the serum/plasma digoxin. Given its extensive tissue distribution (requiring several hours) serum/plasma for digoxin analysis should be obtained no sooner than 8 hours after the last orally administered dose. Otherwise the concentrations will be spuriously elevated. When quinidine is coadministered with digoxin, the concentrations of digoxin become elevated due to quinidine's displacement of digoxin from its receptors in skeletal muscle. Also, quinidine diminishes the renal clearance of digoxin. Amiodarone also decreases the renal clearance of digoxin, elevating the serum/plasma digoxin concentration.

C.1.2.4 Present case

The patient in the present case was not known to have been medicated with either amiodarone or quinidine. It is probable that the patient's impaired renal function was the cause of the elevated serum/plasma digoxin concentration. The timing of the sample collection relative to the last dose of digoxin should be monitored to assure that a trough concentration was obtained. If this sample was collected appropriately, the dose of digoxin should be decreased.

C.1.3 Glycosuria without hyperglycemia

C.1.3.1 Case

A 25-year-old woman presented to clinic with a chief complaint of urinary frequency and urgency. Urinalysis showed 4+ glycosuria, while her serum/plasma glucose was 109 mg/dL.

C.1.3.2 Signs, symptoms & findings

Glycosuria without hyperglycemia is usually asymptomatic.

C.1.3.3 Differential diagnosis

Glycosuria is usually found when the serum/plasma glucose exceeds the renal threshold for reabsorption of glucose (160-180 mg/dL in nondiabetic individuals). Nondiabetic causes of glycosuria with normal serum/plasma glucose concentrations include familial renal glycosuria (impaired renal tubular reabsorption of glucose), Fanconi syndrome, and pregnancy.

C.1.3.4 Present case

It is conceivable that the patient (being of child bearing age) may have been pregnant, and a pregnancy test should be performed.

C.1.4 Hypercalcemia

C.1.4.1 Case

A 46-year-old woman with metastatic breast carcinoma was found to have a serum/plasma calcium of 14.7 mg/dL.

C.1.4.2 Signs, symptoms & findings

Hypercalcemia can cause kidney stones, constipation, polyuria, nausea, vomiting, anorexia, weakness, stupor, and coma. Of course, these findings can be variable depending on the cause(s) of hypercalcemia and other coexisting conditions.

C.1.4.3 Differential diagnosis

Hypercalcemia can be caused by primary hyperparathyroidism (autonomous production of parathyroid hormone by an adenoma, hyperplasia, or carcinoma), tertiary hyperparathyroidism (due to hyperplasia of the parathyroid glands with longstanding hypocalcemia), malignancy (bone metastases, elaboration of PTH related proteins), hypothyroidism (decreased metabolism of 1,25-dihydroxyvitamin D), hyperthyroidism (increased bone turnover), granulomatous diseases (enhanced conversion of 25-hydroxyvitamin D to 1,25-dihydroxyvitamin D by macrophages), excessive vitamin D ingestion, excessive vitamin A ingestion (bone resorption), thiazide diuretics (increased tubular reabsorption of calcium), excessive ingestion of calcium with alkali (milk alkali syndrome), chronic lithium therapy (raises the parathyroid gland set point for negative feedback by calcium), prolonged immobilization, familial hypocalciuric hypercalcemia, hyperalbuminemia, and multiple endocrine neoplasia I syndrome.

C.1.4.4 Present case

In the present case, the metastatic breast carcinoma has caused the hypercalcemia via the mechanisms described above.

C.1.5 Hyperglycemia

C.1.5.1 Case

A 37-year-old diabetic woman presents with a random serum/plasma glucose concentration of 578 mg/dL.

C.1.5.2 Signs, symptoms & findings

Depending on the severity of the hyperglycemia, patients may have polyuria, polydipsia, blurred vision, hypotension, and weight loss, since all of these can be seen with diabetes mellitus.

C.1.5.3 Differential diagnosis

Causes of hyperglycemia include diabetes mellitus type I and type II (fasting serum/plasma glucose >126 mg/dL and/or 2 hour postprandial glucose >200 mg/dL), destruction of the pancreas (pancreatectomy, pancreatic carcinoma, pancreatic cysts, chronic pancreatitis, hemochromatosis), acromegaly (growth hormone excess), glucagonoma (glucagon excess), hyperthyroidism (thyroxine excess), pheochromocytoma (epinephrine excess), hypercortisolism (cortisol excess), somatostatinoma (somatostatin excess), theophylline overdose (stimulation of catecholamine production), and drugs (eg, glucocorticoids, levothyroxine).

C.1.5.4 Present case

In the present case, the patient is a known diabetic, obviously poorly controlled.

C.1.6 Hyperkalemia

C.1.6.1 Case

A 68-year-old man with chronic kidney disease due to diabetic nephropathy and hypertension was admitted to the hospital for removal of a right ureteral stent for recurrent obstruction. His serum/plasma potassium at admission was 6.1 mMol/L (mEq/L).

C.1.6.2 Signs, symptoms & findings

Muscle weakness, flaccid paralysis, and ileus may be seen with hyperkalemia due to impairment of neuromuscular transmission. Electrocardiographic findings may include prolongation of the PR interval, QRS widening, and bradycardia. Of course, these findings can be variable depending on the cause(s) of hyperkalemia and other coexisting conditions.

C.1.6.3 Differential diagnosis

Hyperkalemia can be caused by dehydration, hypocortisolism (potassium retention due to decreased mineralocorticoid effect), metabolic acidosis (shift of potassium from erythrocytes into the plasma), tumor lysis (potassium release), rhabdomyolysis (potassium release), shock (decreased glomerular filtration rate), and renal failure (potassium retention). Excessive use of digoxin (inhibition of sodium-potassium ATPase pump), use of angiotensin converting enzyme inhibitors and antiotensin receptor blockers (inhibition of aldosterone release), transfusion of old blood (elevated potassium in banked blood), and use of potassium chloride may cause hyperkalemia as well.

Spurious increases in potassium can be due to hemolysis (liberation of potassium from the erythrocyte), prolonged tourniquet application and/or fist pumping during phlebotomy (hemoconcentration), refrigeration of an intact whole blood sample (inhibition of the sodium-potassium ATPase pump), essential thrombocytosis and polycythemia vera (release of potassium from platelets during clotting), drawing the electrolyte sample after drawing a tube containing the potassium salt of ethylenediaminetetraacetate (EDTA; carryover contamination), and allowing whole blood samples to sit for prolonged periods of time before centrifugation (glycolysis of glucose needed to drive the sodium-potassium ATPase pump). Finally, serum potassium is elevated in normal neonates due to lower glomerular filtration rate and decreased clearance of potassium.

C.1.6.4 Present case
In the present case, the hyperkalemia was caused by the patient's chronic renal failure.

C.1.7 Hypernatremia
C.1.7.1 Case
A 68-year-old woman is found to have a serum/plasma sodium of 160 mMol/L (mEq/L), chloride of 120 mMol/L (mEq/L), bicarbonate of 28 mMol/L (mEq/L), and potassium of 4.8 mMol/L (mEq/L). She is hypotensive (blood pressure is 90/43 mm Hg), and her urine output is negligible.

C.1.7.2 Signs, symptoms & findings
Lethargy, irritability, weakness, hyperthermia, oliguria, and hypotension can be seen with hypernatremia. These findings may be variable depending on the specific causes(s) of hypernatremia and other coexisting conditions.

C.1.7.3 Differential diagnosis
The major causes of hypernatremia include dehydration, hypercortisolism (retention of sodium), primary hyperaldosteronism (retention of sodium), and diarrhea (with water loss).

C.1.7.4 Present case
The finding of hypotension and oliguria in the patient strongly suggests dehydration as the cause of her hypernatremia. The chloride is increased for the same reason. She has maintained a normal bicarbonate due to pulmonary compensatory mechanisms (hyperventilation).

C.1.8 Hyperphosphatemia
C.1.8.1 Case
A 46-year-old man with chronic kidney disease, hypertension, and diabetes mellitus was noted to have a serum phosphate concentration of 10.7 mg/dL.

C.1.8.2 Signs, symptoms & findings
The signs, symptoms, and findings are those of the underlying condition producing the hyperphosphatemia, the most common cause being chronic kidney disease.

C.1.8.3 Differential diagnosis

Hyperphosphatemia can be caused by renal failure (retention of phosphate), ingestion of phosphate salts, transfusion of outdated blood, hypoparathyroidism, pseudohypoparathyroidism, acromegaly (growth hormone increases the tubular reabsorption of phosphate), prolonged immobilization, milk alkali syndrome, excessive vitamin D ingestion (enhanced intestinal absorption of phosphate), and increased cellular release of phosphate (eg, tumor lysis, metabolic acidosis, thyrotoxicosis due to phosphate release from bone, rhabdomyolysis, infection, and hemolysis).

C.1.8.4 Present case

In the present case, the patient is retaining phosphate due to his chronic kidney disease.

C.1.9 Hypocalcemia

C.1.9.1 Case

A 41-year-old man with acute and chronic renal failure due to a congenital obstructive uropathy is found to have a serum/plasma calcium of 7.2 mg/dL, a urea nitrogen of 80 mg/dL, a creatinine of 8.1 mg/dL, and an albumin of 2.5 g/dL.

C.1.9.2 Signs, symptoms & findings

Hyperreflexia, seizures, cramps, paresthesias, and cardiac conduction defects may be noted with hypocalcemia. Of course, these findings can be variable depending on the cause(s) of hypocalcemia and other coexisting conditions.

C.1.9.3 Differential diagnosis

Hypocalcemia can be caused by chronic renal failure (phosphate retention, loss of albumin into the urine, decreased conversion of 25-hydroxyvitamin D to 1,25-dihydroxyvitamin D by the diseased kidney, and peripheral resistance to the effects of parathyroid hormone), primary hypoparathyroidism, pseudohypoparathyroidism, pseudohypohyperparathyroidism, secondary hyperparathyroidism, vitamin D deficiency, healing bone, drugs that bind calcium (eg, bisphosphonates), acute pancreatitis (saponification of calcium), thyroidectomy/parathyroidectomy with inadequate replacement therapy, hypoalbuminemia, ethylene glycol poisoning (binding of calcium by the oxalate metabolite), fluoride poisoning (binding of calcium), massive blood transfusion (binding of calcium by citrate), and metabolic alkalosis (ionized calcium is decreased).

Spurious hypocalcemia can result when the blood sample is contaminated with ethylenediaminetetraacetate (EDTA), the anticoagulant used in the blood collection tube for complete blood counts. Since the potassium salt of EDTA is utilized, the plasma potassium will be very elevated while the plasma calcium will be very low or even negligible.

C.1.9.4 Present case

In the present case the patient's acute and chronic renal failure led to the observed hypocalcemia due to the mechanisms articulated above.

C.1.10 **Hypoglycemia**

C.1.10.1 **Case**
A 37-year-old woman undergoing evaluation to be a kidney donor was found to have a random serum/plasma glucose of 50 mg/dL. The next morning, her fasting glucose was 100 mg/dL.

C.1.10.2 **Signs, symptoms & findings**
Hypoglycemia may cause confusion, blurred vision, anxiety, diaphoresis, difficulty in concentrating, palpitations, and tremulousness. These findings may be variable depending on the specific cause(s) of the hypoglycemia and other coexisting conditions.

C.1.10.3 **Differential diagnosis**
Hypoglycemia can be caused by malnutrition, insulinoma (excessive insulin), primary and central hypocortisolism (deficiency in glucocorticoids), hypothyroidism (thyroxine promotes glycogenolysis and increased intestinal absorption of glucose), liver failure (deficient gluconeogenesis), and reactive (postprandial) hypoglycemia.

Spurious hypoglycemia can be caused by allowing the intact, uncentrifuged blood sample to sit for several hours before centrifugation so that glycolysis by erythrocytes and leukocytes occurs.

Surreptitious use of insulin (detected by negligible C peptide with high insulin concentrations) and oral antidiabetic use are other causes. Profound leukocytosis has also been reported to cause hypoglycemia due to glycolysis by leukocytes.

C.1.10.4 **Present case**
In the present case, the whole blood sample had sat uncentrifuged for 6 hours prior to analysis by an offsite laboratory. It was apparent that in vitro glycolysis had occurred. The sample should have been centrifuged before delivery to the laboratory or collected into a collection vessel containing sodium fluoride as an inhibitor of glycolysis.

C.1.11 **Hypokalemia**

C.1.11.1 **Case**
A 61-year-old woman on highly active antiretroviral therapy for human immunodeficiency virus (HIV) infection came to the clinic for routine follow-up. Her serum/plasma potassium was found to be 2.7 mMol/L (mEq/L).

C.1.11.2 **Signs, symptoms & findings**
Patients with hypokalemia can manifest muscular weakness, fatigue, muscle cramps, hyporeflexia, and rhabdomyolysis. (Note: Rhabdomyolysis can cause hyperkalemia, which can mask hypokalemia). These findings may be variable depending on the specific cause(s) of the hypokalemia and other coexisting conditions.

C.1.11.3 Differential diagnosis

Hypokalemia can be caused by malnutrition (inadequate potassium intake), diarrhea (loss of potassium in stool), hypercortisolism (mineralocorticoid stimulation of potassium loss into urine), hyperaldosteronism (urinary potassium loss), use of thiazide diuretics (urinary potassium loss), renin producing tumors (stimulation of aldosterone production with loss of potassium into the urine), vomiting, theophylline overdose (stimulation of sodium-potassium ATPase pump), and familial periodic paralysis (extracellular potassium leaking into the myocytes).

C.1.11.4 Present case

In the present case, it is conceivable that the patient had nausea, vomiting, or diarrhea associated with her HIV infection and therapy. There is no history of other conditions that might lead to hypokalemia.

C.1.12 Hypomagnesemia

C.1.12.1 Case

A 39-year-old man with a history of primary IgA nephropathy was found to have a serum/plasma magnesium of 0.7 mg/dL, a creatinine of 2.4 mg/dL, and an estimated glomerular filtration rate of <60 mL/min.

C.1.12.2 Signs, symptoms & findings

Hypomagnesemia may be associated with muscle cramps, muscle weakness, cardiac arrhythmias, nystagmus, and hypertension. These findings may be variable depending on the specific cause(s) of hypomagnesemia and other coexisting conditions.

C.1.12.3 Differential diagnosis

The causes of hypomagnesemia include intestinal malabsorption, malnutrition, alcoholism (poor nutrition as well as alcohol induced impairment of magnesium renal tubular reabsorption), renal magnesium wasting from drugs (eg, thiazide diuretics), gastrointestinal loss of magnesium due to drugs (eg, proton pump inhibitors), prolonged nasogastric suction, primary hyperaldosteronism (the resulting volume expansion causes decreased renal tubular reabsorption of magnesium), hyperthyroidism (causes increased renal excretion of magnesium), vomiting, nephrotoxic drugs (eg, amphotericin, aminoglycoside antibiotics), nondrug related impairment of renal tubular reabsorption of magnesium, diarrhea, "hungry bone" syndrome (increased magnesium uptake into bone due to parathyroidectomy), and osmotic diuresis.

C.1.12.4 Present case

The hypomagnesemia noted in the present case was due to decreased renal tubular reabsorption of magnesium caused by the patient's nephropathy secondary to deposition of IgA antibodies in the glomerular basement membrane. The increased serum/plasma creatinine and decreased glomerular filtration rate reflect this nephropathy.

C.1.13 Hyponatremia

C.1.13.1 Case

A 42-year-old woman with alcoholic cirrhosis and ascites had a serum/plasma sodium of 129 mMol/L (mEq/L); 1 month earlier it was 136 mMol/L (mEq/L).

C.1.13.2 Signs, symptoms & findings

Hyponatremia can cause nausea, vomiting, and disorientation. The findings may be variable depending on the specific cause(s) of the hyponatremia and other coexisting conditions.

C.1.13.3 Differential diagnosis

Hyponatremia can be caused by overhydration, hypocortisolism (diminished mineralocorticoid activity leading to renal sodium loss), renal tubular defects, diabetic ketoacidosis (urinary loss of sodium with the ketoacids), syndrome of inappropriate antidiuretic hormone (due to retention of water), excessive use of potassium sparing diuretics (eg, spironolactone), compulsive water drinking (dilutional hyponatremia), hypothyroidism (impairment of free water excretion), use of angiotensin converting enzyme inhibitors and aldosterone receptor blockers (causing renal loss of sodium), and secondary hyperaldosteronism (decreased renal perfusion causing release of renin and leading to retention of sodium with water and release of antidiuretic hormone).

Spurious hyponatremia can be caused by hyperlipidemia if indirect ion selective electrode measurements are used for sodium analysis (displacement of plasma water by lipid) and can also be caused by hyperglycemia (so called "dilutional hyponatremia").

C.1.13.4 Present case

In the present case, the patient had alcoholic cirrhosis causing decreased serum/plasma albumin and portal hypertension leading to ascites. The ascites caused decreased renal blood flow, leading to secondary hyperaldosteronism.

C.1.14 Hypophosphatemia

C.1.14.1 Case

An 84-year-old man with Alzheimer disease was found to have a serum/plasma phosphate of 1.6 mg/dL; 3 years earlier it was 2.8 mg/dL.

C.1.14.2 Signs, symptoms & findings

Hypophosphatemia can cause rhabdomyolysis (decreased 2,3-diphosphoglycerate concentrations), paresthesias, hemolytic anemia (increased erythrocyte fragility), diaphragmatic weakness, impaired leukocyte chemotaxis, and cardiac arrhythmias. Of course, these findings may be variable depending on the specific cause(s) of hypophosphatemia and other coexisting conditions.

C.1.14.3 Differential diagnosis

Hypophosphatemia can be caused by malnutrition, vitamin D deficiency (inadequate intestinal absorption of phosphate), phosphate redistribution from serum/plasma into cells (due to insulin administration, respiratory alkalosis, healing bone), renal loss (hyperparathyroidism, Fanconi syndrome), and gastrointestinal loss (vomiting, diarrhea, phosphate binding antacids, intestinal malabsorption).

C.1.14.4 Present case

In the present case the cause of the hypophosphatemia was not apparent from the clinical history.

C.1.15 Neonatal laboratory results

C.1.15.1 Case

A 1-month-old baby born to a mother who was infected with human immunodeficiency virus (HIV) had the following serum/plasma concentrations: potassium 5.9 mMol/L (mEq/L), bicarbonate 15 mMol/L (mEq/L), alkaline phosphatase 231 IU/L, amylase 18 U/L.

C.1.15.2 Signs, symptoms & findings

Not applicable.

C.1.15.3 Differential diagnosis

Not applicable.

C.1.15.4 Present case

Reference ranges for some analytes in neonates are very different from those in adults. Serum/plasma potassium is usually higher due to decreased urinary clearance and decreased glomerular filtration rate in neonates. Bicarbonate is usually lower due to decreased renal reabsorption of bicarbonate in the neonate. Alkaline phosphatase activity is higher due to increased osteoclastic activity, and amylase activity is lower in neonates because they produce minimal pancreatic amylase. Thus the patient in this case had analyte concentrations within the neonatal reference ranges.

C.2 Specific interesting cases

C.2.1 Chronic hepatitis C

C.2.1.1 Case

A 25-year-old alcoholic man with hepatitis C has the following abnormal laboratory results: serum/plasma sodium 126 mMol/L (mEq/L), potassium 3.6 mMol/L (mEq/L), chloride 96 mMol/L (mEq/L), bicarbonate 17 mMol/L (mEq/L), calcium 8.0 mg/dL, creatinine 1.2 mg/dL, urea nitrogen 28 mg/dL, total bilirubin 7.8 mg/dL, ferritin 1875 ng/mL, alanine aminotransferase (ALT) 70 U/L, and hepatitis C antibody positive.

C.2.1.2 Discussion

The chronic hepatitis C infection has likely decreased the synthetic capability of the liver, causing decreased albumin synthesis and resulting in a low serum/plasma calcium concentration. Liver damage has caused the increased total bilirubin. The elevated ALT and ferritin are due to hepatic inflammation. The elevated urea nitrogen with normal creatinine suggests prerenal azotemia, which could be due to gastrointestinal bleeding if the patient has varices, or due to decreased renal blood flow if the patient has ascites. Ascites could also explain the low sodium because it may cause secondary hyperaldosteronism and release of antidiuretic hormone, causing dilutional hyponatremia; it could also explain the low bicarbonate if the patient were hyperventilating due to inability to mobilize his diaphragm.

C.2.2 Poorly controlled diabetic patient

C.2.2.1 Case

A 63-year-old woman with type II diabetes mellitus and hypertension is found to have a serum/plasma potassium of 2.9 mMol/L (mEq/L), glucose of 333 mg/dL, and bicarbonate of 33 mMol/L (mEq/L).

C.2.2.2 Discussion

If the patient was not known to have diabetes mellitus, this presentation might be explained by hypercortisolism (including ingestion of exogenous steroid), which is manifested by a metabolic alkalosis, urinary loss of potassium, and stimulation of gluconeogenesis. However, in the context of diabetes mellitus, this presentation could be due to vomiting with loss of potassium and hydrogen ion concentration.

C.2.3 Hyperlipidemia & hyponatremia

C.2.3.1 Case

A 38-year-old diabetic man is found to have the following: serum/plasma glucose 590 mg/dL, triglycerides 2,136 mg/dL, cholesterol 315 mg/dL, sodium 130 mMol/L (mEq/L), potassium 4.3 mMol/L (mEq/L), chloride 90 mMol/L (mEq/L), and bicarbonate 23 mMol/L (mEq/L).

C.2.3.2 Discussion

The hyperlipidemia in this patient is likely secondary to his diabetes mellitus, although he could also have a primary type IIb (familial combined hyperlipidemia) as well. The extreme lipid concentration causes spurious hyponatremia due to displacement of serum/plasma water by lipid with measurements made using indirect ion selective electrode potentiometry because electrolytes are not soluble in lipid. The chloride is low for the same reason. In addition, hyperglycemia can cause dilutional hyponatremia due to its osmotic effect.

C.2.4 Low thyroxine, low thyroid stimulating hormone & elevated triiodothyronine

C.2.4.1 Case

A 61-year-old woman with a history of hypothyroidism is found to have a serum/plasma total thyroxine of 0.4 ng/dL, triiodothyronine of 275 ng/dL, and thyroid stimulating hormone (TSH) of <0.03 mIU/L. Her clinical findings include weakness and fatigue.

C.2.4.2 Discussion

Upon investigation, it was discovered that the patient was being treated by an outside provider with triiodothyronine alone. Thus the TSH was suppressed while the triiodothyronine was elevated. Due to the low TSH, the thyroid produced relatively little thyroxine.

C.2.5 Renal failure

C.2.5.1 Case

A 68-year-old man was found to have a serum/plasma urea nitrogen of 106 mg/dL, creatinine of 2.1 mg/dL, albumin of 3.0 mg/dL, alkaline phosphatase of 257 U/L, and potassium of 6.4 mMol/L (mEq/L).

C.2.5.2 Discussion

The elevation of urea nitrogen and creatinine with an elevated urea nitrogen:creatinine ratio suggests the possibility of acute glomerulonephritis transitioning into chronic glomerulonephritis. The low albumin may be due to albumin loss into the urine caused by the damaged glomeruli. Low albumin would lead to low serum/plasma calcium, stimulating alkaline phosphatase activity. The potassium is elevated due to renal retention.

index

*Note: *f* indicates a figure, and *t* indicates a table.

A

Absence seizure, 177, 180
Accuracy, 1, 8f, 9
Acetaminophen, 162-164, 163f, 164f
Acetoacetic acid, 56
Acetone, 56, 160
Acetylcholine, 156
Acetylcholinesterase, 156, 169, 170
Achlorhydria, 25
Acid-base map, 74, 74f
Acidosis, 66
Acromegaly, 202, 204
ACTH stimulation test, 218-219
Acute coronary syndrome, 16, 17
Acute glomerulonephritis, 43, 52
Acute myocardial infarction, 16
Acute pancreatitis, 101, 102, 104
Acute phase reactants, 127, 130
Acute respiratory acidosis, 72-73
Acute respiratory alkalosis, 73
Addison crisis, 220
Addison disease (primary hypocortisolism), 214
Addisonian crisis, 214
Adenoma, 214, 216
Adrenocortical disease, laboratory diagnosis of, 213-224
    Addison disease, 214
    congenital adrenal hyperplasia, 220-221
    CRH stimulation test, 219
    Cushing syndrome, 214
    dexamethasone, 218
    hyperaldosteronism, 221
    hypercortisolism, 214-215, 216, 218-219
    hypothalamic-pituitary-adrenal cortex axis, 215, 215f
    imaging studies, 221
    long ACTH stimulation test, 219
    metapyrone, 219-220, 220f
    serum/plasma cortisol, 216-217
    short ACTH stimulation test, 219
    urine free cortisol, 217
Adrenocorticotrophic hormone (ACTH), 214, 215
Adrenogenital syndrome, 214, 221
A:G ratio, 112
Alanine aminotransferase (ALT), 109, 113-114
Albumin, 14, 127, 128, 131t
Albuminuria, 37
Alcohol dehydrogenase, 159
Alcohol use, 232

Aldehyde dehydrogenase, 159
Aldosterone, 66, 69, 214, 215, 220
Aldosteronism, 66, 69
Alkaline phosphatase (ALP), 14, 109, 114
Alkaline phosphatase elevation, 239
Alkalosis, 66
Alloimmunization, 149, 152-154
Alveolar cells, 149
Amenorrhea, 214
Amikacin, 181
Aminoglycosides, 177, 181-182
Aminotransferase elevation, 239
Ammonia, 14, 113
    detoxification of, 39
Ammonium biurates, 52
Amniocentesis, 149, 152
Amniotic fluid, 149, 152
Amorphous phosphates, 52
Amphetamines, 166-167
Amylase, 14, 101, 102-103
    reference range for, 103
Amylase:creatinine clearance ratio, 103-104
Amylase elevation, 239
Amyloidosis, 25, 28
Analgesic, 156
Analytes, 11, 12
Analytical variation, 1, 3, 7-8
Anemia, 44
    hemolytic, 209
    iron deficiency, 96
    megaloblastic, 30
    pernicious, 27, 28, 30
Angiotensin, 66, 68
Angiotensin I, 68
Angiotensin II, 68, 69
Angiotensinogen, 66
Anion gap, 66, 69-70, 69f
    depression, 240
    elevation, 240
Anions, 66, 69
Antabuse, 159-160
Antibiotics
    aminoglycosides, 181-182
    glycopeptides, 182
Anticholinergic effects, 156, 164
Anticonvulsants
    carbamazepine, 180
    ethosuximide, 180
    phenobarbital, 179
    phenytoin, 179
    primidone, 179
    valproic acid, 180
Antidiuretic hormone (ADH), 20, 66, 68
Antipyretics, 156
Anxiolytic, 156
Apnea, 156, 165
Apoferritin, 95, 98
Apolipoproteins, 225, 226
Apotransferrin, 95, 96
Arcus senilis, 225, 230

Arginine vasopressin (AVP), 20
Arias syndrome, 109, 111
Arrhythmias, 156, 164
Artifacts, 11, 13
Ascitic fluid, 55, 60
Ascorbic acid, 50, 56
Aspartate aminotransferase (AST), 12, 14, 109, 113-114
    elevation, 240
Aspirin, 50, 161-162
Ataxia, 156, 167, 177, 179
Atheroma, 225, 227
Atherosclerosis, 202, 205, 225, 229
ATPase pump, 68
Atrial fibrillation, 190, 191
Azotemia, 37
    postrenal, 43
    prerenal, 42
    renal, 42

B
Barbiturates, 167, 179
Basal gastric secretion, 27
Benzodiazepines, 165
Bicarbonate, 14, 74-75
Bilirubin, 14, 51, 109, 111-112
    direct, 111
    indirect, 111
    unconjugated, 111
Bilirubin elevation
    conjugated plus unconjugated, 240
    unconjugated, 240
Bilirubinuria, 47, 48
Biomarkers
    cardiac, 20
    cellular location and, 17
    for congestive heart failure, 21
    molecular size and, 17
    for myocardial infarction, 21
    tissue specificity and, 17
    usefulness of cellular constituents as, 17
Blastocyst, 149
Blastula, 119
Blind loop syndrome, 25, 28
Blood-brain barrier, 55, 57
Blood coagulation, 112-113
Blood drawing laboratory, 235-237, 236f
Blood transfusions, 89
Blood urea nitrogen (BUN), 39
B natriuretic peptide (BNP), 16, 20-21
Body fluids, laboratory examination of, 55-64
    cell count in, 58-59
    cerebrospinal fluid, 57, 58
    effusions in, 60
    exudates in, 60
    glucose and protein in, 58
    lumbar puncture, 57
    microbiology studies, 58
    pressure in, 58
    special effusions in, 61
    specialized studies in, 59-60
    synovial fluid in, 61
    transudates in, 60

Bound drugs, 177, 178
Bradycardia, 190, 191
Breath tests, 25
Bronchodilators, theophylline as, 180-181

C

Calcidiol, 86, 87, 88
Calcitonin, 86, 87, 88, 124
Calcitriol, 86, 88
Calcium
    deficiency of, 89
    laboratory diagnosis of disorders of, 87-91
Calcium homeostasis, 87-88
Cancer antigen 15-3, 122
Cancer antigen 19-9, 120, 125
Cancer antigen 27.29, 122
Cancer antigen 125, 120
Cannabinoids, 167
    synthetic, 167
Carbamate insecticides, 169-170
Carbamazepine, 180
Carbon monoxide poisoning, 168
Carcinoembryonic antigen, 121
Carcinoid syndrome, 26, 28
Cardiac biomarkers, 16, 20
Cardiac troponins I (cTnI) and T (cTnT), 16, 17-18
Cardioactive drugs, digoxin as, 181
Carboxyhemoglobin, 167
Casts, 37, 47
    hyaline, 52
Cathartic, 156, 158
Cation, 66, 69
Celiac disease (gluten sensitive enteropathy), 26, 28, 29
Cells
    alveolar, 149
    antral G, 27
    ischemic injury to, 17
    juxtaglomerular, 66, 69
    parietal, 27
    peptic, 27
    plasma, 128, 129
    renal tubular epithelial, 52
    surface epithelial, 27
    syncytiotrophoblast, 119, 121
Central hypothyroidism, 190, 193
Cerebral angiitis, 59
Cerebral infections, 59
Cerebral venous sinus thrombosis, 56, 58
Cerebrospinal fluid (CSF), 56, 57, 58, 240
    proteins in, 14
Chemical chemistry
    pediatric, 14
    reproductive (See Reproductive clinical chemistry)
Chemical examination
    of urine, 47, 49
China White, 167
Chloride, 75
Cholestasis, 109, 112
Cholesterol, 14, 225, 226
    screening guidelines for, 228

Cholesterol effusions, 61
Choriocarcinoma, 119, 121
Choroid plexus, 56, 57
Chromogranins, 123
Chronic glomerulonephritis, 43-44
Chronic kidney disease, 38, 232
Chronic Kidney Disease Epidemiology (CKD-EPI) formula, 42
Chronic lithium therapy, 90
Chronic pancreatitis, 101, 102
Chronic renal failure, 89
Chronic respiratory acidosis, 73
Chronic respiratory alkalosis, 73
Chylomicron, 225, 227, 227t
Chylous effusions, 56, 61
Cirrhosis, 66, 110, 111
    hepatic, 135
    nonendstage, 112
    primary biliary, 114, 135
Clinical laboratory statistics, 1-10
    accuracy and precision, 8f, 9
    analytical variation, 7-8
    background/significance, 3
    clinical sensitivity and specificity, 6-7
    efficiency, 7, 8t
    establishing reference ranges, 3-5, 4f
    false positives, 6
    patterns of test results, 6
    predictive values, 7
    receiver operating characteristics, 9-10, 9f
    sources of variation, 3
Clinical toxicology, 156-176
    acetaminophen, 162-164, 163f, 164f
    amphetamines, 166-167
    aspirin, 161-162
    barbiturates, 167
    benzodiazepines, 165
    cannabinoids, 167
    carbamate insecticides, 169-170
    carbon monoxide poisoning, 168
    cocaine, 166
    defined, 157
    designer drugs, 168
    drug overdoses and, 158
    drug screens in, 158
    ethanol, 159-160, 160f
    ethylene glycol, 161, 161f
    first order kinetics in, 158
    hallucinogens, 167
    iron poisoning, 168-169
    isopropanol, 160, 160f
    lead intoxication, 169
    methanol, 160, 160f
    nitrites, 168
    opiates, 165
    organophosphates, 169-170
    pharmacokinetics in, 158-159, 159f
    steady state drug concentrations in, 158, 159f
    tricyclic antidepressants, 164-165
    zero order kinetics in, 158

Cocaine, 166
Cockcroft-Gault formula, 41, 237
Coefficient of variation, 1, 9
Colorectal cancer, 122
Complement, 128
Congenital adrenal hyperplasia (adrenogenital syndrome), 214, 216, 220
Congenital immunodeficiencies, 134-136
Congestive heart failure, 17, 20-21
    biomarkers for, 21
Congestive heart failure, laboratory diagnosis of, 16-24
    biomarkers in, 21
    copeptin in, 20
    creatine kinase in, 18-20
    myoglobin in, 19f, 20
    troponin in, 17-18
Conjugated bilirubin, 110
Copeptin, 17, 20
Copper, 14
Copper reduction test, 50
Coronary insufficiency, elevation of CKMB in, 20
Corticosteroid binding globulin, 216
Corticotropin-releasing hormone (CRH), 214, 215
Cortisol, 202, 204, 214
C peptides, 207-208
Creatine kinase (CK), 14, 17, 18-20
Creatine kinase (CK) elevation, 240-241
Creatine kinase index, 17, 19
Creatine kinase MB (CKMB), 17, 18-20
Creatinine, 37, 39, 39f
Creatinine clearance, 37, 40
Creatinine elevation, 241
CRH stimulation test, 219
Crigler-Najjar syndrome, 110, 111
Crohn disease, 26, 28
Cryoglobulin, 128, 135
Cryptococcosis, 90
Crystals, 52
    cystine, 52
^{14}C-triolein breath test, 29
Cushing syndrome, 214, 216
Cystatin C, 38, 42
Cystine, 52
Cystinosis, 52

D

Data, interpretation of, 3
Decidua, 149, 154
Densitometer, 128
De Ritis ratio, 110, 114
Dermatomyositis, elevation of CKMB in, 20
Designer drugs, 168
Dexamethasone, 218
Diabetes insipidus, 66, 68

Diabetes mellitus, 52, 232
    laboratory diagnosis of, 201-212
        cortisol, 204
        C peptides, 207-208
        diseases producing hyperglycemia, 204
        epinephrine, 204
        gestational diabetes, 206
        glucagon, 203
        glycated hemoglobin, 208-209
        glycated proteins, 209
        glycosuria, 208
        growth hormone, 204
        impaired glucose tolerance, 206
        insulin, 203
        islets of Langerhans, 203
        ketone bodies, 207, 207f
        maturity onset diabetes of the young, 206
        monitoring of glucose, 204-205
        somatostatin, 203
        thyroxine, 204
        Type I, 205
        Type II, 205
        urinary albumin, 209
Diaphoresis, 156, 166
Digoxin, 181
Digoxin elevation, 241
Dipstick test, 47, 49
Direct bilirubin, 110, 111
Disaccharidase deficiencies, 28, 29
Disulfiram (Antabuse), 159-160
Diurnal variation, 11, 13
Drugs. See also Therapeutic drug monitoring; specific
    bound, 177, 178
    cardioactive, 181
    designer, 168
    free, 177, 178
    interactions with, 158
    overdoses, 158
    screens, 158
    semisynthetic, 165
    total, 178
Dubin-Johnson syndrome, 110, 112
Duodenal ulcers, 27
Dysarthria, 156, 161
Dyslipidemias, 202, 205, 226
Dysphoria, 156, 167
Dyspnea, 17, 190, 191

E
Eclampsia, 86, 92
Ectopic pregnancy, 149, 151
Efficiency, 1, 7
Effusions, 56, 60
    chylous, 61
    pseudochylous, 61
Ehrlich reaction, 51
Electrolyte and acid-base disturbances, laboratory diagnosis of, 65-84
Electrophoresis, 128
Embryo, 149
Emesis, 156, 158

Encephalopathy, hepatic, 113
Endometrium, 119
    cancers of the, 120, 121
Epinephrine, 202, 204
Errors
    random, 7
    systematic, 7
Erythroblastosis fetalis, 150, 152-154
Erythrocytes, 51
Escherichia coli, 51
Ethanol, 57, 159-160, 160f
Ethosuximide, 180
Ethylene glycol, 161, 161f
Euthyroid, 190, 193
Euthyroid hyperthyroxinemia, 190, 193
Euthyroid hypothyroxinemia, 190, 194
Exophthalmos, 190, 193
Exudate, 56, 60

F

Falling drop method, 49
False positives, 5, 6
Familial hypocalciuric hypercalcemia, 86, 90
Familial hypokalemic periodic paralysis, 66, 76
Fanconi syndrome, 86, 202, 208
Fecal fat concentration, 29
Ferritin, 95, 96, 98
Ferroportin, 95, 96
Fetal fibronectin, 154
Fetal lung maturity, 152
Fibroblast growth factor 23, 86, 91
Fibronectins, 154
    fetal, 154
First order kinetics, 158
Folate, 12
Fredrickson classification, 226, 231t
Free drugs, 177, 178
Free light chain, 128, 129
Frequency histograms, 3, 4f
Friedewald formula, 228-229
Froin syndrome, 56, 58
Fructosamine, 209
Fructose, 50

G

Galactose, 50
Gamblegram, 69, 69f, 70
Gastric carcinoma, 27
Gastric lavage, 156, 158
Gastric output, measurement of, 27
Gastric ulcers, 27
Gastrin, 26
Gastrointestinal disease, laboratory diagnosis of
    Helicobacter pylori in, 27-28
    malabsorption in, 28-30
    measurement of gastric acid output in, 27
    Zollinger-Ellison syndrome in, 27
Gaussian distribution, 2, 4, 5, 5f
Gentamicin, 181
Gestation, 150, 151

Gestational diabetes, 206
Gestational trophoblastic disease, 150
Giardiasis, 128, 134
Gilbert syndrome, 110, 111
Gingival hyperplasia, 177, 179
Globulins, 128
Glomerular filtration rate (GFR), 38, 40-42
Glomerulonephritis, 38
    acute, 43, 52
    chronic, 43-44
Glomerulus, 38
Glucagon, 101, 104, 202, 203
Glucagonoma, 202, 204
Glucocorticoid, 214, 215
Gluconeogenesis, 202, 203
Glucose, 49-50
    impaired tolerance, 206
    monitoring of, 204-205
Gluten, 26, 29
Glycated albumin, 209
Glycated hemoglobin, 202, 208-209
Glycated proteins, 209
Glycogenolysis, 177, 181, 202
Glycopeptides, 177, 182
Glycoprotein, 119, 120
Glycoside, 177, 181
Glycosuria, 202, 208, 241
Goiter, 190, 193
Gold paint effusion, 61
Goodpasture syndrome, 52
Gout, 52, 56, 61
Granulomatous diseases, 90
Grave disease, 190, 193, 195
Growth hormone, 13, 202, 204

H

Hallucinogens, 156, 167
Haptoglobin, 14
Hashimoto thyroiditis, 190, 193, 195
Hashish, 167
Helicobacter pylori, 26, 27-28
    tests for, 28
Hematemesis, 157, 169
Hematuria, 38, 43
Heme proteins, 50
Hemochromatosis, 95, 202, 204
    hereditary, 96
Hemoconcentration, 66, 68
Hemoglobin
    glycated, 208-209
Hemoglobin A_{1c}, 202, 205
Hemolysis, 11, 12, 13
Hemolytic anemia, 209
Hemolytic disease of the newborn, 110, 113
Hemorrhage, subarachnoid, 58
Hemosiderin, 95
Hemp oil, 167
Henderson-Hasselbalch equation, 66, 72
Hepatic encephalopathy, 110, 113
Hepatitis, 110

acute, 112
chronic active, 135
Hepatobiliary disorders, 115
Hepatocytes, 157, 163
Hepcidin, 95, 96
Hereditary hemochromatosis, 96
High density lipoproteins (HDL), 226, 227
High dose dexamethasone suppression test, 218
Hirsutism, 214
Histoplasmosis, 90
Homogentisic acid, 50
Human chorionic gonadotropin, 120, 150, 193
Human epididymis protein 4, 123
Human immunodeficiency virus infection, 7
Human leukocyte antigen (HLA) DO2 or DO8 haplotype, 29
Hyaline cast, 47, 52
Hyaluronic acid, 56, 61
Hydatidiform mole, 119, 121
Hydrochloric acid (HCI), 27
Hydrogen breath test, 29
Hydrometer, 47, 49
Hyperaldosteronism, 214
    primary, 214, 221
    secondary, 221
Hyperbaric oxygen therapy, 167
Hyperbilirubinemia, 104
Hypercalcemia, 90, 241
Hypercapnia, 241
Hypercortisolism, 66, 202, 204, 214-215, 216, 218, 232, 242
Hyperglycemia, 104, 202, 204, 205, 242
Hyperhidrosis, 190, 191
Hyper IgM syndromes, 134
Hyperkalemia, 242
Hyperlipidemia, 28, 43, 183, 242-243
    laboratory testing for, 228-229
    primary, 229-230, 231t
    secondary, 232
Hypermagnesemia, 92, 243
Hypernatremia, 243
Hyperparathyroidism
    primary, 90
    secondary, 89
    tertiary, 90
Hyperphosphatemia, 91-92, 243
Hyperthermia, 157, 162
Hyperthyroidism, 204
    primary, 193
    secondary, 193
    subclinical, 196
Hyperthyroxinemia, 243
Hypertriglyceridemia, 104
Hypoalbuminemia, 43
Hypocalcemia, 44, 89, 244
Hypocapnia, 244
Hypocortisolism, 66, 215, 216, 217, 218-219, 244
    primary, 214
Hypoglycemia, 215, 244
Hypokalemia, 177, 181, 244
Hypomagnesemia, 92, 245
Hyponatremia, 245

spurious, 67, 76
Hypoparathyroidism, 86
    primary, 89
Hypophosphatemia, 91, 245
Hypothalamic-pituitary-adrenal cortex axis, 215, 215f
Hypothermia, 167
Hypothyroidism, 90, 232
    central, 193
    primary, 194
    secondary, 193, 194
    subclinical, 196
    tertiary, 193
Hypothyroxinemia, 245
Hypovolemia, 66, 69, 157, 169
Hypoxia, 157, 167

I

Icterus, 11, 12
IgA endomysial antibody, 30
IgG antitissue transglutaminase antibody, 30
IgG deficiency, 134
IgG index, 56, 59
IgG synthesis rate, 56, 59
IgM deficiency, 134
Immunochromatography, 150
Immunofixation electrophoresis, 128, 129
Immunoglobulins, 128, 129, 132
    IgA, 14, 28
    IgE, 14, 28
    IgG, 14
    IgM, 14, 28
Immunosuppressives
    cyclosporine A, 182
    tacrolimus, 184
Impaired glucose tolerance, 206
Indirect bilirubin, 110, 111
Infantile X linked (Bruton) agammaglobulinemia, 134
Insulin, 101, 104, 202, 203
Insulinoma, 202, 208
Interindividual variation, 2, 3
Intermediate density lipoproteins (IDL), 226, 227, 227f
Intestinal resection, 28
Intrahepatic cholestasis, 114, 226, 232
Intraindividual variation, 2, 3
Intrathecal, 56
Intrauterine infection, 135
Intrinsic factor, 26
Iron deficiency, 97, 98
Iron deficiency anemia, 96
Iron elevation, 246
Iron homeostasis, 96
Iron overload, 97
Iron poisoning, 168-169
Islet cell antibodies, 202, 205
Islet of Langerhans, 101, 202, 203
Isoenzyme, 17
Isoform, 150
Isopropanol, 160, 160f
Isosthenuria, 38

J

Jaundice, 111

K

Keratolytic compounds, 157, 162
Kernicterus, 150, 153
Ketone bodies, 48, 50, 56, 207, 207f
Ketonemia, 202, 205
Ketonuria, 202, 205
Kinetics
    first order, 158
    zero order, 158, 159
Kurtosis, 2, 4

L

Laboratory diagnosis
    of adrenocortical disease, 213-224
        Addison disease, 214
        congenital adrenal hyperplasia, 220-221
        CRH stimulation test, 219
        Cushing syndrome, 214
        dexamethasone, 218
        hyperaldosteronism, 221
        hypercortisolism, 214-215, 216
        hypocortisolism, 218-219
        hypothalamic-pituitary-adrenal cortex axis, 215, 215f
        imaging studies, 221
        long ACTH stimulation test, 219
        metapyrone, 219-220, 220f
        serum/plasma cortisol, 216-217
        short ACTH stimulation test, 219
        urine free cortisol, 217
    of calcium disorders, 87-91
        hypercalcemia, 90
        hypocalcemia, 89
    of diabetes mellitus, 201-212
        cortisol, 204
        C peptides, 207-208
        diseases producing hyperglycemia, 204
        epinephrine, 204
        gestational diabetes, 206
        glucagon, 203
        glycated hemoglobin, 208-209
        glycated proteins, 209
        glycosuria, 208
        growth hormone, 204
        impaired glucose tolerance, 206
        insulin, 203
        islets of Langerhans, 203
        ketone bodies, 207, 207f
        maturity onset diabetes of the young, 206
        monitoring of glucose, 204-205
        somatostatin, 203
        thyroxine, 204
        Type I, 205
        Type II, 205
        urinary albumin, 209

Laboratory diagnosis (continued)
    of electrolyte and acid-base disturbances, 65-84
        anion gap in, 69-70, 69f
        bicarbonates in, 74-75
        chloride in, 75
        Henderson-Hasselbalch equation in, 72
        hormones and, 68-69
        metabolic acidosis in, 73-74, 74f, 75f
        metabolic alkalosis in, 73-74, 74f, 75f
        osmolality in, 71-72
        potassium in, 76
        respiratory acidosis in, 72-73
        sample collection, 67-68
        sodium in, 76
    of gastrointestinal disease, 25-36
        Helicobacter pylori in, 27-28
        malabsorption in, 28-30
        measurement of gastric acid output in, 27
        Zollinger-Ellison syndrome in, 27
    of iron disorders, 95-100
    of lipid disorders, 225-234
        cholesterol screening guidelines, 228
        circulating lipoproteins, 226-227, 227t
        Friedewald formula, 228-229, 231t
        hyperlipidemias, 229-231
        laboratory testing for hyperlipidemias, 228-229
        primary, 229-230
        secondary, 232
    of liver disease, 109-118
        alkaline phosphatase in, 114
        ammonia in, 113
        bilirubin in, 111-112
        blood coagulation in, 112-113
        plasma/serum proteins in, 112
        γ glutamyl transferase in, 115
    of myocardial infarction and congestive heart failure, 16-24
        biomarkers in, 21
        copeptin in, 20
        creatine kinase in, 18-20
        myoglobin in, 19f, 20
        troponin in, 17-18
    of pancreatic disease, 101-108
        acute pancreatitis in, 102
        amylase:creatinine clearance ratio in, 103-104
        amylase in, 102-103
        lipase in, 103
        nonspecific biochemical changes in, 104
    of phosphorus disorders, 91-92
    of protein abnormalities, 127-148
        acute phase reactants, 130, 131-132t, 133
        analytical approach, 128-130, 129f, 130f
        congenital immunodeficiencies, 134
        serum protein electrophoretic pattern, 136, 136f, 137f, 138f
    of renal disease, 37-46
        azotemia in, 42-43
        creatinine in, 39, 39f
        cystatin C in, 42
        glomerular filtration rate in, 40-42
        glomerulonephritis in, 43-44
        nephrotic syndrome in, 43

　　　　nonprotein nitrogenous compounds in, 38
　　　　pyelonephritis in, 43
　　　　serum urea-nitrogen to serum creatine ratio in, 40
　　　　tests of tubular function in, 42
　　　　urea nitrogen in, 39, 39f
　　of thyroid disease, 189-200
　　　　antithyroid antibodies, 195
　　　　congenital hypothyroidism, 196
　　　　hypothalamic-pituitary-thyroid gland axis, 192, 192f
　　　　nonspecific findings, 196
　　　　sick euthyroid syndrome, 195
　　　　signs and symptoms of hyperthyroidism and hypothyroidism, 191
　　　　subclinical hypothyroidism, 196
　　　　subclinical hyperthyroidism, 196
　　　　thyroid stimulating hormones, 191, 194
　　　　thyroid stimulating immunoglobulins, 195
　　　　thyrotropin release hormones, 191
　　　　thyroxine, 194-195
　　　　thyroxine binding globulin, 193
Laboratory examination of body fluids, 55-64
　　cell count in, 58-59
　　cerebrospinal fluid, 57, 58
　　effusions in, 60
　　exudates in, 60
　　glucose and protein in, 58
　　lumbar puncture, 57
　　microbiology studies, 58
　　pressure in, 58
　　special effusions in, 61
　　specialized studies in, 59-60
　　synovial fluid in, 61
　　transudates in, 60
Laboratory tests
　　accuracy and precision of, 8f, 9
　　patterns of results, 6
Lacrimation, 56, 60, 157, 170
Lactase deficiency, 29
Lactose, 29, 50
Lead intoxication, 169
Leprosy, 90
Leucine, 52
Leukocyte esterase, 51
Leukocytes, 51
Leukopenia, 177, 183
Liley Prognostication Chart, 153, 153f
Lipase, 101, 103
　　reference range for, 103
Lipase elevation, 246
Lipemia, 11, 13
Lipemia retinalis, 226, 229
Lipids, 226
　　laboratory diagnosis of disorders of, 225-234
Lipoprotein lipase, 226, 227
Lipoproteins, 226, 227t
Lipoprotein X, 226, 232
Low density lipoproteins (LDLs), 226, 227
Low dose dexamethasone suppression test, 218
Lumbar puncture, 56, 57
Lupus nephritis, 52
Lymphoma, 28, 122
Lysergic acid diethylamide (LSD), 167

M

Macroamylasemia, 101, 103
Macroscopic examination of urine, 48
Magnesium, 92
    laboratory diagnosis of disorders, 92
Malabsorption, 26, 28
    general, 28
    specific, 28
    tests used in evaluation of, 29-30
Maldigestion, 26, 28
Malignant hyperthermia
    elevation of CKMB in, 20
Malignant nephrosclerosis, 38
Maltase deficiency, 29
Maltose, 29
Marijuana, 167
Maturity onset diabetes of the young, 206
Maximal acid output, 27
Mean, 2, 4
Meconium, 150, 152
Median, 2, 4
Medullary thyroid carcinoma, 124
Megaloblastic anemia, 30
Melanocytes, 214, 215
Meninges, 56
Meningitis, 58
    tuberculous, 58
    viral, 58
Menstrual disorders, 214
Mescaline, 167
Metabolic acidosis, 66, 73-74, 74f, 75f
Metabolic alkalosis, 67, 73-74, 74f, 75f
Metapyrone, 219-220, 220f
Methanol, 160, 160f
Methicillin resistant *Staphylococcus aureus,* 182
Methylenedioxy-methamphetamine, 167
Methylmalonic acid, 30
Microinfarctions, 18, 19f
Microscopic examination, 48
Milk alkali syndrome, 86, 90
Mineralocorticoids, 214, 215
Miosis, 157, 165
Mode, 2, 4
Modification of Diet in Renal Disease (MDRD) formula, 41
Monoclonal gammopathies of undetermined significance (MGUS), 135-136
Monoclonal gammopathy, 128, 129, 135
Mucin clot (ROPES) test, 56, 61
Multiday high dose dexamethasone suppression test, 218
Multiple endocrine neoplasia (MEN) 1 & 2 syndromes, 86, 90-91
Multiple myeloma, 119, 122, 128, 135
Muscarinic receptor, 157, 170
Muscle trauma, elevation of CKMB in, 20
Muscular dystrophies, elevation of CKMB in, 20
Mydriasis, 157, 164
Myelin basic protein, 56, 59
Myeloma, multiple, 128, 135
Myocardial infarction, 18
    biomarkers for, 21
Myocardial infarction, laboratory diagnosis of, 16-24
    biomarkers in, 21

practical laboratory **DIAGNOSIS OF DISEASE** CLINICAL CHEMISTRY

copeptin in, 20
creatine kinase in, 18-20
myoglobin in, 19f, 20
troponin in, 17-18
Myocarditis, elevation of CKMB in, 20
Myoglobin, 17, 20
Myoglobinuria, 48, 50

N

Narcolepsy, 157, 166
National Institute of Standards and Technology, 9
Negative predictive value, 2, 7
Nephrolithiasis, 86, 90
Nephrotic syndrome, 38, 43, 52, 76, 232
Nephrotoxicity, 177, 181, 183
Neuroblastoma, 119, 123
Neuropathic pain, 177, 180
Neurophysin II, 20
Neurosarcoidosis, 59
Neurosyphilis, 58
Nicotinic receptor, 157, 170
Nitrites, 167, 168
    in urine, 51
Nonglucose reducing substance in urine, 246
Nonparametric reference range calculation, 2, 5
Nonprotein nitrogen (NPN), 38
Nonseminomatous germ cell tumor of the testes, 119, 120, 121
NT pro-BNP, 17
Nystagmus, 157, 167, 177, 179

O

Oligoclonal banding, 56, 59
Oliguria, 38, 43
Oncofetal protein, 119, 122
Opiates, 165
Organophosphate, 169-170
Osmolal gap, 67, 72
Osmolality, 67, 68, 71-72
Osteoclasts, 86, 87
Otorrhea, 56, 60
Ototoxicity, 177
Ovarian cancer, 120, 121

P

Paget disease of bone, 110, 114
Pancreatic cancer, 120, 121
Pancreatic disease, 28
    laboratory diagnosis of, 101-108
        acute pancreatitis in, 102
        amylase:creatinine clearance ratio in, 103-104
        amylase in, 102-103
        lipase in, 103
        nonspecific biochemical changes in, 104
Pancreatitis
    acute, 102, 104
    chronic, 102
Paracentesis, 56
Parametric reference range calculation, 2, 5
Paraprotein, 128, 135
Parasitic infestations, 28

Parathyroid hormone (PTH), 86, 87
Paresthesia, 177, 180
Parietal cells, 27
Peak acid output, 27
Peak concentration, 177, 182
Pentose, 50
Pernicious anemia, 26, 27, 28, 30
Peyote, 167
Pharmacobezoars, 162
Pharmacogenomics, 177, 183
Pharmacokinetics, 157, 158-159, 159f, 180
Phenobarbital, 179
Phenytoin, 179
Pheochromocytoma, 119, 123, 202, 204
Phlebotomy, 235
pH of urine, 49
Phosphate, 91
Phospholipids, 226
Phosphorus, 14, 91
    laboratory diagnosis of disorders of, 91-92
Phosphorus homeostasis, 91
Placental α microglobulin 1, 154
Plasma cells, 128, 129
Plethora, 214
Poisoning
    carbon monoxide, 168
    iron, 168-169
Polyclonal hypergammaglobulinemia, 135
Polycystic ovary syndrome, 214, 216
Polycythemia vera, 67, 202, 208
Polydipsia, 67, 68, 202, 205
Polymyositis, elevation of CKMB in, 20
Polyphagia, 202, 205
Polyuria, 67, 68, 202, 205
Positive predictive value, 2, 7
Postantibiotic effect, 181
Postrenal azotemia, 38, 43
Potassium, 12, 14, 76
Preanalytical variation, 2, 3
Precision, 2, 8f, 9
Predictive values, 7
    negative, 7
    positive, 7
Pre-eclampsia, 86, 92
Pregnancy
    ectopic, 151
    testing in, 150-151
Prerenal azotemia, 38, 42
Pressor agents, 157, 158
Preterm births, 154
Priapism, 128, 135
Primary biliary cirrhosis, 114
Primary hyperaldosteronism, 86, 90, 92, 214, 221
Primary hyperparathyroidism, 86
Primary hyperthyroidism, 190, 193
Primary hypocortisolism, 214
Primary hypoparathyroidism, 86, 89
Primary hypothyroidism, 190, 194
Primidone, 179
Proinsulin, 202, 207
Prolonged immobilization, 90
Prostate specific antigen, 124

Protein losing enteropathy, 28
Proteins
 in cerebrospinal fluid (CSF), 14
 glycated, 209
 heme, 50
 myelin basic, 56
 oncofetal, 119, 122
 PTH related, 87, 90
 Tamm-Horsfall, 48, 51-52
 in urinalysis, 49, 50
Pseudochylous effusion, 56, 61
Pseudogout, 56, 61
Pseudohyperkalemia, 67, 68
Pseudohypohyperparathyroidism, 86, 89
Pseudohypoparathyroidism, 86, 89
Pseudo Zollinger-Ellison syndrome, 26, 27
Psilocybin, 167
PTH related protein, 87, 90
Pulmonary surfactant, 150, 152
Puncture, 203
Pyelonephritis, 38, 43

R

Random error, 2, 7
Receiver operating characteristic, 2, 9-10, 9f
Reference range, 2, 3
 establishing, 3-5, 4f
Refractive index, 48, 49
Refractometry, 48, 49
Refrigeration of uncentrifuged samples, 13
Regan isoenzyme, 114
Renal azotemia, 38, 42
Renal disease, laboratory diagnosis of, 37-46
 azotemia in, 42-43
 creatinine in, 39, 39f
 cystatin C in, 42
 glomerular filtration rate in, 40-42
 glomerulonephritis in, 43-44
 nephrotic syndrome in, 43
 nonprotein nitrogenous compounds in, 38
 pyelonephritis in, 43
 serum urea-nitrogen to serum creatine ratio in, 40
 tests of tubular function in, 42
 urea nitrogen in, 39, 39f
Renal failure, 102
Renal tubular epithelial cells, 52
Renin, 67, 68
Renin-angiotensin-aldosterone system, 214, 221
Reproductive clinical chemistry, 149-155
 alloimmunization, 152-154
 amniotic fluid, 152
 ectopic pregnancy and, 151
 erythroblastosis fetalis, 152-154
 fetal fibronectin, 154
 fetal lung maturity, 152
 Human chorionic gonadotropin, 150
 Liley Prognostication Chart, 153, 153f
 placental α microglobulin I, 154
 pregnancy testing, 150-151
 preterm births, 154
 semen analysis in, 151
 semen reference ranges, 151

 ISBN 978-089189-6548

Respiratory acidosis, 67
    acute, 72-73
    chronic, 73
Respiratory alkalosis, 67
    acute, 73
    chronic, 73
Respiratory distress syndrome, 150, 152
Reverse triiodothyronine, 190
Reye syndrome, 110, 113
Rhabdomyolysis, 48, 50, 67, 76, 87, 92, 157, 166
    elevation of CKMB in, 20
Rhinorrhea, 56, 60
rosebud, 278
Rotor syndrome, 110, 112
Rule in a disease diagnosis, 7
Rumack nomograms, 163

S
Salicylates, 179
Saponification, 101, 104
Sarcoidosis, 90
Schilling test, 30
Scleroderma, 26, 28
Secondary hyperaldosteronism, 221
Secondary hyperparathyroidism, 87, 89
Secondary hyperthyroidism, 190, 193
Secondary hypocortisolism, 216
Secondary hypothyroidism, 190, 193, 194
Second immunodeficiencies, 135
Selective IgA deficiency, 134
Semen analysis, 151
Semen reference ranges, 151
Semisynthetic drugs, 165
Sensitivity, 2, 6
Serum ascites albumin gradient (SAAG), 56, 60
Serum globulins, 128
Serum half-life, 157, 158, 177, 179
Serum hyperosmolality, 71
Serum hypoosmolality, 72
Serum indices, 13
Serum urea-nitrogen to serum creatine (SUN:CR), 40, 43
Severe anemia, elevation of CKMB in, 20
Severe combined immunodeficiency (SCID), 134-135
Shock, elevation of CKMB in, 20
Short (overnight) dexamethasone suppression test, 218
Sick euthyroid syndrome, 190, 194
Sirolimus, 182-183
Skewness, 2, 4
SLUD, 170
Smoking, 232
Sodium, 76
Sodium-potassium ATPase pump, 67, 68
Somatostatin, 203, 204
Somatostatinoma, 203
Specific gravity of urine, 48, 49
Specificity, 2, 6
Spurious hyponatremia, 67, 76
Squamous epithelial cells, 51

Standard deviation, 2, 9
Steady state drug concentrations, 158, 159f
Steatorrhea, 26, 29
Stenosis, 157, 169
Striae, 214
Subacute bacterial endocarditis, 52
Subarachnoid cistern, 56, 57
Subarachnoid hemorrhage, 56, 58
Subclinical hyperthyroidism, 190, 196
Subclinical hypothyroidism, 190, 196
Sucrose, 29
Sulfosalicylic acid test, 49
Surface epithelial cells, 27
Sympathomimetic effects, 157, 166
Syncytiotrophoblast cell, 119, 121
Syndrome of inappropriate antidiuretic hormone (SIADH), 67, 68
Synovial fluid, 56, 61
    leukocyte count in, 61
Synthetic cannabinoids, 167
Systematic error, 3, 7
Systemic lupus erythematosus, 59

T

T_3 thyrotoxicosis, 195
Tachycardia, 157, 161, 166, 190, 191
Tacrolimus, 184
Tamm-Horsfall protein, 48, 51-52
Tertiary hyperparathyroidism, 87, 90
Tertiary hypothyroidism, 190, 193
Testis
    nonseminomatous germ cell tumor of the, 120, 121
Tetrahydrocannabinol, 167
Theophylline, 180-181
Therapeutic drug monitoring, 157, 177-183
    antibiotics
        aminoglycosides, 181-182
        glycopeptides, 182
    anticonvulsants
        carbamazepine, 180
        ethosuximide, 180
        phenobarbital, 179
        phenytoin, 179
        primidone, 179
        valproic acid, 180
    bronchodilators
        theophylline, 180-181
    cardioactive drugs
        digoxin, 181
    defined, 178
    future directions, 184
    immunosuppressives
        cyclosporine A, 182
        sirolimus, 182-183
        tacrolimus, 184
    principles of, 178-179
Thiazide diuretics, 90
Thoracentesis, 56
Thrombocytopenia, 110, 113, 178, 183
Thyroglobulin, 123, 190, 196

Thyroid disease, laboratory diagnosis of, 189-200
    antithyroid antibodies, 195
    congenital hypothyroidism, 196
    hypothalamic-pituitary-thyroid gland axis, 192, 192f
    nonspecific findings, 196
    sick euthyroid syndrome, 195
    signs and symptoms of hyperthyroidism and hypothyroidism, 191
    subclinical hyperthyroidism, 196
    subclinical hypothyroidism, 196
    thyroid stimulating hormones, 191, 194
    thyroid stimulating immunoglobulins, 195
    thyrotropin release hormones, 191
    thyroxine, 194-195
    thyroxine binding globulin, 193
Thyroid stimulating hormone (TSH), 14, 190
Thyroid stimulating immunoglobulins (TSIs), 191, 195
Thyroperoxidase, 191, 195
Thyrotropin releasing hormone (TRH), 191
Thyroxine, 191, 194, 203, 204
Thyroxine binding globulin, 191, 193
Tinnitus, 157, 162
Tobramycin, 181
Total bilirubin, 110
Total drugs, 178
Total iron binding capacity, 97
Toxicology
    clinical (*See* Clinical toxicology)
    forensic, 158
Transferrin, 43, 56, 60, 95, 96
Transudates, 57, 60
Traumatic tap, 57, 58
Tricyclic antidepressants, 164-165
Triglycerides, 101, 103, 226
Triiodothyronine, 191
Triolein, 29
Triple phosphates, 52
Trophoblast, 119, 121, 150
Tropical sprue, 26
Tropin, 17-18
Trough concentration, 178, 182
True negative, 6
True positives, 6-7
Tuberculous meningitis, 58
Tumor markers, 119-126
    calcitonin, 124
    cancer antigen 15-3, 122
    cancer antigen 19-9, 120, 125
    cancer antigen 27.29, 122
    cancer antigen 125, 120
    carcinoembryonic antigen, 121
    chromogranins, 123
    combination of, 125
    defined, 120
    Human chorionic gonadotropin, 120
    Human epididymis protein 4, 123
    monitoring, 125
    prostate specific antigen, 124
    thyroglobulin, 123
    uses of, 120
    α fetoprotein, 120
    β microglobulin, 122
Type I diabetes, 205
Type II diabetes, 205

U

Ulcerative colitis, 26, 28
Ulcers
    duodenal, 27
    gastric, 27
Uncentrifuged samples, refrigeration of, 13
Unconjugated bilirubin, 110, 111
Unsaturated iron binding capacity, 97
Urea, 38
Urea nitrogen, 39
Urea-nitrogen elevation, 246
Urinalysis, 47-54, 48
    background/significance, 48
    bilirubin in, 51
    casts in, 51-52
    cells in, 51
    chemical examination of urine in, 49
    crystals in, 52
    defined, 48
    heme proteins in, 50
    ketone bodies in, 50
    leukocyte esterase in, 51
    macroscopic examination of urine in, 48
    microscopic examination of urine in, 51
    nitrite in, 51
    proteins in, 49
    specific gravity of urine in, 49
    urine pH in, 49
    urobilinogen in, 51
Urinalysis laboratory, 237-238
Urinary albumin, 209
Urine
    chemical examination of, 49
    macroscopic examination of, 48
    microscopic examination of, 51
    nonglucose reducing substance in, 246
    pH, 49
    specific gravity of, 49
Urine osmolality, 38, 42
Urine specific gravity, 38, 42
    osmolality depression, 246
    osmolality elevation, 246
Urobilinogen, 48, 51
Urticaria, 178, 180

V

Valproic acid, 179, 180
Vancomycin, 182
Variance, 3
Variation
    analytical, 3, 7-8
    coefficient, 9
    diurnal, 13
    interindividual, 3
    intraindividual, 3
    preanalytical, 3
Varices, 110, 113
Vasopressin, 20, 68
Venipuncture, 205
Ventricles, 57

Very low density lipoprotein (VLD), 226, 227
Viral meningitis, 58
Vitamin A, 90
Vitamin B_{12} deficiency, 30
Vitamin C, 50
Vitamin D, 88
    deficiency of, 89
    ingestion of, 90
Vitamin D_2, 87, 88
Vitamin D_3, 87, 88
Vitamin K, 28, 112
Vitiligo, 191
Von Willebrand factor, 112

W
Waldenström macroglobulinemia, 135
Whipple disease, 26, 28

X
Xanthelasma, 226, 230
Xanthochromia, 57, 58
Xanthoma, 226, 229

Z
Zero order kinetics, 158, 159
Zollinger-Ellison (ZE) syndrome, 26, 27, 28
    pseudo, 27
11-β-hydroxylase deficiency, 221
^{14}C-triolein breath test, 29
21-hydroxylase deficiency, 220
α_1-antitrypsin deficiency, 127
α_1 globulins, 131, 133
α_2 globulins, 131, 133
β globulins, 132, 133
β-hydroxybutyric acid, 50
β_1 transferrin, 60
β_2 microglobulin, 122
β_2 transferrin, 60
α fetoprotein, 14, 120
γ aminobutyric acid, 157, 165, 178, 179
γ globulins, 132, 133
γ glutamyl transferase, 14, 110, 115
δ bilirubin, 110, 111
κ and λ light chains, 128, 129